ANNUAL REVIEW OF NURSING RESEARCH

Volume 17, 1999

ANNUAL REVIEW OF NURSING RESEARCH

Volume 17, 1999

Focus on
Complementary Health and Pain Management

Joyce J. Fitzpatrick, PhD
Editor

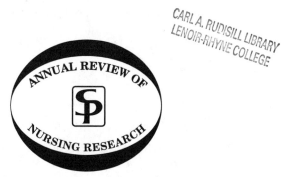

SPRINGER PUBLISHING COMPANY
New York

Order ANNUAL REVIEW OF NURSING RESEARCH, Volume 18, 2000, prior to publication and receive a 10% discount. An order coupon can be found at the back of this volume.

Springer Publishing Company, Inc.
536 Broadway
New York, NY 10012

ISBN-0-8261-8236-4
ISSN-0739-6686

ANNUAL REVIEW OF NURSING RESEARCH is indexed in *Cumulative Index to Nursing and Allied Health Literature* and *Index Medicus*.

Printed in the United States of America.

Contents

Preface

This seventeenth volume of the Annual Review of Nursing Research (ARNR) marks the completion of a second phase in the development of the ARNR Series. In this volume, as in previous volumes, there is special emphasis on selected content areas of clinical nursing practice and additional chapters covering a wide range of other research topics. In the nursing practice area this volume includes a special emphasis on both complementary therapies and pain research.

In Part I, focused on complementary therapies, Mariah Snyder and Linda Chlan review the research on music therapy. Judith Floyd's chapter includes review of sleep promotion in adults. Lucille Eller describes the research on guided imagery interventions for symptom management, and Sarah Jo Brown analyzes research on patient-centered communication.

Part II includes three chapters focused on pain research. Marion Good reviews research on acute pain; Susan Auvil-Novak analyzes the chronobiology, chronopharmacology, and chronotherapeutics of pain; and Julia Faucett reports on early interventions with chronic low back pain.

Part III includes other research in nursing. Two of these chapters are focused on the elderly: Donna Algase reviews the research on wandering in dementia and Graham McDougall analyzes the research on cognitive interventions among older adults. In Chapter 10 Beverly McElmurry and Gwen Keeney report on research on primary health care, and in Chapter 11 Merle Mishel analyzes research on uncertainty in chronic illness. The final chapter in this volume is authored by Renzo Zanotti and is focused on nursing research in Italy. This follows the pattern of previous volumes of including an international nursing research chapter in this final section.

Volume 18 of the ARNR Series will begin a new phase. The content will be more focused around a general theme. Volume 18 will be focused on chronic illness, and will include a range of research topics related to nursing research in this area.

As with previous volumes, this monumental work could not have been accomplished without the involvement of several others. I would like to thank the chapter authors, reviewers, and the Advisory Board members for their continued contributions to the ARNR Series.

Joyce J. Fitzpatrick
Editor

Contributors

Donna L. Algase
School of Nursing
University of Michigan
Ann Arbor, MI

Susan E. Auvil-Novak, PhD
Case Western Reserve University
Cleveland, OH

Sarah Jo Brown, PhD
Principal & Consultant
Practice-Research Integrations
Norwich, VT

Gwen Brumbaugh Keeney, PhD
College of Nursing
University of Illinois
Chicago, IL

Linda Chlan, PhD
College of Nursing
University of Iowa
Iowa City, IA

Lucille Sanzero Eller, PhD
College of Nursing
Rutgers University
Newark, NJ

Julia Faucett, PhD
School of Nursing
University of California
San Francisco, CA

Judith A. Floyd, PhD
College of Nursing
Wayne State University
Detroit, MI

Marion Good, PhD
Frances Payne Bolton School of
Nursing
Case Western Reserve University
Cleveland, OH

Merle H. Mishel, PhD
School of Nursing
University of North Carolina
Chapel Hill, NC

Graham J. McDougall, Jr., PhD
School of Nursing
University of Texas
Austin, TX

Beverly J. McElmurry, EdD
College of Nursing
University of Illinois
Chicago, IL

Mariah Snyder, PhD
School of Nursing
University of Minnesota
Minneapolis, MN

Renzo Zanotti
International Institute of Nursing
Research (ISIRI)
Padua, Italy

PART I

Complementary Therapies

Chapter 1

Music Therapy

MARIAH SNYDER
LINDA CHLAN

ABSTRACT

Nurses have used music as an intervention for many years. A sizeable number of investigations to determine the efficacy of music in managing pain, in decreasing anxiety and aggressive behaviors, and in improving performance and well-being have been conducted by nurses and other health professionals. Nursing and non-nursing research reports published between the years 1980–1997 were reviewed. Great variation existed in the type of musical selection used, the dose of the intervention (number of sessions and length exposure), the populations studied, and the methodologies used. Overall, music was found to be effective in producing positive outcomes.

Keywords: Music Therapy, Music, Stress Management, Pain Management

Music has been an integral component of societies since the beginning of time. Music is unique in that it is not only a cultural medium of expression, but it is also recognized as a powerful medium that affects human health. A recent review by Maranto (1993) details how music has influenced health from the time of the ancient Egyptians, who used music for healing incantations, to the emergence of empirical investigations into the physiological and psychological responses to music in the 19th and 20th century. Nursing's pioneering leader, Florence Nightingale, recognized the power of music to aid the sick. Nightingale (1860/1969) noted the effects of different types of music, recommending wind instrumental pieces with continuous sound or an air as generally having a beneficent effect for the sick.

Music has been defined as the science or art of ordering tones or sounds in succession, in combination, and in temporal relationships to produce a composition having unity and continuity (Woolf, 1979). Music therapy is the application of music to bring about positive patient outcomes. According to Munro and Mount (1978) music therapy is

> The controlled use of music and its influence on the human being to aid in physiologic, psychologic, and emotional integration of individual during treatment of an illness or disability. (p. 1029)

Since the articles reviewed in this chapter are related to the application of music, the focus of this chapter is on music therapy.

While the therapeutic application of music in various healthcare settings has evolved over time into a distinct profession of music therapy (Maranto, 1993), investigations into the effectiveness of music on health have not been limited to music therapists. Members from many disciplines, including nursing, medicine, and psychology, have conducted research on the effectiveness of music therapy with a variety of patient populations to achieve numerous health outcomes. In some studies music has been tested singularly, while in other studies it has been combined with other interventions.

SEARCH PROCESS AND ARTICLES REVIEWED

For this review, a search of Cumulative Index of Nursing and Allied Health (CINAHL) and Medline using the key word "music" was carried out for the years 1980 to mid-1997. Research reports in nursing and non-nursing English-language journals were retrieved and reviewed. The authors eliminated reports that focused on non-clinical aspects of music therapy (e.g., tiredness of music students). The studies reviewed were almost evenly divided between nursing and non-nursing journals. The number of published research studies increased almost exponentially from 1980 through 1996. Only one research report on music was published in 1981. The number increased to eight in 1990 and 17 in 1995. This increase indicates the growing interest in music and other complementary therapies in nursing and other disciplines and an increase in investigations to determine the efficacy of music in achieving patient outcomes.

Research studies on music have been grouped according to the purpose(s) for which they were implemented: anxiety/stress reduction, pain reduction, improved performance, decrease in aggressive/agitation behaviors, desired outcomes, imagery and music, and impact on psychoneuroimmunological variables. Conceptual and methodological issues identified in these studies and future directions for research on music are addressed in subsequent sections.

USES OF MUSIC

Anxiety/Stress Reduction

Music therapy has been tested extensively alone or in conjunction with other interventions for purposes of anxiety/stress reduction and relaxation promotion. A variety of physiological and psychological outcome variables were used to measure the achievement of this outcome.

Music therapy tested alone: Anxiety. Numerous conceptualizations of anxiety exist. Anxiety is a common response of many patients receiving health care. Music has been used in many settings to attempt to decrease or allay the anxiety patients experience. In particular, strong evidence exists for music therapy's effectiveness in decreasing state anxiety in patients in coronary care units (CCU) and for patients undergoing a variety of surgical procedures. A large number of investigators selected Spielberger's (1983) conceptualization of state anxiety (subjective feelings of tension, apprehension, nervousness, and worry), assuming that anxiety indeed is amenable to intervention. However, findings were not consistent across all studies reviewed, as music did not always decrease anxiety or produce relaxation.

Decreases in state anxiety (i.e., anxiety level which changes) have been reported in two studies after CCU subjects listened to investigator-selected pieces of classical music for 22 minutes (Bolwerk, 1990) or 25 minutes (White, 1992). However, other investigators reported non-significant changes in anxiety measures in subjects' responses after listening to self-selected tapes of instrumental music or video with New Age music with a similar population (Barnason, Zimmerman, & Nieveen, 1995; Zimmerman, Pierson, & Marker, 1988).

Music therapy has been used to allay anxiety in surgical patients, particularly ambulatory surgery patients. Music therapy was effective in reducing pre-operative state anxiety in subjects awaiting surgical procedures at one ambulatory surgery center (Augustin & Hains, 1996). Subjects selected a preferred tape from a variety of musical choices and listened to the tapes for 15 to 30 minutes prior to the operative procedure. Likewise, state anxiety was reduced in subjects awaiting gynecological procedures who listened to self-selected music tapes for an average of 50 minutes in the surgical holding area (Winter, Paskin, & Baker, 1994). Gaberson (1995) reported a reduction in pre-operative anxiety in subjects awaiting ambulatory surgery; subjects listened to music for a single 20-minute period of investigator-selected "tranquil" music. However, positive findings were not found in all studies in which music was used pre-operatively. Despite listening to "tranquil" music, state anxiety in subjects undergoing hand or wrist surgery was not reduced in a study by Steelman (1990). Subjects undergoing surgical procedures generally found music helpful for relaxation, for distraction from the surgical procedure, and also for pain reduction (Heitz, Symreng, & Scamman, 1992; Steelman, 1990; Stevens, 1990). Despite being offered choices from a tape collection, a number of subjects would have preferred bringing their own tapes to listen to before or during a surgical procedure (Stevens, 1990).

The impact of music on state anxiety associated with diagnostic proce-dures (i.e., colposcopy examination or flexible sigmoidoscopy) or other stress-ful experiences (i.e., test-taking) has been examined by a number of investigators. Adolescent females viewing rock and roll music videos while undergoing colposcopy examinations were found to be less anxious and re-quired less physician reassurance than those in a routine care group (Rickert, Kozlowski, Warren, Hendon, & Davis, 1994). Use of music therapy with subject-selected tapes during flexible sigmoidoscopy, which is highly stressful, reduced state anxiety during this procedure for adults (Palakanis, DeNobile, Sweeney, & Blankenship, 1994). In a study by Summers, Hoffman, Newf, Hanson, and Pierce (1990), 60-beat-per-minute background music played for nursing students was not an effective intervention in reducing state or test anxiety during an examination. One-third of the students found the music to be too loud and distracting.

Music therapy to promote relaxation.   Various physiological measures (heart rate, respiratory rate, blood pressure) have been used to determine if music therapy produces relaxation and stress reduction. Blood pressure de-creased and mood improved following subject-selected music listening in a small sample of intensive care unit patients (Updike, 1990). Heart rate and respiratory rate decreased and mood improved in response to the music inter-vention of subject-selected tapes in a small sample of critically ill patients receiving mechanical ventilatory support (Chlan, 1995). In a case study design, Burke, Walsh, Oehler, and Gingras (1995) documented an improvement in oxygen saturation and less agitation in four neonates for whom an audiocassette (*Transitions*, intrauterine sounds blended with a female voice) was played either through a mattress with speakers or via tape recording. Collins and Kuck (1991) reported similar findings of improved oxygen saturation and behavior state for intubated neonates exposed to *Transitions*. Not surprisingly, a decrease occurred in noise annoyance, heart rate, and blood pressure in subjects who had undergone coronary artery bypass and were provided with investigator-selected music intervention with classical music blended with ocean sounds (Byers & Smyth, 1997). One team of investigators pronounced music to be a safe intervention without clinically dangerous side effects for 24 coronary care patients who listened to 36 minutes of investigator-selected classical music (Davis-Rollans & Cunningham, 1987). Heart rate varied across the listening time with both increases and decreases noted. No statistically significant changes in the respiratory rate were found.

Varying degrees of effectiveness were reported in investigations on the use of music therapy specifically for stress reduction. In a study by Hatta and Nakamura (1991), university students exposed to an experimental mental stress situation were found to have reduced stress as indicated by decreases on the Stress Arousal Adjective Checklist (Mackay, Cox, Burrow, & Lazzerini, 1978) in response to listening to three types of investigator-selected music (classical, music with nature sounds, and pop tunes) as opposed to those who did not experience music listening. Another group of 58 university students who listened to three tapes of investigator-selected New Age or classical music reported less perceived stress than after listening to student-selected pop music (Mornhinweg, 1992). Interestingly, subjects preferred the less effective pop music and expressed a dislike for the New Age music, which proved to produce the most relaxation.

Music therapy was not found to be effective in reducing stress in blood donors, particularly in those with previous donation experience (Ferguson, Singh, & Cunningham-Snell, 1997). Easy-listening music was played free-field in the background at the donor center. Music was found to have a detrimental effect on the environmental appraisal for those with two previous blood donations. Music was not found to impact mood. The investigators concluded that music was not a beneficial stress management technique for blood donors.

Music therapy used in conjunction with other relaxation techniques. Music therapy has been tested in conjunction with other techniques for purposes of relaxation in a variety of patient populations. Results from these studies do not provide clear guidance for the use of music with these populations. Benson's relaxation technique was found to produce more positive results in anxiety and pain ratings than investigator-selected contemporary instrumental music in patients undergoing femoral angiography (Mandle et al., 1990). No significant differences in heart rate were detected between Benson's relaxation technique and subject-selected music therapy in a sample of coronary care unit subjects (Guzzetta, 1989). However, skin temperature was higher posttest in the music condition than in the relaxation condition, suggesting music produced greater relaxation. In a single group, quasi-experimental design study, when music was used as one of four components in a relaxation exercise for inpatient psychiatric subjects, the combined relaxation regimen was found to decrease anxiety post-intervention (Weber, 1996). Although a sample of CCU subjects reported music therapy (investigator-selected classical music) and muscle relaxation beneficial, no significant differences in heart rate, blood pressure, anxiety, or depression were detected between these two groups (Elliott, 1994). The investigator reported the findings to be of low statistical power with effect sizes ranging from 0.19–0.22, thus contributing to the non-significance of the findings (Elliott, 1994).

Conclusions.   Overall, there is evidence that music therapy is an effective intervention for reducing state anxiety and promoting relaxation across divergent patient populations from coronary care patients to premature neonates. Music therapy was also an effective anxiolytic for those undergoing stressful procedures such as sigmoidoscopy or colposcopy. In some studies, subject-selected relaxing music promoted physiological relaxation, as indicated by decreased heart rate and respiratory rate. Mood improvement in response to music therapy occurred in most studies. In general, subjects reported that they enjoyed the music listening and felt it should be offered to other patients experiencing similar situations.

The effectiveness of music therapy however, over and above a control condition or other relaxation interventions, has not been consistently demonstrated. Non-significant findings may be due to the lack of enough effect size or sample size to capture statistical and/or clinical significance. Although music therapy is an effective intervention for promoting relaxation, no clear benefit of one relaxation technique over another is apparent. Patient preference may be a key to the effectiveness of any intervention. Perhaps what investigators deem to be relaxing music is not received as such by all listeners. Additional research is needed to support these contentions.

Pain Reduction

Management of pain is a major care concern of nurses. A growing body of knowledge on the efficacy of complementary therapies in the management of pain is evolving. The use of music to decrease of pain was explored in 18 studies. Studies addressed the management of postoperative pain (7), pain

associated with chronic conditions such as cancer (5), and pain during procedures and labor.

A variety of research designs, measurements, and music selections were
used in the seven studies in which the impact of music on post-surgical patients
was examined. In one of the first reported studies on the use of music postoperatively, Locsin (1981) noted that music had an impact on musculo-skeletal
and verbal pain reactors of 24 obstetric or gynecologic patients. Locsin played
music for 15 minutes every 2 hours. Using a similar population (women who
had had hysterectomies), Mullooly, Levin, and Feldman (1988) reported that
anxiety was decreased on the first and second postoperative days while pain
decreases were present on the second postoperative day. Subjects listened to
easy listening music for 10 minutes. Good (1995) compared the effectiveness
of music, jaw relaxation, and a combination of these two interventions with
84 persons who had had abdominal surgery. Music did not result in any
significant changes in pain during the first ambulation after surgery. However,
on the third postoperative check 89% of the subjects indicated that music
helped to decrease both the sensation and distress of pain. The tape recorder
had been left for their use at the bedside. The efficiency of music and music
videos in decreasing pain and improving sleep in a sample of 96 adults was
explored by Zimmerman, Barnason, and Schmaderer (1996). Decreases in
pain were found with the use of music, music videos, and use during a rest
period. Interestingly, subjects receiving videos with music reported better
sleep than those who only received music.

Use of music to decrease pain was also examined. Marchette and colleagues (Marchette, Main, & Redick, 1989; Marchette, Main, Redick, Bagg, &
Leatherland, 1991) examined the impact music had on decreasing pain associated with circumcision when no anesthetic agent was used. Music was not
effective in reducing the observed manifestations of pain during circumcisions.

To determine the effect of music on pain in the immediate postoperative
period, Heiser, Chiles, Fudge, and Gray (1997) played country, instrumental,
or classical music during the final 30 minutes of surgical procedures and
during the first hour in the postanesthesia care unit. They found that music
had no impact on pain, anxiety, satisfaction, heart rate, blood pressure, or
respiratory rate as compared to a control group, but patients who listened to
music reported that the music served as a distractor and helped them to relax.

The efficacy of music in decreasing pain in persons with cancer was
explored in two studies (Beck, 1991; Zimmerman, Pozehl, Duncan, & Schmitz,
1989). Subjects in the study by Beck selected the type of music to which they
wished to listen; three-fourths of the subjects reported that music decreased
their pain to some extent, with 47% having a moderate or "great" response
to the music. Similarly, subjects in the study by Zimmerman et al. (1989)

reported that music helped to decrease their perception of pain. Curtis (1986) used music with nine persons who were terminally ill; no significant differences in the perception of pain were found between the time music was played and during the control period. The investigators noted, however, that individual subjects did have a positive response to music.

The efficacy of music to decrease pain in patients with severe pain was examined in several studies. Miller, Hickman, and Lemasters (1992) explored the efficacy of a music video with 17 burn patients undergoing dressing changes. The investigators found that pain intensity and anxiety were significantly decreased when subjects used the music video. In a study using Newman's health as expanding consciousness model (1994) as the theoretical basis for the efficacy of music, Schorr (1993) reported that the pain threshold increased in persons with chronic pain who listened to their favorite music piece for 20 minutes a day as compared to the level reported during the baseline period. Menegazzi, Paris, Kersteen, Flynn, and Trautman (1991), using a randomized controlled trial, examined the use of patient-selected music in patients receiving laceration repair in an emergency department. Pain scores in the music group were significantly lower than scores in the control group.

Studies by Arts et al. (1994), Dubois, Bartter, and Pratter (1995), and Fowler-Kerry and Lander (1987) examined the effect that music had on pain during medical procedures. During bronchoscopy, patients reported greater comfort while listening to music, but no effects on dyspnea were noted (Dubois et al., 1995). Children reported less pain during injections when music was played (Fowler-Kerry & Lander, 1987). In contrast, Arts and colleagues (1994) found that music had no impact on reducing pain in children undergoing intravenous cannulation. Due to differences in the types of music and the duration for listening to the selections, it is difficult to compare outcomes across these three studies.

The effect that music had on pain perception was examined in two laboratory studies. Geden, Lower, Beattie, and Beck (1989) used a sophisticated design to examine the effects of music and imagery on physiological and psychological variables. Easy listening and rock and roll selections could be selected by the subjects. Music had an effect on heart rate and blood pressure. Interestingly, there was no difference in outcomes when subjects listened to the various types of musical selection. Whipple and Glynn (1992) attempted to identify the basis for music decreasing pain. Soothing music selections elevated the pain threshold of subjects while stimulating music elevated both the pain and tactile thresholds. However, neither type of music had a significant impact on autonomic responses.

Overall, music was an effective intervention for reducing pain in the studies reviewed. Sample sizes in the pain studies ranged from 20 to 200 subjects and were relatively larger than those used in studying the effect of music on behavioral and performance outcomes. However, great variation existed in the type of music selection, length and frequency of the intervention, and outcome measures. Thus, it is difficult to make specific recommendations about the type of music and length of exposure for use in pain management.

Improved Performance

Many persons routinely use music while walking, jogging, or exercising. Does listening to music enhance performance in these and other activities? Twenty studies were conducted for the aim of improving performance outcomes. Music was used to improve outcomes associated with exercise (Brownley, McMurray, & Hackney, 1995; Copeland & Franks, 1991; Landrieu-Seiter, French, Silliman, & Tynan, 1995; Macnay, 1995; Seath & Thow, 1991; Thaut et al., 1996; Thornby, Haas, & Axen, 1995), compliance in a blind child (Silliman, French, & Tynan, 1992), rate of speech in an adolescent with brain damage (Cohen, 1988), behaviors in pre-schoolers (Godeli, Santana, Souza, & Marquetti, 1996) and adolescents (McIntyre & Cowell, 1991; Weidinger & Demi, 1991), trust and cooperation (Anshel & Kipper, 1988), schizophrenia (Tang, Yao, & Zheng, 1994), pulmonary function in adults with asthma (Lehrer et al., 1994), food intake in persons with dementia (Ragneskog, Brane, Karlsson, & Kihlgren, 1996; Ragneskog, Kihlgren, Karlsson, & Norberg, 1996), memory in persons with dementia (Norberg, Melin, & Asplund, 1986; Prickett & Moore, 1991), and mobility in persons with dementia (Pomeroy, 1993).

Exercise. Use of music during exercise resulted in subjects perceiving decreased exertion, increased exercise tolerance, and more positive experiences (Copeland & Franks, 1991; Macnay, 1995; Seath & Thow, 1991; Thornby et al., 1995). Easy listening, hymns, classical, and pop music were used in these four studies. Copland and Franks compared the efficacy of easy listening music with loud, fast music and no music in 24 college students; heart rate was lower and perceived exertion less when easy listening was provided. The time to exhaustion was longer when subjects listened to easy listening music. This finding raises questions about a common myth that loud, stimulating music is conducive to productive exercise workouts. Although the findings from these studies were quite similar, the sample sizes were small (4–36) and the studies examined the efficacy of music with two distinct age groups: college students and adults with chronic obstructive pulmonary disease or cardiac conditions.

Cognitive functioning.   Numerous articles in clinical nursing journals advocate using music with elders, particularly those with cognitive impairments. In five studies, the impact of music on improving performance in persons with dementia was explored. Pomeroy (1993) used a cross-over design to examine the effect music had on improving the mobility of eight elders with dementia who were unable to walk independently. Music was used in conjunction with physiotherapy. Improvement was found with the use of music as compared to the baseline period; however, no improvement occurred in elders who had severe mobility problems. Ragneskog, Brane et al. (1996) compared the effects of romantic, '20s and '30s, pop, and rock and roll music on mood and food intake. Intake was poorer when '20s and '30s music was played. Staff served more food, and subjects ate more food, particularly desserts, when pop music was played. A second study by Ragneskog, Kihlgren, et al. (1996) validated that staff fed patients more when pop and '30s music was played. Prickett and Moore (1991) reported that in the 10 subjects they studied, greater recall of words (61.9%) occurred when these words were sung by the elder as compared to when the words had been spoken to the subjects (37.4%). In an early study (1986), Norberg and colleagues explored if music would increase responsiveness in two persons in advanced stages of dementia. One became more peaceful when music was played, while the second subject became more responsive.

Behavior functioning.   Interventions other than medications have been sought by clinicians caring for children, adolescents, adults, and elders who manifest aggressive or aberrant behaviors. In five studies, the impact that music had on behaviors of children or adolescents was explored. In a case study design, Silliman et al. (1992) examined the efficacy of music as a reinforcer to improve motor skills in a child who was blind and mentally retarded. Although initial improvement was found in walking, stair climbing, standing, and sitting, the increased skills began to decline over 3 months. Regina, Santana, Souza, and Marquetti (1996) found that social interaction skills improved in a sample of 27 Brazilian pre-schoolers who had background rock and roll and folk music played during the observation sessions.

Use of music to improve behaviors in adolescents was examined in three studies. Use of a superimposed musical rhythm was found to decrease the rate of speech in an adolescent with Kleever-Bucy syndrome (Cohen, 1988). Although the use of music did not result in a normal rate of speech, a 28% reduction in speed of speaking was found in this case study. Weidinger and Demi (1991) explored the impact of two types of music on behaviors of institutionalized adolescents. Adolescents listening to heavy metal music and songs with negative lyrics displayed more dysfunctional behaviors than those who listened to country and western, pop, or blues music. However, McIntyre and Cowell (1991) observed no differences in the behaviors of adolescents in a residential facility during the playing of sedative, stimulating, and no music. Because of the varying results and small sizes, considerably more research on the use of music to alter problem behaviors in adolescents is needed.

Although music therapy encompasses both active participation in and listening to music, the majority of studies used the latter approach. Active participation was examined in only a few studies. Tang and colleagues (1994) provided both active and passive involvement in music for patients with schizophrenia. A decrease in negative symptoms, an increase in ability to converse, and an increased interest in external events was found after subjects had participated in 19 music therapy sessions which involved listening to music and singing songs as compared to findings in a control group. Likewise, Anshel and Kipper (1988) found that cooperation was higher when subjects actively participated in singing or reading poetry aloud in a group as opposed to passive involvement. Subjects in these two studies were recruited in China and Israel, respectively.

Overall, music was helpful in improving performance in a variety of areas. The basis for selecting music as the intervention to use was not specifically addressed in the majority of studies. However, Godeli et al. (1996), Lehrer et al. (1994), and Ragneskog, Brane, et al. (1996) noted that reduction of stress was the hypothesized mechanism underlying improved performance. This could well have been the basis for the improvement of performance in many of the other studies. The purposes for using music to improve performance varied, so it was not surprising that a wide variety of musical selections were used.

Behaviors

Because of the increasing number of elders with dementia and the high percentage of this population who display aggressive or agitated behaviors, explorations in the use of therapies other than physical and chemical restraints for managing these behaviors is an important area of investigation. Likewise, effective complementary therapies that can be used in the treatment of mental illnesses address a major health problem. Music was used in nine studies to improve mood or decrease aggressive or agitated behaviors.

The use of music to produce relaxation and decrease aggressive behaviors in persons with dementia was explored in five studies (Broton & Pickett-Cooper, 1996; Casby & Holm, 1994; Gerdner & Swanson, 1993; Sambandham & Schirm, 1995; Snyder & Olson, 1996). Positive results were found in all five studies. Casby and Holm (1994) reported that vocalizations decreased in three subjects who had routinely demonstrated repetitive vocalizations when classical or favorite music was played as compared to during the baseline period. In a study conducted by Sambandham and Schirm (1995), less talking occurred during the playing of music. Using a sample of 20 subjects who had displayed agitated behaviors, Broton and Pickett-Cooper (1996) noted that less agitation was observed during and after music was played. Persons who reported to have liked music showed the most decline in agitated behaviors in a small study (*n* = 5) conducted by Gerdner and Swanson (1993). Snyder and Olson (1996) reported that classical, New Age, or hymns delivered via a Spinoza bear (tape player in huggable bear) produced greater relaxation in five elderly women as compared to behaviors observed during the baseline period. The different designs and musical selections used in these five studies in elders with dementia preclude comparisons across the studies. Likewise, small sample sizes (2 to 20 subjects) limit the clinical applications that can be recommended. However, the positive outcomes suggest the need for further validation.

Reduction of aggressive behaviors in persons with mental illness through the use of musical selections was explored by Courtright, Johnson, Baumgartner, Jordan, and Webster (1990). The musical selection was *Sea Gulls*, a composition developed for relaxation and rest. Use of this selection twice a week for 4 weeks resulted in a dramatic decline in aggressive behaviors during meals. Janelli and Kanski (1997) used a case study to examine the effect that music had on improving positive behaviors when restraints were removed on an elderly male. Band, classical, country and western, and popular music styles were played. A slight increase in positive behaviors occurred during the playing of music as compared to the behaviors observed during the baseline period.

Depression is a major health problem in all age groups. Hanser and Thompson (1994) reported improvement in depressive mood, distress, self-esteem, and mood when a multiple relaxation therapy comprise of music, exercise, facial massage, imagery, and progressive muscle relaxation was employed for 8 weeks with a group of elderly females. Most notably, these changes were maintained over a 9-month period. Music was found to be effective in the management of aggressive behaviors and in the improvement in mood. Additional studies with larger sample sizes are needed to validate these findings.

Desired Outcomes

Music has been explored as an intervention to promote desired patient outcomes in such divergent populations as newborns, elders, persons with brain injuries, and during childbirth. Soothing, lyrical music was found to induce newborns in one nursery to have fewer arousal states and spend less time in arousal states when music was played in the isolette (Kaminski & Hall, 1996). Inconsistent results were found when lullabies with a mother's voice were played over a 3-day period for babies in a neonatal intensive care unit (Standley & Moore, 1995). Oxygen saturation increased the first day, but not on days 2 or 3. Neonates receiving music therapy had a fewer number of oxygenation alarms over the 3 days; depressive effects of oxygen saturation levels occurred after the music was discontinued.

Elders are another age group who have benefited from the music therapy. Patient satisfaction in elderly populations undergoing cataract surgery was enhanced by music listening during the procedures as compared to a group not receiving music (Cruise, Chung, Yogendran, & Little, 1997). Those subjects who listened to music reported being more satisfied with their experience, were more relaxed, and stated they would use music again if needed. Ninety-six percent of community-based elders in a study by Mornhinweg and Voignier (1995) reported improved quality of sleep when listening to classical or New Age music prior to bedtime.

In two studies researchers found that music tapes were not effective in producing desired outcomes. A tape of classical piano music was not found to have a statistically or clinically impact on cerebral perfusion pressure in a small sample ($n = 15$) of traumatic brain injured subjects (Schinner et al., 1995). Popular or self-selected music was not found to influence the frequency of medications used during prepared childbirth (Durham & Collins, 1986).

Although positive findings were presented in the majority of studies reviewed in this section, the diversity of patient populations precludes making meaningful comparisons across studies. The negative findings in several studies suggest careful attention to the type of music used in future studies.

Imagery With Music Interventions

A number of investigations tested guided imagery and music (GIM) or music with imagery. Investigators proposed that music-induced relaxation facilitated the imagery process. Guided imagery and music (GIM) is a specific psychotherapy technique that was developed by Helen Bonny (1978). GIM utilizes carefully selected and sequenced music to induce deep relaxation to aid an individual in retrieving unconscious thought through guided imagery with a trained therapist (Bonny, 1978). In a study of two subjects with fibroid tumors, Bonny's GIM method was found to provide physiological and psychological healing of the tumors over an extensive course of therapy for two females (Pickett, 1987). Other investigators have used background music concurrently with taped suggestions to facilitate imagery in order to minimize perceived degree of nausea, vomiting, and anxiety associated with chemotherapy treatments in those subjects exposed to the tape condition (Frank, 1985). In an anecdotal report, another sample of subjects undergoing chemotherapy who listened to a personal physician message with background music had less anxiety and felt better than those who did not listen to a tape (Sabo & Michael, 1996).

Psychoneuroimmunology-based Investigations With Music

The relatively new and emerging field of psychoneuroimmunology (PNI) and its salient variables has been investigated in response to music therapy, both alone and with imagery-based interventions. In a study by Miluk-Kolasa, Obminski, Stupnicki, and Golec (1994), decreased salivary cortisol was found in subjects who listened to individualized music for 60 minutes prior to surgery as compared to those who did not listen to music. In another study of well adults, serum measures of interleukin-1 (cortisol generating hormone) and cortisol decreased in response to 15 minutes of subject-selected music therapy and perceived sensory experiences (subjects articulated what they felt, saw, or heard while music listening) (Bartlett, Kaufman, & Smeltekop, 1993). However, no differences were noted on anxiety among the treatment conditions. Lastly, healthy adults who participated in a 13-week trial of Bonny's GIM method reported improved mood, with decreases in depression, fatigue, and serum cortisol levels (McKinney, Antoni, Kumar, Tims, & McCabe, 1997). The positive results found in these studies suggest the need for continued explanations.

CONCEPTUAL AND METHODOLOGICAL ISSUES

Few programs of study on the use of music were found. Three studies on the use of music with several different populations were published by Zimmerman and colleagues (Zimmerman et al., 1988, 1989, 1996). A number of authors had two reports on the use of music (Janelli, Kanski, Jones, & Kennedy, 1995; Janelli & Kanski, 1997; Marchette et al., 1989, 1991; Mornhinweg, 1992; Mornhinweg & Voignier, 1995; Ragneskog, Brane, et al., 1996; Ragneskog, Kihlgren, et al., 1996). Although many authors reviewed past research on the use of music therapy, few investigators provided links on how they incorporated findings and suggestions from past studies into their investigations; for example, were the music selections offered ones that had produced positive results in a previous study, or were new selections employed. The majority of nurse investigators published their findings in clinical journals. Because many of the studies had comparatively small sample sizes, research-focused journals with more stringent publication guidelines may have found that these reports did not fit the specifications of their journal. Another possible reason for the preponderance of studies on music being published in clinical journals may be that investigators may have wished to share their findings with audiences who could apply the findings in practice sites.

Great diversity existed in the types of musical selections offered to subjects, and many investigators provided subjects with a choice in selections. Providing subjects with choices is preferable as music likes and dislikes vary greatly across individuals. Even when selection choices were available, some subjects indicated that they would have preferred listening to their own selections. Gerdner and Swanson (1993) found the best responses in subjects who had enjoyed listening to music before inclusion in the study. More consistency in the musical selections offered across studies or consistency in allowing patients to use their own selections would allow for more definitive conclusions to be made about the comparative efficacy of music in the achievement of specific outcomes.

Variation existed across the studies in the length of exposure to the musical selection during a session and the number of sessions used. The length of a session ranged from 10 minutes to 60 minutes. The purpose for which music was implemented may have influenced the length of exposure chosen by an investigator. However, considerable variation was found in the length of time music was played for the achievement of similar outcomes. For example, in the management of postoperative pain, exposure to music varied from 10 minutes to 60 minutes. In addition to differences in the length of the sessions, some studies used only one session while many investigators used multiple sessions. Exploration within and across studies on the dose of the intervention would provide valuable information for practitioners.

Similar to the samples used in studies in which other interventions have been tested, the sample size in the majority of studies were quite small. Only two studies (Barnason et al., 1995; Byers & Smyth, 1997) indicated that they used a power analysis to determine the sample sizes. Although most investigators provided the exclusion criteria for selecting participants, few obtained data about subjects' prior use of music. Larger sample sizes, multiple-site studies, and more homogeneity of subjects would produce findings that would provide more definitive direction for the use of music in clinical practice.

Great diversity existed in the study designs used to examine the impact that music had on health outcomes. Study designs ranged from case studies to multiple groups using repeated measures. The majority of studies used well thought-out designs that provided the investigators with an opportunity to truly determine if the outcomes resulted from the use of music. For example, even though it was a case study, Cohen (1988) employed an ABACAC design. (Period A was used to collect baseline data, musical selections were played during period B, and functional speaking was used during period C.) An overwhelming number of the studies were conducted in clinical sites. However, Geden et al. (1989) and Whipple and Glynn (1992) examined the efficacy of music in laboratories. Because greater control of variables can be achieved in laboratories, investigators need to give careful attention as to whether a laboratory study is needed before testing the intervention with clinical populations.

DIRECTIONS FOR FUTURE RESEARCH

This chapter has reviewed studies on the use of music as a therapeutic intervention to effect human health that have been conducted by nurses, music therapists, psychologists, and other health professionals. Music has been tested with a wide variety of populations in numerous settings. Music was tested alone and in conjunction with other interventions, such as imagery and other relaxation techniques. Music has been found to positively influence outcomes in a broad range of variables: improve exercise performance, increase food intake, allay agitated behaviors in elders with dementia, improve mood, and reduce pain. Music also has been found to decrease anxiety and promote physiological and psychological relaxation in a wide variety of clinical populations, including critically ill adults, in patients undergoing a variety of surgical and diagnostic procedures, and in intubated premature neonates. Despite the documented broad-based effectiveness of music, a number of areas require attention in future studies.

Research on the efficacy of music in achieving positive health outcomes has primarily focused on White populations, particularly White adults. Explorations on the efficacy of music in different cultural groups are needed. Incorporation of the music of the specific cultural group is needed. Studies both within the United States and collaborative efforts with colleagues in other countries would further knowledge about the types of music that are effective with various cultural/ethnic groups and would provide the basis for making generalizations about the overall effectiveness of music.

Replication studies that test the efficacy of specific musical selections are needed. Although most studies noted the general types of music used, the specific selections were often not reported. Using the same selections with larger samples would increase knowledge about the effectiveness of specific selections with populations.

Few studies provided detailed information about subjects beyond age, gender, and type of clinical problem. Avants, Margolin, and Salovey (1990) noted that it is important to examine personality traits when determining the fit of the various relaxation techniques with individuals. Isolating personality characteristics, such as high trait anxiety or absorption (Chlan, 1997), would allow investigators to compare the efficacy of music with persons with high and low personality factors. Another variable is subjects' past experience with music and responses to specific types of music. Obtaining information on this variable and including these data in the analysis would provide valuable information to guide practice.

Overall, positive outcomes were achieved with the use of music. However, few studies specifically examined the basis for why music might produce positive outcomes. Additional studies exploring the mechanisms for "why" music works are needed. Particularly, studies are needed that examine the impact of music on psychoneuroimmunological variables. This is an emerging critical area, and nurse researchers are in a prime position to include this outcome variable.

Synthesis of the findings of research on music is needed. Good (1996) reviewed the effects of relaxation and music on postoperative pain. Meta-analytic techniques can be used not only to correct for various artifacts that can affect findings (i.e., sampling error), but can also be applied to a body of research to synthesize the evidence in a particular area (Hunter & Schmidt, 1990). No recent meta-analysis has been done on the vast and diverse areas of music's effectiveness. Such analyses would provide valuable information for researchers and clinicians.

Investigators are advised to "build on" the findings and recommendations from past studies in order to build the scientific basis for the use of music. With the growing emphasis in health care on cost-effective outcomes and the increasing attention being given to the use of complementary therapies, it is critical that nurses be able to provide a sound basis for the use of music therapy.

ACKNOWLEDGMENT

WenYun Cheng and YuehHsia Tseng assisted with the retrieval and review of the articles.

Supported in part by a research training grant, "Nursing Interventions, Outcomes, and Effectiveness." (5-T32-NR07082, J. McCloskey and M. Maas, Co-Directors).

REFERENCES

Anshel, A., & Kipper, D. A. (1988). The influence of group singing on trust and cooperation. *Journal of Music Therapy, 25,* 145–155.

Arts, S. E., Abu-Saad, H. H., Champion, G. D., Crawford, M. R., Fisher, R. J., Juniper, K. H., & Ziegler, J. B. (1994). Age-related response to lidocaine-prilocaine (EMLA) emulsion and effect of music distraction on the pain of intravenous cannulation. *Pediatrics, 93,* 797–801.

Augustin, P., & Hains, A. (1996). Effect of music on ambulatory surgery patients' preoperative anxiety. *AORN Journal, 63,* 750–758.

Avants, S., Margolin, A., & Salovey, P. (1990). Stress management techniques: Anxiety reduction, appeal, and individual differences. *Imagination, Cognition and Personality, 10,* 3–23.

Barnason, S., Zimmerman, L., & Nieveen, J. (1995). The effects of music intervention on anxiety in the patient after coronary bypass grafting. *Heart & Lung, 24,* 124–132.

Bartlett, D., Kaufman, D., & Smeltekop, R. (1993). The effects of music listening and perceived sensory experiences on the immune system as measured by interleukin-1 and cortisol. *Journal of Music Therapy, 30,* 194–209.

Beck, S. L. (1991). The therapeutic use of music for cancer-related pain. *Oncology Nursing Forum, 18,* 1327–1337.

Bolwerk, C. (1990). Effects of relaxing music on state anxiety in myocardial infarction patients. *Critical Care Nursing Quarterly, 13,* 63–72.

Bonny, H. (1978). *The role of taped music programs in the GIM process.* Salina, KS: Bonny Foundation.

Broton, M., & Pickett-Cooper, P. K. (1996). The effects of music therapy intervention on agitation behaviors of Alzheimer's disease patients. *Journal of Music Therapy, 33,* 2–18.

Brownley, K. A., McMurray, R. G., & Hackney, A. C. (1995). Effects of music on physiological and affective responses to graded treadmill exercise in trained and untrained runners. *International Journal of Psychophysiology, 19,* 193–201.

Burke, M., Walsh, J., Oehler, J., & Gingras, J. (1995). Music therapy following suctioning: Four case studies. *Neonatal Network, 14*(7), 41–49.

Byers, J., & Smyth, K. (1997). Effect of a music intervention on noise annoyance, heart rate, and blood pressure in cardiac surgery patients. *American Journal of Critical Care, 6,* 183–191.

Casby, J. A., & Holm, M. B. (1994). The effect of music on repetitive disruptive vocalizations of persons with dementia. *The American Journal of Occupational Therapy, 48,* 883–889.

Chlan, L. (1995). Psychophysiologic responses of mechanically ventilated patients to music: A pilot study. *American Journal of Critical Care, 4,* 233–238.

Chlan, L. (1997). *The relationship of absorption to the effects of music therapy on anxiety and relaxation for mechanically ventilated patients.* Unpublished doctoral dissertation, University of Minnesota, Minneapolis.

Cohen, N. S. (1988). The use of superimposed rhythm to decrease the rate of speech in a brain-damaged adolescent. *Journal of Music Therapy, 25,* 85–93.

Collins, S., & Kuck, K. (1991). Music therapy in the neonatal intensive care unit. *Neonatal Network, 9*(6), 23–26.

Copeland, B. L., & Franks, B. D. (1991). Effects of types and intensities of background music on treadmill endurance. *The Journal of Sports Medicine and Physical Fitness, 31,* 100–103.

Courtright, P., Johnson, S., Baumgartner, M. A., Jordan, M., & Webster, J. C. (1990). Dinner music: Does it affect the behavior of psychiatric inpatient? *Journal of Psychosocial Nursing, 28,* 37–40.

Cruise, C. J., Chung, F., Yogendran, S., & Little, D. (1997). Music increases satisfaction in elderly out-patients undergoing cataract surgery. *Canadian Journal of Anesthesiology, 44,* 43–48.

Curtis, S. (1986). The effect of music on pain relief and relaxation of the terminally ill. *Journal of Music Therapy, 23,* 10–24.

Davis-Rollans, C., & Cunningham, S. G. (1987). Physiologic responses of coronary care patients to selected music. *Heart & Lung, 16,* 370–378.

Dubois, J. M., Bartter, T., & Pratter, M. R. (1995). Music improves patient comfort level during outpatient bronchoscopy. *Chest, 108,* 129–130.

Durham, L., & Collins, M. (1986). The effect of music as a conditioning aid in prepared childbirth education. *Journal of Obstetric, Gynecologic and Neonatal Nursing, 15,* 268–270.

Elliott, D. (1994). The effects of music and muscle relaxation on patient anxiety in a coronary care unit. *Heart & Lung, 23,* 27–35.

Ferguson, E., Singh, A., & Cunningham-Snell, N. (1997). Stress and blood donation: Effects of music and previous donation experience. *British Journal of Psychology, 88,* 277–294.

Fowler-Kerry, S., & Lander, J. R. (1987). Management of injection pain in children. *Pain, 30,* 169–175.

Frank, J. (1985). The effects of music therapy and guided visual imagery on chemotherapy-induced nausea and vomiting. *Oncology Nursing Forum, 12*(5), 47–51.

Gaberson, K. (1995). The effect of humorous and musical distraction on preoperative anxiety. *AORN Journal, 62,* 784–791.

Geden, E. A., Lower, M., Beattie, S., & Beck, N. (1989). Effects of music and imagery on physiologic and self-report of analogued labor pain. *Nursing Research, 38,* 37–41.

Gerdner, L., & Swanson, E. (1993). Effects of individualized music on confused and agitated elderly patients. *Archives of Psychiatric Nursing, 7,* 284–291.

Godeli, M. R., Santana, P. R., Souza, V. H., & Marquetti, G. P. (1996). Influence of background music on preschoolers behavior: A naturalistic approach. *Perceptual and Motor Skills, 82,* 1123–1129.

Good, M. (1995). A comparison of the effects of jaw relaxation and music on postoperative pain. *Nursing Research, 44,* 52–57.

Good, M. (1996). Effects of relaxation and music on postoperative pain: A review. *Journal of Advanced Nursing, 24,* 905–914.

Guzzetta, C. (1989). Effects of relaxation and music therapy on patients in a coronary care unit with presumptive acute myocardial infarction. *Heart & Lung, 18,* 609–616.

Hanser, S. B., & Thompson, L. W. (1994). Effects of a music therapy strategy on depressed older adults. *Journal of Gerontology: Psychological Sciences, 49,* 265–269.

Hatta, T., & Nakamura, M. (1991). Can antistress music tapes reduce mental stress? *Stress Medicine, 7,* 181–184.

Heiser, R. M., Chiles, K., Fudge, M., & Gray, S. E. (1997). The use of music during the immediate postoperative recovery period. *AORN Journal, 65,* 777–785.

Heitz, L., Symreng, T., & Scamman, F. L. (1992). Effect of music therapy in the postanesthesia care unit: A nursing intervention. *Journal of Post Anesthesia Nursing, 7,* 22–31.

Hunter, J., & Schmidt, F. (1990). *Methods of meta-analysis.* Newbury Park, CA: Sage.

Janelli, L. M., & Kanski, G. W. (1997). Music intervention with physically restrained patients. *Rehabilitation Nursing, 22,* 14–19.

Janelli, L. M., Kanski, G. W., Jones, H. M, & Kennedy, M. C. (1995). Exploring music intervention with restrained patients. *Nursing Forum, 30,* 12–18.

Kaminski, J., & Hall, W. (1996). The effect of soothing music on neonatal behavioral states in the hospital newborn nursery. *Neonatal Network, 15*(1), 45–54.

Landrieu-Seiter, M., French, R., Silliman, L. M., & Tynan, D. (1995). Influence of video and music reinforcement on strength exercise performance by nonambulatory children who are profoundly mentally retarded. *Clinical Kinesiology: Journal of American Kinesiotherapy Association, 48,* 69–82.

Lehrer, P. M., Hochron, S. M., Mayne, T., Isenber, S., Carlson, V., Lasoski, A. M., Gilchrist, J., Morales, D., & Rausch, L. (1994). Relaxation and music therapies for asthma among patients prestabilized on asthma medication. *Journal of Behavioral Medicine, 17,* 1–24.

Locsin, R. G. R. A. C. (1981). The effect of music on the pain of selected postoperative patients. *Journal of Advanced Nursing, 6,* 19–25.

Mackay, C. J., Cox, T., Burrow, G. C., & Lazzerini, A. J. (1978). An inventory for the measurement of self-reported stress and arousal. *British Journal of Clinical Psychology, 17,* 283–284.

Macnay, S. K. (1995). The influence of preferred music on the perceived exertion, mood, and time estimation scores of patients participating in a cardiac rehabilitation exercise program. *Music Therapy Perspectives, 13,* 91–96.

Mandle, C., Domar, A., Harrington, D., Leserman, J., Bozadjian, E., Friedman, R., & Benson, H. (1990). Relaxation response in femoral angiography. *Radiology, 174*(3), 737–739.

Maranto, C. (1993). Music therapy and stress management. In P. M. Lehrer & R. L. Woolfolk (Eds.), *Principles and practice of stress management* (2nd ed.) (pp. 407–433). New York: Guilford.

Marchette, L., Main, R., & Redick, E. (1989). Pain reduction during neonatal circumcision. *Pediatric Nursing, 15,* 207–210.

Marchette, L., Main, R., Redick, E., Bagg, A., & Leatherland, J. (1991). Pain reduction interventions during neonatal circumcision. *Nursing Research, 40,* 241–244.

McIntyre, T., & Cowell, K. (1991). Effects of various music conditions on multiple dimensions of behavior of emotionally disturbed adolescents. *Psychological Reports, 69,* 1007–1009.

McKinney, C., Antoni, M., Kumar, M., Tims, F., & McCabe, P. (1997). Effects of guided imagery and music (GIM) therapy on mood and cortisol in healthy adults. *Health Psychology, 16,* 390–400.

Menegazzi, J. J., Paris, P. M., Kersteen, C. H., Flynn, B., & Trautman, D. E. (1991). A randomized, controlled trial of the use of music during laceration repair. *Annals of Emergency Medicine, 20,* 348–350.

Miller, A. C., Hickman, L. C., & Lemasters, G. K. (1992). A distraction technique for control of burn pain. *Journal of Burn Care Rehabilitation, 13,* 576–580.

Miluk-Kolasa, B., Obminski, Z., Stupnicki, R., & Golec, L. (1994). Effects of music treatment on salivary cortisol in patients exposed to pre-surgical stress. *Experimental and Clinical Endocrinology, 102,* 118–120.

Mornhinweg, G. (1992). Effects of music preference and selection on stress reduction. *Journal of Holistic Nursing, 10,* 101–109.

Mornhinweg, G., & Voignier, R. (1995). Music for sleep disturbance in the elderly. *Journal of Holistic Nursing, 13,* 248–254.

Mullooly, V. M., Levin, R. F., & Feldman, H. R. (1988). Music for postoperative pain and anxiety. *Journal of New York State Nurses, 19,* 4–7.

Munro, S., & Mount, B. (1978). Music therapy in palliative care. *Canadian Medical Association Journal, 119,* 1029–1034.

Newman, M. A. (1994). *Health as expanding consciousness* (2nd ed.). St. Louis: Mosby.

Nightingale, F. (1969). *Notes on nursing.* New York: Dover. Original work published 1860.

Norberg, A., Melin, E., & Asplund, K. (1986). Reactions to music, touch and object presentation in the final stage of dementia: An exploratory study. *International Journal of Nursing Studies, 23,* 315–323.

Palakanis, K., DeNobile, J., Sweeney, W., & Blankenship, C. (1994). Effect of music therapy on state anxiety in patients undergoing flexible sigmoidoscopy. *Diseases of the Colon and Rectum, 37,* 478–481.

Pickett, E. (1987). Fibroid tumors and response to guided imagery and music: Two case studies. *Imagination, Cognition and Personality, 7,* 165–176.

Pomeroy, V. M. (1993). The effect of physiotherapy input on mobility skills of elderly people with severe dementing illness. *Clinical Rehabilitation, 7,* 163–170.

Prickett, C. A., & Moore, R. S. (1991). The use of music to aid memory of Alzheimer's patients. *Journal of Music Therapy, 28,* 101–110.

Ragneskog, H., Brane, G., Karlsson, I., & Kihlgren, M. (1996). Influence of dinner music on food intake and symptoms common in dementia. *Scandinavian Journal of Caring Sciences, 10,* 11–17.

Ragneskog, H., Kihlgren, M., Karlsson, I., & Norberg, A. (1996). Dinner music for demented patients. *Clinical Nursing Research, 5,* 262–282.

Regina, M., Santana, P. R., Souza, V. H., & Marquetti, G. P. (1996). Influence of background music on preschoolers' behavior: A naturalistic approach. *Perceptual and Motor Skills, 82,* 1123–1129.

Rickert, V., Kozlowski, K., Warren, A., Hendon, A., & Davis, P. (1994). Adolescents and colposcopy: The use of different procedures to reduce anxiety. *American Journal of Obstetrics and Gynecology, 170,* 504–508.

Sabo, C., & Michael, S. (1996). The influence of personal massage with music on anxiety and side effects associated with chemotherapy. *Cancer Nursing, 19,* 283–289.

Sambandham, M., & Schirm, V. (1995). Music as a nursing intervention for residents with Alzheimer's disease in long-term care. *Geriatric Nursing, 16,* 79–83.

Schinner, K., Chisholm, A., Grap, M., Siva, P., Hallinan, M., & LaVoice-Hawkins, A. (1995). Effects of auditory stimuli on intracranial pressure and cerebral perfusion pressure in traumatic brain injury. *Journal of Neuroscience Nursing, 27,* 348–354.

Schorr, J. A. (1993). Music and pattern change in chronic pain. *Advances in Nursing Science, 15,* 27–36.

Seath, L., & Thow, M. (1991). The effect of music on the perception of effort and mood during aerobic type exercise. *Physiotherapy, 81,* 592–596.

Silliman, L. M., French, R., & Tynan, D. (1992). Use of sensory reinforcement to increase compliant behavior of a child who is blind and profoundly mentally retarded. *Clinical Kinesiology: Journal of the American Kinesiotherapy Association, 46,* 3–9.

Snyder, M., & Olson, J. (1996). Music and hand massage interventions to produce relaxation and reduce aggressive behaviors in cognitively impaired elders: A pilot study. *Clinical Gerontologist, 17,* 64–69.

Spielberger, C. (1983). *Manual for the State-Trait Anxiety Inventory.* Palo Alto, CA: Consulting Psychologists Press.

Standley, J., & Moore, R. (1995). Therapeutic effects of music and mother's voice on premature infants. *Pediatric Nursing, 21,* 509–512.

Steelman, V. (1990). Intraoperative music therapy: Effects on anxiety, blood pressure. *AORN Journal, 52,* 1026–1034.

Stevens, K. (1990). Patients' perceptions of music during surgery. *Journal of Advanced Nursing, 15,* 1045–1051.

Summers, S., Hoffman, J., Newf., J., Hanson, S., & Pierce, K. (1990). The effects of 60 beats per minute music on test taking anxiety among nursing students. *Journal of Nursing Education, 29,* 66–70.

Tang, W., Yao, X., & Zheng, Z. (1994). Rehabilitative effect of music therapy for residual schizophrenia: A one-month randomized controlled trial in Shanghai. *British Journal of Psychiatry, 165,* 38–44.

Thaut, M. H., McIntosh, G. C., Rice, R. R., Miller, R. A., Rathbun, M. J., & Brault, J. M. (1996). Rhythmic auditory stimulation in gait training for Parkinson's patients. *Movement Disorders, 11,* 193–200.

Thornby, M. A., Haas, F., & Axen, K. (1995). Effect of distractive auditory stimuli on exercise tolerance in patients with COPD. *Chest, 107,* 1213–1217.

Updike, P. (1990). Music therapy results for ICU patients. *Dimensions of Critical Care Nursing, 9,* 39–45.

Weber, S. (1996). The effects of relaxation exercises on anxiety levels in psychiatric inpatients. *Journal of Holistic Nursing, 14,* 196–205.

Weidinger, C. K., & Demi, A. S. (1991). Music listening preferences and preadmission dysfunctional psychosocial behaviors of adolescents hospitalized on an in-patient psychiatric unit. *Journal of Child & Adolescent Psychiatric & Mental Health Nursing, 4,* 3–8.

Whipple, B., & Glynn, N. J. (1992). Quantification of the effects of listening to music as a noninvasive method of pain control. *Scholarly Inquiry for Nursing Practice: An International Journal, 6,* 43–58.

White, J. (1992). Music therapy: An intervention to reduce anxiety in the myocardial infarction patient. *Clinical Nurse Specialist, 6,* 58–63.

Winter, M., Paskin, S., & Baker, T. (1994). Music reduces stress and anxiety of patients in the surgical holding area. *Journal of Post-Anesthesia Nursing, 9,* 340–343.

Woolf, H. (Ed.). (1979). *New collegiate dictionary.* Springfield, MA: Merriman.

Zimmerman, L., Barnason, S., & Schmaderer, M. (1996). The effects of music interventions on postoperative pain and sleep in coronary artery bypass graft (CABG) patients. *Scholarly Inquiry for Nursing Practice: An International Journal, 10,* 153–170.

Zimmerman, L., Pierson, M., & Marker, J. (1988). Effects of music on patient anxiety in coronary care units. *Heart & Lung, 17,* 560–566.

Zimmerman, L., Pozehl, B., Duncan, K., & Schmitz, R. (1989). Effects of music in patients who had chronic cancer pain. *Western Journal of Nursing Research, 11,* 289–309.

Chapter 2

Sleep Promotion in Adults

JUDITH A. FLOYD

ABSTRACT

Insomnia is among the most frequent health complaints brought to the attention of primary care providers. The prevalence estimates are highest in women, older adults, and patients with medical or psychiatric disorders. Clinical researchers have studied many barriers to sleep as well as some sleep promotion interventions for the ill and aging adult. Environmental, personal, and person-environment rhythm factors have been identified as correlates of poor sleep. All interventions studied by nurse researchers are non-pharmacological and have been classified as interventions that (a) create an environment more conducive to sleep, (b) relax the sleeper, or (c) entrain the circadian sleep-wake rhythm. This chapter summarizes results of published research on correlates of poor sleep and interventions to promote sleep. The chapter includes the relevant studies conducted by researchers in related disciplines as well as nurses' research. The *arcs*© software package was used to facilitate summarization of intervention studies. It was concluded that correlates of poor sleep are well described, but theories of sleep promotion are not well explicated. Also, the research base for sleep promotion interventions for use with clinical populations other than those with chronic insomnia is sparse. Gaps in knowledge are identified and conceptual and methodological issues are discussed as the basis for future directions in sleep promotion research.

Keywords: Sleep, Sleep Promotion, Relaxation Techniques, Sleep-wake Rhythm, Insomnia

Many adults complain of poor sleep. Lack and Thorn (1991) carried out a meta-analysis of the prevalence of insomnia based on 61 surveys published since 1962. Of the respondents surveyed in the 61 studies, 33% reported difficulty sleeping at least sometimes and 11% said they frequently had difficulty sleeping. The Gallup Organization estimates that some aspect of their sleep bothers 38% of the adult population. Half of them considered their problems serious enough to seek professional help (National Sleep Foundation, 1995). For healthy adults over age 60, nearly half report being bothered by some aspect of their sleep (Floyd, 1993).

Also, poor sleep often accompanies medical and psychiatric disorders. Any disorder or its accompanying treatment that leads to fear or worry, pain or discomfort, hyperarousal, respiratory or gastrointestinal distress, or urinary frequency or incontinence can interfere with sleep. Often the treatment of health problems requires hospitalization, other institutionalization, or changes in the home environment that decrease sleep opportunity and increase sleep fragmentation. Finally, many medications have side effects that interfere with sleep. Thus, managing sleep problems resulting from aging and illness is a major challenge facing care providers.

Anyone who has difficulty initiating or maintaining sleep is said to have insomnia. Insomnia is considered "primary" when it is an outcome of environmental or personal factors or "secondary" when it is an outcome of medical, psychiatric, or pharmacological factors. In addition to being classified as primary or secondary, insomnia also is classified by its duration and its presenting symptoms. "Transient insomnia" describes a sleep complaint that has been present for only a few nights. "Short-term insomnia" is the term used when the condition has lasted for up to 6 to 8 weeks, while "long-term" or "chronic insomnia" generally refers to symptoms that have been present for at least 2 months, but in many cases have been occurring for years (Mant & Bearpark, 1990). In terms of presenting symptoms, insomnia is referred to as "sleep onset insomnia" when patients complain of an inability to initiate sleep and "sleep maintenance insomnia" when patients find it difficult to remain asleep.

The prevention and effective treatment of chronic insomnia are important goals. Chronic insomnia is a risk factor for mood disorders (Eaton, Badawi, & Melton, 1995). It also is associated with an increased risk of daytime sleepiness, alcohol consumption, and automobile accidents (Kupfer & Reynolds, 1997). There is some evidence that mismanagement of transient and short-term insomnia leads to chronic difficulty initiating and maintaining sleep. Approximately 75% of adults with chronic insomnia attribute the start of their sleep problems to a stressful life event such as a personal loss, an illness, or moving from one residence to another (Healey et al., 1981; Kales et al., 1984). Bearpark (1994) hypothesized that chronic insomnia frequently develops from transient or short-term insomnia that gives rise to a "fear of not sleeping." As a result, behavior is changed in an attempt to improve sleep. Typical responses are more time in bed in an attempt to increase night-time sleep amount, increased napping in order to make up for lost nighttime sleep, and the use of alcohol to decrease sleep latency (i.e., length of time to fall asleep). These responses often make matters worse.

To assist patients with insomnia, nurses need scientific knowledge about sleep promotion. The remainder of this chapter addresses the research base currently available to nurses interested in promotion of sleep in adults. It also addresses what researchers have learned about barriers to sleep in ill and aging patient populations. First, the methods used for the systematic review are described. Next, the research about factors associated with difficulty initiating and maintaining sleep in the ill or older adult is discussed. Then, research that evaluates the effectiveness of interventions designed to promote sleep is described and analyzed. Finally, gaps in scientific knowledge and conceptual and methodological issues are discussed as the basis for recommendations regarding the future of sleep promotion research.

REVIEW METHODS

The steps taken to identify nursing and related research literature about sleep promotion in ill and aging adults were:

1. Cumulative Index of Nursing and Allied Health Literature (CINAHL) searches using the keyword "sleep," and document type, "research."

2. A search of the Virginia Henderson Library's Registry of Nursing Research (RNR) using the keyword "sleep."

3. Use of nurse sleep researchers who belong to one or more member organizations in the Association of Professional Sleep Societies as key informants about their own and colleagues' published studies of adult sleep.

4. Author searches in Medline and PSYCInfo using author names identified during CINAHL and RNR searches and by key informants.

5. Keyword searches in Medline and PSYCInfo using the terms "sleep" and "sleep disorders" with variations on terms describing each sleep intervention studied by nurse researchers as well as general terms (i.e., "intervention," "treatment," "education").

6. Ancestry searches using reference lists from all articles retrieved by other methods described above.

Nearly 300 citations published from 1958 to 1997 were retrieved and reviewed. Over 100 sleep research reports published by nurses were studied in depth to identify potential interventions for promotion of sleep. The interventions identified were all non-pharmacological in nature. They were categorized according to their presumed mechanism of action: (a) to create an environment more conducive to sleep, (b) to relax the sleeper, or (c) to entrain the personal sleep-wake rhythm to the circadian rhythm of the environment. All interventions studied by nurse researchers were judged to fall within the basic scope of nursing practice. Although specialized interventions exist for the treatment of chronic insomnia, nurses have published no studies of their use.

Research reports about adult sleep were retained in the review if the primary author was identified as a nurse or a member of a nursing faculty/ nursing department. The initial review showed that populations studied by nurses were those with health problems or lifespan developmental changes. The sleep environments studied were homes, hospitals, and residential care facilities. The outcome variables measured typically were related to symptoms of insomnia including sleep latency, waking frequency, waking duration, nighttime sleep amount, and subjective quality of nighttime sleep.

If the primary authors were not identified with nursing, research reports were retained for the review under the following circumstances: (a) The researcher studied initiation or maintenance of sleep in ill or older adults in home, hospital, or residential care settings; or (b) the researcher evaluated non-pharmacological interventions for insomnia that fall within the scope of basic nursing practice. Nursing and related-discipline studies of sleep disorders other than insomnia (e.g., narcolepsy and sleep apnea) were omitted from this review. Studies of sleep during developmental changes due to pregnancy, childbirth, menstrual cycle changes, and menopause also were omitted.

To facilitate detailed analysis of interventions, information about intervention studies was stored in *arcs*©, an experimental software program under development at the Virginia Henderson Library at Sigma Theta Tau International (Graves, 1990, 1997). The program facilitated retrieval of bibliographic information and information about the specific interventions studied including (a) direction and magnitude of treatment effects and (b) design and sampling conditions under which research results were obtained. In addition, the software facilitated examination of the research domain meta-structure.

CORRELATES OF INSOMNIA IN ILL AND AGING ADULTS

Nurse researchers began publishing results of studies of adults' sleep in the early 1970s. From the beginning descriptive studies of adult sleep in clinical settings tended to be of high quality and produced by well-prepared nurse researchers. Although sample sizes were sometimes small, repeated measurements helped assure reliability of measures. *Nursing Research* published the earliest studies (McFadden & Giblin, 1971; Walker, 1972; Woods, 1972). The studies described sleep of cardiac surgery patients in intensive care settings. All three early studies had very small sample sizes (i.e., four subjects each). Data were collected via observation, interviews, and questionnaires. These studies suggested that patients in intensive care settings (ICUs) had little opportunity for uninterrupted periods of sleep longer than 50 to 60 minutes.

Sleep in intensive care settings has continued to interest researchers. Different types of units have been studied including specialized cardiac ICUs (Simpson & Lee, 1996; Simpson, Lee, & Cameron, 1996a, 1996b) and respiratory ICUs (Aaron et al., 1996; Hilton, 1976). General medical and surgical ICUs also have been studied (Aurell & Elmqvist, 1985; Ballard, 1981; Broughton & Baron, 1978; Dlin, Rosen, Dickstein, Lyons, & Fisher, 1971; Edwards & Schuring, 1993; Helton, Gordon, & Nunnery, 1980; Hill, 1989; Orr & Stahl, 1977; Richards & Bairnsfather, 1988; Richards, Curry, Lyons, & Todd, 1996; Wilson, 1987). In the more than 25 years that sleep has been studied in ICUs, sample sizes have increased. Measurement of sleep variables has continued to be done primarily by observation, interviews, and paper-pencil means, but polysomnography also has been used in a number of studies (Aaron et al., 1996; Edwards & Schuring, 1993; Hilton, 1976; Richards & Bairnsfather, 1988; Richards et al., 1996). Cardiac patients have been the most studied patient population. All studies, despite differences in type of ICU or patient population studied, sample sizes obtained, or measurement approaches employed, support the early observations that sleep opportunity is very limited in intensive care settings.

Environmental Factors Associated With Insomnia in Hospitals

Many researchers have described the specific environmental factors that limit sleep opportunity in ICUs and other hospital units. Dlin et al. (1971) and Walker (1972) were the first to report that noise and constant activity of others in the sleep environment were major barriers to sleep in ICU. All studies since the early work have continued to identify noise and activities of others as the two primary deterrents to patients' sleep in hospitals (Ballard, 1981; Closs, 1992a; Edwards & Schuring, 1993; Helton et al., 1980; Hill, 1989; Hilton, 1976; Simpson et al., 1996a, 1996b; Wilson, 1987). Other barriers include lighting (Edell-Gustafsson, Aren, Hamrin, & Hetta, 1994; Hilton, 1976; Southwell & Wistow, 1995; Simpson et al., 1996a, 1996b); temperature

(Closs, 1992a; Dlin et al., 1971; Edell-Gustafsson et al., 1994; Southwell & Wistow, 1995); and uncomfortable or unfamiliar sleeping surfaces (Closs, 1992a; Dlin et al., 1971; Simpson et al., 1996a, 1996b; Southwell & Wistow, 1995; Walker, 1972). Only noise and activities of others have been studied in more depth regarding their impact on sleep in hospitals.

Noise.   High noise levels in ICUs have been shown to have a negative effect on nearly all sleep parameters measured by polysomnography (Aaron et al., 1996; Snyder-Halpern, 1985; Topf, 1992; Topf & Davis, 1993) and self-report measures of sleep quality (Snyder-Halpern, 1985; Topf, Bookman, & Arand, 1996). Specifically, Snyder-Halpern (1985) found self-reported sleep quality was decreased for normal female volunteers attempting to sleep under taped ICU-noise conditions compared with usual-noise conditions in a sleep laboratory. Using similar methods, Topf and her colleagues found normal female volunteers exposed to a taped noise condition had more difficulty falling asleep, awakened more often, had longer awakenings, and reported poorer sleep quality (Topf, 1992; Topf et al., 1996). Another group of researchers examined magnitude of noise and waking frequency in both male and female subjects (Aaron et al., 1996). They reported a strong correlation between the number of sound peaks of greater than or equal to 80 decibels and arousals from sleep for patients sleeping in an intermediate respiratory care unit.

Although most nurse researchers' studies of noise and sleep have examined the impact of ICU noise on sleep, one study compared sleep quality in two hospitals with significantly different mean nocturnal noise levels (Pimental-Souza, Carvalho, & Siqueira, 1996). The researchers found patients had a worse perception of sleep in the noisier hospital, where mean decibels equaled 53.7, than the less noisy hospital where mean decibels equaled 45.5. Only male patients were surveyed.In summary, the six studies that examined sleep and noise in hospital settings document that noise is an environmental factor contributing to poor sleep for hospitalized patients.

Activities of others.   Those studies that describe the nature of activities that disrupt sleep of patients in ICU and other hospital settings have identified many activities related to the direct and indirect care of the patient or other patients in the sleep environment. These include admission and transfer of patients, emergency bedside procedures, monitoring of patient status, and routine bedside care. In addition to direct and indirect care, the interactions among care providers are often identified as disrupters of sleep (Sheely, 1996; Snyder-Halpern, 1985; Walker, 1972; Woods, 1972). As could be expected, the greater the frequency and duration of interruptions, the lower the ratings of sleep quality (Sheely, 1996). In addition, Sheely reported a negative correlation between the amount of participation in care required from patients and their ratings of sleep quality.

Environmental factors associated with insomnia in other settings. Schnelle, Ouslander, Simmons, Alessi, and Gravel (1993) found noise, lights, and activities of others also were the major deterrents to sleep in residential care facilities. In nursing homes, noise and light associated with both general environmental events and more specific nursing care accounted for half of awakenings of 4 or more minutes in length and approximately one-third of awakenings under 2 minutes in length. For older adults in home settings, noise and the activities of others in the environment also have been identified as major correlates of disturbed sleep (Floyd, 1993; Johnson, 1986).

Personal Factors Associated With Insomnia

Although environmental factors play a major role in insomnia in ill and older adults, nurse researchers have identified many personal factors related to poor sleep. The most frequently identified factors for both hospitalized and community-based adults are anxiety, pain and discomfort, and nocturia including nighttime incontinence. In addition age, gender, and use of social drugs including alcohol, caffeine, and nicotine are associated with insomnia.

Anxiety, pain, and nocturia. Essentially all studies of sleep-disturbing factors for ill or older adults have identified anxiety or a related concept (e.g., worry, stress, tension, state of mind) as a major deterrent to initiating and maintaining sleep (Closs, 1992a, 1992b; Cohen, Ferrans, Vizgirda, Kunkle, & Cloninger, 1996; Floyd, 1993; Johnson, 1994; Pacini & Fitzpatrick, 1982; Simpson et al., 1996a, 1996b). Specific sources of anxiety that are sleep-disturbing have been studied very little. In one qualitative study that identified the specific sources of anxiety interfering with sleep in older community-based participants, women reported worries about health, family, and finances (Floyd, 1993).

A second personal factor identified by research as interfering with sleep is pain and other sources of physical discomfort. The relationship between sleep and pain is complex. Patients have reported that sleep is a mechanism for avoiding awareness of pain and that adequate sleep is a factor in coping with subsequent pain (Closs, 1992b). For ICU patients and those recently transferred from the ICU, pain and discomfort were reported as major causes of sleep disturbance. The sources of pain and discomfort were surgical incisions, symptoms of disease, and inability to find a comfortable sleeping position

(Closs, 1992a; Schaefer, Swavely, Rothenberger, Hess, & Williston, 1996; Simpson et al., 1996a, 1996b). Aches, pains, and general discomfort were also a major theme in Floyd's (1993) qualitative work on sleep bothers in community-based older adults.

In addition to pain and general physical discomfort, other frequently identified sources of nighttime discomfort in ill and older adults are nocturia and incontinence (Closs, 1992a; Cohen et al., 1996; Floyd, 1993; Johnson, 1994; Schnelle, Ouslander, & Alessi, 1993). When nocturia or incontinence are not identified as factors interfering with sleep, tubing and drains are identified, suggesting that study participants may have had indwelling catheters. Aside from documenting that anxiety, pain, discomfort, nocturia, and incontinence are perceived by patients as deterrents to sleep, sleep researchers have not studied these relationships further. The one exception is Schnelle et al. (1993) who have documented the relationship between incontinence care and waking frequency in nursing home residents.

Age and gender.   Many narrative summaries addressing research on age, gender, and sleep have been published (Bliwise, 1989, 1993; Dement, Miles, & Carskadon, 1982; Herbert, 1978; Horne, 1992; Jensen & Herr, 1993; Miller & Bartus, 1982; Regestein, 1980; Smallwood, Vitiello, Giblin, & Prinz, 1983). As individuals age, narrative reviewers have concluded that the following changes occur in sleep: (a) sleep latency increases, (b) frequency and duration of waking increase, (c) nighttime sleep amount decreases, and (d) general satisfaction with sleep decreases. The early narrative reviews suggested few gender differences in age-related sleep change other than a tendency for women to report more sleep problems than men as they grow older. A more recent meta-analytic study (Rediehs, Reis, & Creason, 1990) suggests the following gender differences exist between older men and women: (a) a small but consistent finding of longer sleep latency (SL) in women than in men; (b) greater frequency of waking after sleep onset (WASO) in women than in men; (c) longer WASO durations in men than women; and (d) no gender difference in mean nighttime sleep amount (NTSA), although men reported greater variability than women.

Social drugs.   The relationships among alcohol, caffeine, and nicotine use and sleep also have been summarized previously (Zarcone, 1994). Even the moderate use of alcohol, caffeine, and nicotine can affect the ill or older adult's ability to initiate and maintain sleep. Ethyl alcohol, or ethanol, is commonly self-prescribed to initiate sleep (Johnson, 1994); however, it creates sleep maintenance difficulties. After ethanol ingestion equivalent to just one to two drinks, awakening from intense dreaming activity occurs with some frequency. There are many studies in the literature that indicate caffeine also has deleterious effects on sleep. They have been summarized by Curatolo and Robertson (1983). Caffeine produces increases in WASO frequency and decreases in NTSA. Laboratory and survey studies indicate that nicotine has many of the same effects as caffeine on nighttime sleep parameters, especially at moderate blood concentrations (Soldatos, Kales, Scharf, Bixler, & Kales, 1980). Because ethanol, caffeine, and nicotine are typically used in conjunction with one another, the sedating and arousal effects frequently interact, creating multiple sleep disturbances for users of these substances (Zarcone, 1994).

The relationships between age, gender, and social substance use and sleep, respectively, have been well studied by sleep researchers across disciplines. In addition, nurse researchers have established the importance of examining anxiety, pain, discomfort, nocturia, and incontinence in clinical populations.

Person-Environment Interaction Factor

Three other factors described by insomnia researchers focus on the rhythmic interaction between the personal sleep-wake pattern and circadian features of the environment. One factor is the use of bedtime routines to entrain the sleep-wake rhythm to the circadian rhythm of the environment. The second is the role of naps as a possible deterrent to a stable circadian sleep-wake pattern. The third is the circadian type, that is, the sleep-phase orientation of the sleeper.

Bedtime routines.   Simpson et al. (1996a) reported postoperative cardiac patients identified lack of a bedtime routine as one of three major disrupters to their sleep. She noted the reasons for no routine require further study. In three earlier studies of bedtime routines in older adults living outside the hospital setting, use of bedtime routines was associated with shorter SL, fewer and shorter WASOs, longer NTSA, and higher sleep quality ratings (Johnson, 1986, 1988, 1991a). Subjects in all three studies were over 65 years of age with mean ages in the mid-80s. Many of the subjects without bedtime routines reported abandoning routines when they moved out of their own homes to homes with adult children or to residential care facilities. Those with bedtime routines reported simplifying routines whenever they had to relocate. Bedtime routines consisted of bathing and related hygiene activities, watching/listening to television or radio, reading, writing, eating, drinking, talking to someone, praying, having a backrub, doing relaxation exercises, and taking bedtime medication including sleeping pills.

All three studies of bedtime routines currently published are correlational; therefore, bedtime routines may promote sleep in ill and older adults or be mediated by some other variable(s). Also, bedtime routines as practiced by subjects often included other strategies for sleep promotion (e.g., relaxation exercises, sleeping medication). Thus, it is possible that bedtime routines improved sleep parameters by relaxing participants or by pharmacological mechanisms. Also, because all three studies of bedtime routines were of community-based men and women with average ages in the 80s, findings cannot be generalized to younger or hospitalized populations.

Napping.   Ill and older adults have not identified napping during the daytime as a factor in their insomnia, but the relationship between napping and difficulty initiating and maintaining sleep has been the focus of a number of studies. The studies have been limited to community-based rather than hospitalized populations. Although it has been assumed that sleep during the day would decrease sleep-need and thus lead to long SLs and frequent WASOs, some nurse researchers questioned the validity of the assumption for older adults. Hayter was the first to systematically examine the relationship between daytime sleep and nighttime sleep parameters (1983, 1985). Her work suggested no relationship between napping and sleep maintenance. Floyd (1995) conducted a construct replication study that supported most of Hayter's findings but suggested SL and WASO frequency may increase significantly if naps extend beyond 50 minutes in length. Metz and Bunnel (1990) reported a positive trend between nap length and SL for a sample with a mean nap length of 57.5 minutes. In the only experimental study of napping in older adults, Aber and Webb (1986) found no differences between nap and no-nap days for polysomnographic and self-report measures of sleep; however, naps in the Aber and Webb study ranged from 21 to 54 minutes. Two other studies, which examined nap frequency rather than nap duration, found no relationship between naps and nighttime sleep parameters (Buysse et al., 1992; Evans & Rogers, 1994).

Overall, there is no evidence that naps under 50 minutes in duration impede nighttime sleep in community-based elderly. Longer naps may negatively affect SL and WASO frequency. None of the studies found a relationship between daytime napping and WASO duration or NTSA. Because the length of naps was an hour or less in most published studies, and naps were taken in the early afternoon, results cannot be generalized to naps of different lengths or naps taken at different times of day.

Circadian type.   Some attention has been paid to the imposed timing of sleep in hospital settings and its relationship to patients' usual or preferred timing of sleep. Pacini and Fitzpatrick (1982) compared sleep of hospitalized and non-hospitalized adults aged 60 to 82. Significant differences between groups were found on self-reported sleep parameters. Hospitalized patients reported shorter NTSA, more napping, and had earlier bedtimes and times of arising (i.e., were phase-advanced in comparison with non-hospitalized older adults). Circadian type (i.e., whether subjects were "morning types" who preferred to arise and retire early vs. "evening types" who preferred late times of retiring and arising), appeared over-ridden by the sleep-wake schedule imposed by the hospital environment.

Using self-report measures similar to Pacini and Fitzpatrick's (1982) work, Floyd (1983, 1984) studied the sleep of psychiatric inpatients and outpatients. Inpatients and evening circadian types had shorter NTSAs than outpatients and morning types, respectively. Circadian type was a good predictor of times of falling asleep and awakening for outpatients but not for inpatients. The schedules of inpatients were phase-shifted by the hospital's rest-activity schedule such that morning types fell asleep and awakened an hour later than matched morning types who were outpatients. (Patients were matched on age, gender, and psychiatric diagnosis.) Evening types fell asleep 1 1/2 hours earlier and awakened 3 hours earlier than matched outpatients.

Richards and Bairnsfather (1988) found that ICU patients who normally slept days when at home had 86 minutes less NTSA than those who normally slept nights at home. Measurement of sleep was by polysomnography. WASO duration composed 51% of the night for day sleepers compared to 33% of the night for night sleepers. Although home day sleepers had less WASO frequency during hospitalization than home night sleepers, given the long durations of awakenings, opportunities for awakening were limited.

The three published studies of relationships between hospital rest-activity patterns and personal sleep-wake rhythms also are correlational. Studies that vary the environmentally imposed rest-activity schedule are needed to further examine relationships among circadian type, sleep schedule changes, and sleep characteristics. Nevertheless, research in this area suggests adult patients' circadian type has not been accommodated in hospital environments and that the result may be shortened NTSAs.

Summary of research on correlates of insomnia.   Studies of correlates of insomnia in ill and older adults have identified several environmental factors that interfere with sleep. The number of studies of noise and interruptions by others clearly implicate these two factors as major deterrents to sleep in intensive care settings. Studies of light and sleep surfaces are needed to understand their roles in poor sleep in hospital settings. For patients attempting to sleep at home or in residential care facilities, the research base is very sparse, but suggests that similar factors impede sleep.

Age, gender, and use of alcohol, caffeine, and nicotine are generally accepted personal factors affecting sleep. In addition, nurse researchers have identified anxiety, pain, discomfort, nocturia, and incontinence as deterrents to sleep in ill and older adults. They have also explored the relationships between poor sleep in ill and older patients and their bedtime routines, napping, and circadian type.

SLEEP INTERVENTION STUDIES

Much of nurses' published sleep research suggests potential interventions. These could include providing a quiet environment, making the sleep quarters as comfortable as possible, increasing sleep opportunity, minimizing the degree to which patients are engaged in their nighttime care, helping the patient relax, improving pain management, encouraging bedtime routines, monitoring napping, and facilitating circadian phase shifts. However, relatively few interventions have been studied systematically. The interventions that have been studied are discussed in sections based on their presumed mechanisms for influencing sleep: (a) altering the environment, (b) relaxing the person, or (c) re-patterning the rhythmic person-environment interaction.

Noise Management

Clinical settings have been shown to have many features that disturb sleep. Noise, activity of others, uncomfortable sleep surfaces, and lighting have all been identified as problematic. With regard to creating an environment more conducive to sleep, the published intervention studies focus exclusively on noise management.

In an exceptionally well-designed experimental study, Topf (1992) examined the effects of personal control over hospital noise on sleep. She compared the sleep of three groups of female volunteers sleeping in a laboratory environment. Subjects were randomly assigned to one of three conditions: quiet, simulated coronary care unit (CCU) noise, and simulated CCU noise plus instruction in personal control over noise. Sleep variables were measured by polysomnography. Personal control over noise consisted of instruction on the use of a sound conditioner or "white noise" machine. Subjects were instructed about how to turn on the sound conditioner, and switch channels to select different types of white noise (e.g., ocean sounds or sounds of a waterfall), how to adjust volume, and how to add more base or treble. Subjects in the two noise conditions heard audio-taped nighttime sounds recorded in a CCU.

Personal control over noise had no significant effect on sleep characteristics when analyzed by multiple *t*-tests. On inspection the mean values of sleep outcome variables for the treatment group were consistently more negative than the control group's. This suggests that a trend for personal control over noise to negatively affect sleep parameters might have been detected had a multivariate statistical test been used.

Topf (1992) suggested the most obvious interpretation for the failure of the personal control intervention was that the aversiveness of CCU sounds outweighed the masking effect of the sound conditioner. She also noted that other researchers contend personal control interventions are not always positive because they may facilitate added attention to the negative aspects of a stressor. She further speculated that the degree of effort required to exercise control could negatively affect outcomes, given that participants in the study were required to turn over in bed to turn up the volume or make other adjustments to the sound.

In addition to personal control over noise via use of a sound conditioner, other interventions designed to promote sleep through noise management also have focused on the use of a sound conditioner. In a study by Williamson (1992), the use of white noise was examined in 60 coronary artery bypass graft (CABG) patients. Subjects were systematically assigned to treatment and control conditions. The treatment group heard ocean sounds played on a sound conditioner for 3 consecutive nights post-transfer from an intensive care unit. The sound machine was turned on when subjects retired for the night and was left on until it was time to awaken in the morning. No control of environment, except for the absence of the sound conditioner, was done for the control group. When the treatment group was compared to the control group, WASO frequency and WASO duration were decreased ($p < .05$). SL was not affected. NTSA was not reported. Subjective quality of sleep was increased ($p < .05$).

White noise also has been studied as a method to promote sleep in Alzheimer's patients (Young, Muir-Nash, & Ninos, 1988). The sound of "the roll of slow surf" was randomly selected from the various sounds available on the sound conditioner. A convenience sample of eight subjects was selected from a gerontological research unit in an inpatient setting. The study included four males and four females ranging from 60 to 82 years old ($M = 70$ years). All were classified in the moderately advanced stage of Alzheimer's disease and had a history of nocturnal wandering behavior. Persons who were not able to hear the sound generator, who had mobility problems requiring assistance, or who had precipitate micturation were excluded from the study. The study period was 12 nights for each subject. The first 4 nights were baseline nights. A crossover design was used to randomly alter treatment exposure. No differences were found between treatment and control nights for NTSA or amount of wandering. SL, WASO frequency, and WASO duration were not reported. Because the use of white noise was effective for increasing sleep maintenance of CABG patients when provided for the entire sleep period, Young and colleagues' negative results suggest cognitive functioning may be an important mediating variable. Differences also may be due to the fact that different sleep outcome variables were examined.

Another approach to noise management, the use of earplugs, was studied by Haddock (1994). Large positive effects were reported by women surgical and gynecological patients for NTSA and perceived quality of sleep. Participants in the study self-selected to use earplugs. Because of failure to control for reactivity and demand effects, it may be that only those patients who choose to wear earplugs will report them effective.

Overall, the intervention research involving environmental alteration is very limited. Of all the environmental correlates of poor sleep, only a few studies of noise management have been published. The one study of personal control over noise suggests it may not be an effective strategy as operationalized in the study. The three other studies published to date suggest that noise-masking or noise-muffling interventions may be effective in some patient populations. Whether or not noise-masking/muffling approaches, such as using a sound conditioner or wearing earplugs, can improve some sleep parameters if provided continuously during the sleep period awaits further study. A strength of the few studies conducted on noise management is their experimental designs. Except for the study by Haddock (1994), they are well-controlled studies.

Relaxation Strategies

Relaxation approaches are designed to alleviate somatic or cognitive arousal. Relaxation procedures, such as progressive muscle relaxation and autogenic training, focus primarily on somatic arousal (e.g., muscle tension), while attention-focusing procedures, such as imagery training, meditation, and thought stopping, target cognitive arousal (e.g., intrusive thoughts, racing mind) (Morin, Culbert, & Schwartz, 1994). Given that many ill and older adults report anxiety, tension, and worries as barriers to sleep, relaxation approaches may be effective for sleep promotion in patient populations.

Both somatic and cognitive relaxation have been studied extensively in samples of individuals with chronic insomnia, that is, individuals who routinely need longer than 30 minutes to fall asleep, are awake 30 minutes or more during the night, and who average less than 6.5 hours of sleep per night. The results of these studies have been summarized in two published meta-analyses. Both meta-analyses used recommended quantitative methods for research synthesis (Cooper & Hedges, 1994).

Meta-analytic studies.   In the first meta-analysis, Morin et al. (1994) published the results of 59 studies of non-pharmacological sleep interventions on the self-reported values for SL, WASO frequency and duration, and NTSA. The mean age of the 2,102 patients represented in the meta-analysis was 44.2 years (SD = 12.6). Slightly less than 60% (59.9) of the subjects were women. The mean length of time the subjects had experienced insomnia was 11.2 years (SD = 3.7). Their symptoms were severe: The mean SL was 64.3 minutes (SD = 23.2); the mean WASO frequency was 1.9 (SD = 0.6); the mean WASO duration was 70.3 minutes (SD = 31.3); the mean NTSA was 5.82 hours (SD = .73). The typical non-pharmacological intervention in the meta-analysis consisted of 5 contact hours. On average, somatic relaxation strategies had a large positive effect (d = .83) on SL, a medium effect (d = .56) on WASO frequency, negligible effect (d = .06) effect on WASO duration, and a small effect (d = .25) on NTSA. Cognitive relaxation strategies also had significant impact on decreasing some symptoms of insomnia: a large effect (d = 1.20) for decreasing SL, a medium effect (d = .56) for decreasing WASO frequency, a small effect (d = .28) for decreasing WASO duration, and a small effect (d = .28) for increasing NTSA. The clinical gains achieved by the end of treatment were well maintained at the follow-ups, which averaged 6 months in duration. For SL and NTSA, additional improvements were made from end of treatment to follow-up.

In a second meta-analytic study (Murtagh & Greenwood, 1995), somatic and cognitive relaxation also had large effects for decreasing SL in individuals with chronic insomnia by end of treatment. The effect size for somatic relaxation was large (d = .81). It was somewhat larger for cognitive relaxation (d = .93). At 8 months follow-up, improvement in SL was further enhanced. For all other sleep variables, results were reported at end-of-treatment or at 8 months follow-up but not both. Somatic and cognitive relaxation strategies had a moderate (d = .57) and small (d = .33) impact on decreasing WASO frequency, respectively, at 8 months post-treatment. For increasing NTSA, somatic and cognitive relaxation strategies had moderate effect sizes: d was .52 and .57, respectively, at end of treatment. Both types of relaxation approaches had a large impact on subjective reports of sleep quality at end-of-treatment, d = .97 for somatic relaxation and d = 1.08 for cognitive strategies. Murtagh and Greenwood did not study WASO duration.

Murtaugh and Greenwood's (1995) meta-analysis integrated results from 66 studies published from 1973 to 1993. Although Morin et al. (1994) did not identify references used in the meta-analysis in the published reference list, it is likely that the two meta-analyses included many of the same studies. On average, the 1,538 subjects in Murtagh and Greenwood's synthesis were slightly younger than Morin and colleagues' with a mean of 41.6 years (SD = 12.6) and included a slightly higher percentage of women, 61.5%. The mean length of time subjects had experienced insomnia was similar at 11.1 years (SD = 4.0). Their symptoms were equally severe prior to treatment: The mean SL was 61.4 minutes (SD = 31.4); the mean WASO frequency was 1.6 (SD = 1.9); the mean WASO duration was not reported; the mean NTSA was 5.65 hours (SD = 1.12).

The results summarized by both Morin et al. (1994) and Murtagh and Greenwood (1995) were based on self-report measures. Patients with insomnia tend to overestimate SL and WASO duration and to underestimate WASO frequency and NTSA (Coates et al., 1982). Nevertheless, as authors of both meta-analytic reports note, the few studies that have used polysomnography to evaluate outcomes have shown that relaxation approaches are effective not only in altering sleep perceptions but also in improving objective sleep measures. The magnitude of recorded improvements when measured by polysomnography is somewhat smaller, but in the same direction, as the magnitude of changes shown in sleep diaries (Jacobs, Benson, & Friedman, 1993; Morin, Kowatch, Barry, & Walton, 1993). Self-reported improvements in sleep patterns also have been validated by data obtained from behavioral assessment devices and by collateral reports from significant others (Morin & Azrin, 1987, 1988; Morin et al., 1993).

Primary relaxation studies.   Because the two meta-analytic studies summarized research about non-pharmacological interventions in patients with chronic insomnia through 1993, they were reviewed in lieu of the 60+ studies involved. To supplement the meta-analyses, studies of relaxation interventions used to treat chronic insomnia published since 1993 were sought. Also sought were studies published between 1970 and 1997 that used relaxation interventions to manage sleep in other clinical populations. Five studies were found. All five studies examined somatic relaxation using some form of progressive muscle relaxation (PMR). In one study, PMR was supplemented by a component of cognitive relaxation.

Going in order of publication, the first study (DeBerry, 1981–1982), examined PMR in 10 highly anxious women between the ages of 69 and 84. The subjects had experienced the death of a husband within the past 5 years, but had no prior psychiatric history. Except for their anxiety and tension, they reported no outstanding physical symptoms. Participants responded to an offer extended to nervous senior citizens to participate in a relaxation study. Subjects were randomly assigned to treatment and control groups ($n = 5$). The treatment group received 2 weeks of baseline evaluation, 10 weeks of 1 hour/week relaxation training based on methods of Wolpe (1969) and Lazarus (1966), and 10 weeks of home practice using taped instructions. Specifically, the first three sessions were purely muscle relaxation, while the remaining five consisted of muscle relaxation and visual imagery. At the end of the training, participants in the treatment group received personalized relaxation tapes and were asked to practice daily. Both groups were evaluated prior to training, at the end of training, and 10 weeks after training, but no sleep outcome data were reported for the final data collection period.

In addition to two sleep outcomes of interest, SL and WASO frequency, participants were measured on state and trait anxiety, self-reported muscle tension, and frequency of headaches. With the exception of trait anxiety, the treatment group reported significant ($p < .05$) improvement in all symptoms from baseline to end of training. Baseline measures of SL and WASO frequency were extreme for these 10 women (i.e., approximately 5 hours to fall asleep and 12 awakenings per night). Following treatment, the PMR group reported 1.2 hours to fall asleep and an average of 6 awakenings per night. Although the treatment group improved dramatically, their sleep disturbance remained severe by most standards.

In the second relaxation study, Cannici, Malcolm, and Peek (1983) evaluated PMR using a two-group design ($n = 15$). Subjects were patients at a university medical center who were under treatment for cancer and who reported SLs of at least 30 minutes duration. Nearly half had genito-urinary cancers; others had gastrointestinal or breast cancer or lymphomas, leukemias, or carcinomas. The mean number of years that cancer had been diagnosed was 6.4. At the time of the study the patients were receiving radiation, chemotherapy, pre-surgery, post-surgery, or follow-up treatment. Of the patients, 16 were experiencing pain and 11 of these were receiving pain medications. The mean number of years of insomnia reported was 9.4.

In the Cannici et al. (1983) study participants were randomly assigned to PMR and routine care. The PMR program consisted of three sessions of unreported length presented on consecutive days. The sessions involve sequential instructions to focus attention, tense, and relax 16 muscle groups throughout the body (Bernstein & Borkovec, 1973), and indirect suggestions of relaxation by the therapist during training. Treatment subjects were given a sheet containing instructions for home practice of the relaxation training (twice daily was recommended). SL was significantly reduced from 124 minutes to 29 minutes in the treatment group ($p < .05$), while the control group SL decreased from 116 to 109 minutes. At 3 months follow-up the treatment group had maintained its improvement in SL ($M = 33$ minutes; SD not reported) while the control group continued to report long SLs (M = 104 minutes; SD not reported). Similar, but much less dramatic and non-significant, patterns were found for decreasing WASO frequency and increasing NTSA.

The third study (Lutz, 1990) examined the effect of relaxation teaching on sleep, anxiety, and sick call in a prison population. The relaxation teaching was based on Benson's (1975, 1987) methods. Forty-two male prisoners aged 19 to 51 were randomly assigned to treatment and control groups. Post-assignment analysis found no significant differences between groups on background variable other than race. Groups were significantly different on race despite random assignment. Fifty-five percent of the control group and 25% of the treatment group were Caucasian. Prisoners showing signs of drug withdrawal or who could not answer questions on the Mini-Mental exam were excluded from the study. According to the author, the treatment group was given the relaxation training and asked to practice it every day for 2 weeks. The training was not described. At the end of 2 weeks, the investigator found a non-significant trend toward better sleep quality in the treatment group.

Johnson (1991b, 1993) published the final two primary studies of relaxation approaches located. Both used a pretest-posttest design with no control group. Subjects in both studies received instruction in Benson's (1975) method of progressive relaxation. The intervention used controlled breathing and alternating contractions and relaxation of muscle groups involving the whole body. Subjects also were provided with a tape guiding them through the process so they could practice at home. In Johnson's first study (1991b), data were collected from 55 noninstitutionalized women ages 65 to 84 before and after 2 days of instruction and home practice. Subjects were referred by physicians from randomly selected practices. The subjects were being treated for one or more of the following: angina, congestive heart failure, hypertension, or arthritis. Sleep parameters were measured by polysomnography as well as self-report. Results did not vary by measurement approach. PMR significantly decreased SL ($p < .001$) and WASO frequency ($p < .01$). PMR did not increase NTSA. A number of indicators of sleep quality also were measured. After PMR, subjects reported a better state of mind at bedtime, being more refreshed upon awakening, sounder sleep, and more satisfaction with their sleep. Reported significance levels were all between .05 and .01 for these variables.

In Johnson's second study of PMR (1993), data were collected from 176 men and women ages 65 to over 99 following 5 days of instruction and at-home practice. Subjects were individuals who responded to newspaper advertisements and other community notices. All of the subjects had complaints about their sleep prior to participating in the study. The majority of subjects was using either prescription or over-the-counter drugs to promote sleep. All subjects underwent drug wash-out periods before entering the study.

Because no measurement difference was noted in the first study, only self-report measures were obtained. Reported results were nearly identical to those reported in the first study. The only differences were that (a) the decrease in WASO frequency was significant at the .05 level rather than the .01 level, and (b) no difference was found in the second study on feeling more refreshed upon awakening.

Overall, the meta-analytic studies suggest that both somatic and cognitive relaxation strategies are very effective for decreasing SL and increasing sleep quality in patients with long-term insomnia who are otherwise healthy. Meta-analysis also indicates that relaxation strategies are moderately effective for decreasing WASO frequency and have a small-to-moderate positive effect on NTSA in this population. Less is known about the effectiveness of relaxation strategies in other clinical populations. Taken as a set, the five primary studies of PMR suggest improved SL and WASO frequency despite variations in PMR theory and techniques employed, amount of instruction, sample characteristics, and measurement strategies. In the one study reporting only a trend in improved sleep quality, it is unclear if subjects had guided participation or simply had PMR described to them. Given that two of the four primary studies that found an improvement in sleep used random assignment of treatment to groups, there is some evidence that it is something about the PMR intervention that accounts for the variation. Given uncontrolled demand characteristics in all studies, the combination of somatic and cognitive relaxation approaches in the DeBerry (1981–1982) study, and probable inadequate operationalization of PMR in the study by Lutz (1990), there are construct validity issues. Finally, generalizability is limited because few of the subjects in the clinical studies were acutely ill. The other clinical groups studied ranged from relatively healthy to chronically ill. The extent to which relaxation interventions might improve the sleep of other populations, especially the acutely ill, requires exploration. Although additional research is needed with patients experiencing transient and short-term insomnia secondary to illness or its treatment, there is evidence from the existing studies that a variety of relaxation approaches do improve the sleep of individuals with chronic insomnia and may be effective in helping ill adults initiate and maintain sleep.

One other study focused on relaxation indirectly. Zimmerman, Nieveen, Barnason, and Schmaderer (1996) examined the effects of music therapy on pain and sleep in postoperative patients. The investigators randomly assigned 96 patients having CABG surgery to one of three groups: music, music video, and a control group who rested quietly. The mean age of the sample was 67 (SD = 9.9) with a range of 37 to 84 years. Subjects in the music intervention group selected one of five audiotapes that investigators judged as a soothing type that facilitates sleep. The music video group chose from among three videos that combined soft instrumental music with visual images of different scenes from nature. The control group participated in an undisturbed rest period. All sessions were 30 minutes in length and were provided the second and third days post-operatively during the afternoon or early evening. The three groups were not significantly different on pain, but were significantly different on sleep quality (p < .05); post-hoc Tukey tests revealed that the video group had significantly higher sleep quality scores than the resting group. In addition, the difference between the music group and the resting group approached statistical significance (p < .06). Based on the gate-control theory of pain, the researchers hypothesized that daytime pain would be decreased by the intervention. They further surmised that better daytime pain management would improve nighttime sleep quality. Given results showing no effect on pain but an improvement in sleep quality, the researchers suggested daytime music had a long acting relaxation effect. Additional research is needed to determine the relationships among music, relaxation, pain, and sleep.

Circadian Re-patterning

Any intervention designed to help establish a regular sleep-wake rhythm was placed in this category. The use of bedtime routines, regular bedtimes and times of arising, and regular or restricted naptimes are potential circadian re-patterning interventions, but they have not been studied separately as interventions to promote sleep. They are traditional elements of sleep education, that is, "sleep hygiene" programs. Such programs also typically advise no use of caffeine after midday and limited use of alcohol. Because of the variation in sleep hygiene instruction, it is difficult to know what aspects may account for improvement in sleep patterns. Studies of the effectiveness of sleep hygiene education were included in the Morin et al. (1994) meta-analysis. No additional studies of sleep hygiene were located. Morin et al. reported that on average patients with chronic insomnia who were taught sleep hygiene practices had a moderate improvement in SL ($d = .71$), no change in WASO frequency, but a very large improvement in NTSA ($d = 1.16$.). Only one study measured WASO duration, but Morin et al. reported a decrease in mean WASO duration from 81.1 to 59.0 minutes for that study.

Because of an established link between the core body temperature rhythm and the sleep-wake rhythm (Kryger, Roth, & Dement, 1994), interventions that alter body temperature can be used to entrain the sleep-wake rhythm. One well-controlled intervention study was found that evaluated the use of passive body heating via hot baths as a treatment for sleep maintenance insomnia in older women (Dorsey et al., 1996). The subjects were nine healthy women volunteers with a mean age of 65.1 (SD = 3.3) years. Initially, they reported: (a) three awakenings of greater than 30 minutes in duration at least three times per week, and/or (b) more than three awakenings per night at least three times per week. Subjects were medication- and drug-free as determined by both self-report and drug screens. Potential subjects who napped more than one time per week or reported irregular sleep schedules (bedtimes or wake times that varied by more than 2 hours in range) were excluded from the study.

Dorsey et al. (1996) used a crossover design to examine the effect of hot baths (40–40.5° C) and luke-warm baths (37.5–38.5° C). The baths were 30 minutes long. Subjects were immersed in water to mid-thorax. The baths were taken 1.5 hours before the participant's regular bedtime. The purpose of the luke-warm baths was to control for the possible soporific effect achieved simply by sitting in bath water without the concurrent rise in core body temperature. Core body temperatures were increased an average of nearly 1° C by the hot baths, but on average less than .2° C by the luke-warm baths. Participants in the study drank 50 to 100 ml of water to ensure adequate hydration following the hot baths. All subjects had their sleep measured by polysomnography for one baseline night and two nights each following luke-warm and hot baths, respectively, for a total of five nights in a sleep laboratory. Order of luke-warm versus hot baths was randomly assigned. Participants were also instructed to urinate immediately before bedtime on all five laboratory nights to avoid the potentially sleep-disruptive effects of increased urinary frequency due to water intake on bath nights.

Significant improvements were found in WASO duration as measured by polysomnography for hot bath nights versus the baseline night ($p < .05$). Polysomnography results for SL, WASO frequency, and NTSA were not reported. Trends ($p < .06$) in self-reported improvement in SL and WASO frequency were reported for hot bath nights versus the baseline night. Participants also reported significantly "deeper" and "more restful" sleep after hot bath nights versus the baseline night ($p < .05$). No significant polysomnography or self-reported effects were found for luke-warm bath nights versus the baseline nights. Although only Dorsey and her colleagues' study (1996), which has limited generalizability, has been published to date, interventions that improve sleep maintenance through the manipulation of the circadian temperature rhythm may prove useful, especially for environments or populations where noise management and relaxation strategies are difficult to implement.

Overall, very few circadian re-patterning interventions have been studied. The use of different components of bedtime rituals, regular bed- and arise-times, and key aspects of naps (e.g., frequency, timing, duration) need to be evaluated for use in clinical populations. Also, the various elements of sleep hygiene education need to be systematically varied to determine which aspects of circadian re-patterning instruction are helpful. Interventions that improve sleep through manipulation of other circadian rhythms also require further study.

THEORETICAL AND METHODOLOGICAL ISSUES

The theoretical frameworks used by sleep promotion researchers have been derived primarily from stress-and-coping theories. This is especially true for intervention studies that evaluate relaxation approaches. No one stress-and-coping framework dominates the field. Physiological models of arousal underpin most studies of noise and noise management. Circadian rhythm theories have served to organize most studies of person-environment interaction correlates and circadian re-patterning interventions. Two mid-range frameworks for the conceptualization of sleep in natural (i.e., non-laboratory) settings have been developed: Floyd (1983) presented a model of interacting rhythms and Topf (1984) presented a framework for studying aversive aspects of the environment. Nurses' studies occasionally link the mid-range theory used to a more abstract nursing conceptual framework such as Levine (Schaefer et al., 1996), Neuman (Wilson, 1987), and Rogers (Floyd, 1983, 1984). More work is needed to further explicate mid-range theories of sleep in settings where nurses care for patients. Increasingly, this means homes as well as hospitals and residential care facilities.

The use of *arcs*© to examine the meta-structure (Graves, 1997) of sleep promotion research showed that the greatest emphasis has been on the measurement of variables related to the construct of person. Less focus has been placed on measurement of variables that represent the environment or person-environment interaction constructs. Examination of the meta-structure for the sleep promotion domain also showed that nurses' research on interventions and potential interventions is nearly equally divided between facilitation of sleep in the hospitalized ill and the community-based older adult whose health status is stable.

Measurement Issues

Sleep researchers in nursing have used the wide variety of measurement approaches available to sleep researchers in all disciplines. These include biophysical, observational, and self-report methods. Nevertheless, only a small proportion of sleep promotion research by nurse researchers and investigators in related disciplines has used polysomnography or other instrumentation.

Other available instrumentation includes (a) actigraphy, which correlates well with the inactivity of sleep (Hauri & Wisbey, 1993); and (b) the Sleep Assessment Device, which records participants' responses to faint tones during the night to provide estimates of sleep parameters (Lichstein & Johnson, 1991; Lichstein, Nickel, Hoelscher, & Kelley, 1982). With the advent of instrumentation that can be used to measure sleep in natural settings, practical obstacles that prevented more common use of objective measures in sleep promotion studies in the past should abate.

Although polysomnography traditionally has been considered the most reliable method for measurement of objective symptoms of insomnia, there is some evidence that self-reports of these variables approximate polysomnography for community-based adults with transient and short-term insomnia (Johnson, 1991b), even though reports from individuals with chronic insomnia are less reliable. Little is known about the reliability of self-reported sleep characteristics obtained from other patient populations, especially the acutely ill. To determine the best approaches for measurement of sleep in clinical populations, additional research is needed that establishes the reliability and validity of measures for populations cared for by nurses in settings where care is provided.

Measurement of the quantitative aspects of sleep is not the only goal in clinical sleep research, because success as defined by patients often is dependent on more favorable perceptions of sleep than on objective changes. To create a full understanding of sleep promotion, studies employing reliable and valid measures of both objective and subjective aspects of sleep are needed. And, measurement approaches must take into consideration the needs of patients and care delivery environments.

Nurse researchers have developed two questionnaires that supplement existing approaches to the measurement of sleep quality. Each was designed with the compromised physical functioning of inpatient populations in mind. The Verran and Snyder-Halpern (VSH) Sleep Scale is composed of 13 visual analog scales (VAS) (Snyder-Halpern & Verran, 1987). It was designed to measure a number of sleep factors including sleep length, disturbance, effectiveness, supplementation, and satisfaction. Although the extent to which some scales are considered relevant for different clinical populations is an important consideration, the instrument shows promise for use with many clinical populations. The Richards-Campbell Sleep Questionnaire (Richards, 1987) also was developed for use in hospitalized patients, especially those in critical care with very limited energy but the ability to mark visual analog scales. Like the VSH Sleep Scale, it uses the VAS format. The five scales address sleep depth, falling asleep, awakenings, returning to sleep, and global quality of sleep.

Evaluation Research

Many potential interventions have not been studied at all; others have not been subjected to experimental study. Still other interventions have been studied using experimental designs, but have not been replicated. More focus on the systematic evaluation of sleep promotion strategies is needed to strengthen the research base underpinning practice.

A number of factors suggest that relatively small, purposively selected samples will continue to be the norm in sleep promotion research. These factors include the need for both objective and subjective measures of sleep, the current expense and complexity of measuring sleep objectively, and the variation in night-to-night sleep, which requires repeated measurements. Purposive sampling—and continued careful description of subject characteristics when convenience samples are used—will provide information that facilitates decisions about generalizability of results. Repeated measures will assure adequate power despite small sample sizes as well as assist in the understanding of night-to-night variability in sleep in clinical populations. In addition, evaluation studies would benefit from concurrent replications using multiple sites to more quickly establish the efficacy and effectiveness of sleep promotion interventions.

SUMMARY

Sleep research conducted in nursing over nearly three decades has established the study of sleep promotion as an important domain of inquiry in nursing. Much has been achieved and much more awaits attention. Many sleep researchers in nursing have used sophisticated approaches to the measurement of objective characteristics of sleep. Others have contributed to instrument development for measurement of sleep quality in medical care settings. Correlates of poor sleep are well described for patients in critical care settings and have begun to be described in other settings. Although theories of sleep promotion are not well explicated, potentially useful concepts and conceptual models have been identified. Models that emphasize the environment and person-environment interaction need more use to provide a balance of perspectives and develop a full array of intervention strategies.

Currently, there is strong evidence to suggest that relaxation interventions are generally effective for improving many features of poor sleep in those with chronic insomnia. PMR appears effective for improving sleep initiation and increasing perceived sleep quality in selected clinical populations with transient or short-term sleep problems. Other interventions designed to relax the sleeper need identification and study. Interventions that mask or muffle noise also need additional study and research on environmental factors and their management must expand beyond noise management. The limited number of studies and design limitations decrease confidence in circadian re-patterning strategies; however, these are promising areas for future research on sleep promotion in adults.

ACKNOWLEDGMENTS

The preparation of this paper was supported in part by 1996–97 and 1997–98 Fuld Research Scholar Awards from Sigma Theta Tau International (STTI) and by the National Institutes of Health: National Institute of Nursing Research under grant RO1 NR03880, "Aging-Related Sleep Changes: A Meta-Analysis."

The author thanks Margaret L. Falahee, MS, RN, Fuld Clinical Scholar and Rigolea H. Fhobir, Fuld Undergraduate Research Assistant for their assistance in research report retrieval and data entry using arcs©, and Judith R. Graves, Ph.D., FAAN, creator of arcs© for guidance in using the software system. The examination of sleep promotion interventions was part of the STTI research project, "A New Learning Paradigm for Nursing," funded by the Helene Fuld Health Trust.

REFERENCES

Aaron, J. N., Carlisle, C. C., Carskadon, M. A., Meyer, T. J., Hill, N. S., & Millman, R. P. (1996). Environmental noise as a cause of sleep disruption in an intermediate respiratory care unit. *Sleep, 19*(9), 707–710.

Aber, R., & Webb, W. B. (1986). Effects of a limited nap on night sleep in older subjects. *Psychology and Aging, 1,* 300–302.

Aurell, J., & Elmqvist, D. (1985). Sleep in the surgical ICU: Continuous polygraphic recording of sleep in nine patients receiving postoperative care. *British Medical Journal, 290,* 1029–1032.

Ballard, K. S. (1981). Identification of environmental stressors for patients in a surgical intensive care unit. *Issues in Mental Health Nursing, 3,* 89–108.

Bearpark, H. M. (1994). Insomnia: Causes, effects and treatment. In R. Cooper (Ed.), *Sleep* (pp. 587–613). London: Chapman and Hall Medical.

Benson, H. (1975). *The relaxation response.* New York: Avon.

Benson, H. (1987). *Your maximum mind.* New York: Random House.

Bernstein, D. A., & Borkovec, T. D. (1973). *Progressive relaxation training.* Champaign, IL: Research Press.

Bliwise, D. L. (1989). Neuropsychological function and sleep. *Clinical Geriatric Medicine, 5,* 381–394.

Bliwise, D. L. (1993). Sleep in normal aging and dementia. *Sleep, 16*(1), 40–81.

Broughton, R., & Baron, R. (1978). Sleep patterns in the intensive care unit and on the ward after acute myocardial infarction. *Electroencephalography and Clinical Neurophysiology, 45,* 348–360.

Buysse, D. J., Browman, K. E., Monk, T. H., Reynolds, C. F., III, Fasiczka, A. L., & Kupfer, D. J. (1992). Napping and 24-hour sleep/wake patterns in healthy elderly and young adults. *Journal of the American Geriatrics Society, 40*(8), 779–786.

Cannici, J., Malcolm, R., & Peek, L. A. (1983). Treatment of insomnia in cancer patients using muscle relaxation training. *Journal of Behavior Therapy & Experimental Psychiatry, 14*(3), 251–256.

Closs, S. J. (1992a). Patients' night-time pain, analgesic provision and sleep after surgery. *International Journal of Nursing Studies, 29*(4), 381–392.

Closs, S. J. (1992b). Post-operative patients' views of sleep, pain and recovery. *Journal of Clinical Nursing, 1,* 83–88.

Coates, T. J., Killen, J. D., George, J., Silverman, S., Marchini, E., & Thoresen, C. E. (1982). Estimating sleep parameters: A multitrait-multimethod analysis. *Journal of Consulting and Clinical Psychology, 50,* 345–352.

Cohen, F. L., Ferrans, C. E., Vizgirda, V., Kunkle, V., & Cloninger, L. (1996). Sleep in men and women infected with human immunodeficiency virus. *Holistic Nursing Practice, 10*(4), 33–43.

Cooper, H., & Hedges, L. V. (1994). *The handbook of research synthesis.* New York: Russell Sage.

Curatolo, P. W., & Robertson, D. (1983). The health consequences of caffeine. *Annals of Internal Medicine, 98,* 641–653.

DeBerry, S. (1981–1982). An evaluation of progressive muscle relaxation on stress related symptoms in a geriatric population. *International Journal of Aging & Human Development, 14*(4), 255–269.

Dement, W. C., Miles, L. E., & Carskadon, M. A. (1982). "White paper" on sleep and aging. *Journal of the American Geriatric Society, 30,* 25–50.

Dlin, B. M., Rosen, H., Dickstein, K., Lyons, J., & Fisher, G. (1971). The problems of sleep and rest in the intensive care unit. *Psychosomatics, 12*(3), 155–163.

Dorsey, C. M., Lukas, S. E., Teicher, M. H., Harper, D., Winkelman, J. W., Cunningham, S. L., & Satlin, A. (1996). Effects of passive body heating on the sleep of older female insomniacs. *Journal of Geriatric Psychiatry & Neurology, 9*(2), 83–90.

Eaton, W. E., Badawi, M., & Melton, B. (1995). Prodromes and precursors: Epidemiologic data for primary prevention of disorders with slow onset. *American Journal of Psychiatry, 152,* 967–972.

Edell-Gustafsson, U., Aren, C., Hamrin, E., & Hetta, J. (1994). Nurses' notes on sleep patterns in patients undergoing coronary artery bypass surgery: A retrospective evaluation of patient records. *Journal of Advanced Nursing, 20,* 331–336.

Edwards, G. B., & Schuring, L. M. (1993). Pilot study: Validating staff nurses' observations of sleep and wake states among critically ill patients, using polysomnography. *American Journal of Critical Care, 2*(2), 125–131.

Evans, B. D., & Rogers, A. E. (1994). 24-hour sleep/wake patterns in healthy elderly persons. *Applied Nursing Research, 7*(2), 75–83.

Floyd, J. A. (1983). Research using Rogers' conceptual system: Development of a testable theorem. *Advances in Nursing Science, 5*(2), 37–48.

Floyd, J. A. (1984). Interaction between personal sleep-wake rhythms and psychiatric hospital rest-activity schedule. *Nursing Research, 33*(5), 255–259.

Floyd, J. A. (1993). The use of across-method triangulation in the study of sleep concerns in healthy older adults. *Advances in Nursing Science, 16*(2), 70–80.

Floyd, J. A. (1995). Another look at napping in older adults. *Geriatric Nursing, 16*(1), 136–138.

Graves, J. R. (1990). A research-knowledge system (ARKS) for storing, managing, and modeling knowledge from the scientific literature. *Advances in Nursing Science, 13*(2), 34–45.

Graves, J. R. (1997). *arcs©* manual. Indianapolis: Sigma Theta Tau International.

Haddock, J. (1994). Reducing the effects of noise in hospital. *Clinical Sleep, 8*(43), 25–28.

Hauri, P. J., & Wisbey, J. (1993). Wrist actigraphy in insomnia. *Sleep, 15,* 293–301.

Hayter, J. (1983). Sleep behaviors of older persons. *Nursing Research, 32*(4), 242–246.

Hayter, J. (1985). Sleep apnea cause for concern. *Journal of Gerontological Nursing, 10*(9), 26–29.

Healey, E. S., Kales, A., Monroe, L. J., Bixler, E. O., Chamberlin, C., & Soldatos, C. R. (1981). Onset of insomnia: Role of life-stress events. *Psychosomatic Medicine, 45,* 341–356.

Helton, M. C., Gordon, S. H., & Nunnery, S. L. (1980). The correlation between sleep deprivation and the intensive care unit syndrome. *Heart & Lung, 9*(3), 464–468.

Herbert, M. (1978). Studies of sleep in the elderly. *Age and Ageing, 7*(Supplement), 41–45.

Hill, J. (1989). A good night's sleep. *Senior Nurse, 9*(5), 17–19.

Hilton, B. A. (1976). Quantity and quality of patients' sleep and sleep-disturbing factors in a respiratory intensive care unit. *Journal of Advanced Nursing, 1,* 453–467.

Horne, J. (1992). Human slow wave sleep: A review and appraisal of recent findings, with implications for sleep functions, and psychiatric illness. *Experientia, 48,* 941–954.

Jacobs, G. D., Benson, H., & Friedman, R. (1993). Home-based central nervous system assessment of a multifactor behavioral intervention for chronic sleep-onset insomnia. *Behavior Therapy, 24*(1), 159–174.

Jensen, D. P., & Herr, K. A. (1993). Sleeplessness. *Nursing Clinics of North America, 28*(2), 385–405.

Johnson, J. E. (1986). Sleep and bedtime routines of non-institutionalized aged women. *Journal of Community Health Nursing, 3*(3), 117–125.

Johnson, J. E. (1988). Bedtime routines: Do they influence the sleep of elderly women? *Journal of Applied Gerontology, 7*(1), 97–110.

Johnson, J. E. (1991a). A comparative study of the bedtime routines and sleep of older adults. *Journal of Community Health Nursing, 8*(3), 129–136.

Johnson, J. E. (1991b). Progressive relaxation and the sleep of older noninstitutionalized women. *Applied Nursing Research, 4*(4), 165–170.

Johnson, J. E. (1993). Progressive relaxation and the sleep of older men and women. *Journal of Community Health Nursing, 10*(1), 31–38.

Johnson, J. E. (1994). Sleep and alcohol use in rural old-old women. *Journal of Community Health Nursing, 11*(4), 211–218.

Kales, J. D., Kales, A., Bixler, E. O., Soldatos, C. R., Cadieux, R. J., Kashuba, G. J., & Vela-Bueno, A. (1984). Biopsychobehavioral correlates of insomnia: V. Clinical characteristics and behavioral correlates. *American Journal of Psychiatry, 141*, 1371–1376.

Kryger, M. H., Roth, T., & Dement, W. C. (1994). *Principles and practice of sleep medicine* (2nd ed.). Philadelphia: Saunders.

Kupfer, D. J., & Reynolds, C. F., III. (1997). Management of insomnia. *New England Journal of Medicine, 336*(5), 341–346.

Lack, L. C., & Thorn, S. J. (1991). Sleep disorders: Their prevalence and behavioral treatment. In D. G. Byrne & G. R. Caddy (Eds.), *International perspectives in behavioral medicine* (Vol. 2). Norwood, NJ: Ablex.

Lazarus, R. S. (1966). *Psychological stress and the coping process.* New York: McGraw-Hill.

Lichstein, K. L., & Johnson, R. S. (1991). Older adults' objective self-recording of sleep in the home. *Behavior Therapy, 22*, 531–548.

Lichstein, K. L., Nickel, R., Hoelscher, T. J., & Kelley, J. E. (1982). Clinical validation of a sleep assessment device. *Behaviour Research and Therapy, 20*, 292–297.

Lutz, S. J. (1990). The effect of relaxation training on sleep, state anxiety, and sick call in a jail population. *Journal of Prison & Jail Health, 9*(1), 55–71.

Mant, A., & Bearpark. (1990). Management of insomnia. *Australian Prescriber, 13*, 51–54.

McFadden, E. H., & Giblin, E. C. (1971). Sleep deprivation in patients having open-heart surgery. *Nursing Research, 20*(3), 249–254.

Metz, M. E., & Bunnell, D. E. (1990). Napping and sleep disturbances in the elderly. *Family Practice Research Journal, 10*(1), 47–56.

Miller, N. E., & Bartus, R. T. (1982). Sleep, sleep pathology, and psychopathology in later life: A new research frontier. *Neurobiology of Aging, 3*, 283–286.

Morin, C. M., & Azrin, N. H. (1987). Stimulus control and imagery training in treating sleep maintenance insomnia. *Journal of Consulting and Clinical Psychology, 55*, 260–262.

Morin, C. M., & Azrin, N. H. (1988). Behavioral and cognitive treatments of geriatric insomnia. *Journal of Consulting and Clinical Psychology, 56*(5), 748–753.

Morin, C. M., Culbert, J. P., & Schwartz, S. M. (1994). Nonpharmacological interventions for insomnia: A meta-analysis of treatment efficacy. *American Journal of Psychiatry, 151*(8), 1172–1180.

Morin, C. M., Kowatch, R. A., Barry, T., & Walton, E. (1993). Cognitive-behavior therapy for late-life insomnia. *Journal of Consulting and Clinical Psychology, 61*(1), 137–146.

Murtagh, D. R. R., & Greenwood, K. M. (1995). Identifying effective psychological treatments for insomnia: A meta-analysis. *Journal of Consulting and Clinical Psychology, 63*(1), 79–89.

National Sleep Foundation. (1995). *Sleep in America: A national survey of U.S. adults.* Houston: Gallup Organization.

Orr, W. C., & Stahl, M. L. (1977). Sleep disturbances after open heart surgery. *The American Journal of Cardiology, 39,* 196–201.

Pacini, C. M., & Fitzpatrick, J. J. (1982). Sleep patterns of hospitalized and nonhospitalized aged individuals. *Journal of Gerontological Nursing, 8*(6), 327–332.

Pimentel-Souza, F., Carvalho, J. C., & Siqueira, A. L. (1996). Noise and the quality of sleep in two hospitals in the city of Belo Horizonte, Brazil. *Brazil Journal of Medical and Biological Research, 29*(4), 515–520.

Rediehs, M. H., Reis, J. S., & Creason, N. S. (1990). Sleep in old age: Focus on gender differences. *Sleep, 13*(5), 410–424.

Regestein, Q. R. (1980). Insomnia and sleep disturbances in the aged: Sleep and insomnia in the elderly. *Journal of Geriatric Psychiatry, 13,* 153–171.

Richards, K. (1987). Techniques for measurement of sleep in critical care. *Focus on Critical Care, 14*(4), 34–40.

Richards, K. C., & Bairnsfather, L. (1988). A description of night sleep patterns in the critical care unit. *Heart & Lung, 17*(1), 35–42.

Richards, K. C., Curry, N., Lyons, W., & Todd, B. (1996). Cardiac dysrhythmia during sleep in the critically ill: A pilot study. *American Journal of Critical Care, 5*(1), 26–33.

Schaefer, K. M., Swavely, D., Rothenberger, C., Hess, S., & Williston, D. (1996). Sleep disturbances post coronary artery bypass surgery. *Progress in Cardiovascular Nursing, 11*(1), 5–14.

Schnelle, J. F., Ouslander, J. G., & Alessi, C. A. (1993). Nightime sleep and bed mobility in incontinent nursing home patients. *Journal of the American Geriatrics Society, 41*(9), 903–909.

Schnelle, J. F., Ouslander, J. G., Simmons, S. F., Alessi, C. A., & Gravel, J. G. (1993). The nighttime environment, incontinence care, and sleep disruption in nursing homes. *Journal of the American Geriatrics Society, 41*(9), 910–914.

Sheely, L. C. (1996). Sleep disturbances in hospitalized patients with cancer. *Oncology Nursing Forum, 23*(1), 109–111.

Simpson, T., & Lee, E. R. (1996). Individual factors that influence sleep after cardiac surgery. *American Journal of Critical Care, 5*(3), 182–189.

Simpson, T., Lee, E. R., & Cameron, C. (1996a). Patients' perceptions of environmental factors that disturb sleep after cardiac surgery. *American Journal of Critical Care, 5*(3), 173–181.

Simpson, T., Lee, E. R., & Cameron, C. (1996b). Relationships among sleep dimensions and factors that impair sleep after cardiac surgery. *Research in Nursing & Health, 19*(3), 213–233.

Smallwood, R. G., Vitiello, M. V., Giblin, E. C., & Prinz, P. N. (1983). Sleep apnea: Relationship to age, sex, and Alzheimer's dementia. *Sleep, 6*(1), 16–22.

Snyder-Halpern, R. (1985). The effect of critical care unit noise on patient sleep cycles. *Critical Care Quarterly, 7*(4), 41–51.

Snyder-Halpern, R., & Verran, J. A. (1987). Instrumentation to describe subjective sleep characteristics in healthy subjects. *Research in Nursing and Health, 10*(3), 155–163.

Soldatos, C. R., Kales, J. D., Scharf, M. B., Bixler, E. O., & Kales, A. (1980). Cigarette smoking associated with sleep difficulty. *Science, 207,* 551–552.

Southwell, M. T., & Wistow, G. (1995). Sleep in hospitals at night: Are patients' needs being met? *Journal of Advanced Nursing, 21,* 1101–1109.

Topf, M. (1984). A framework for research on aversive physical aspects of the environment. *Research in Nursing and Health, 7,* 35–42.

Topf, M. (1992). Effects of personal control over hospital noise on sleep. *Research in Nursing and Health, 15*(1), 19–28.

Topf, M., Bookman, M., & Arand, D. (1996). Effects of critical care unit noise on the subjective quality of sleep. *Journal of Advanced Nursing, 24*(3), 545–551.

Topf, M., & Davis, J. E. (1993). Critical care unit noise and rapid eye movement (REM) sleep. *Heart & Lung, 22*(3), 252–258.

Walker, B. B. (1972). The postsurgery heart patient: Amount of uninterrupted time for sleep and rest during the first, second, and third post-operative days in a teaching hospital. *Nursing Research, 21*(2), 164–169.

Williamson, J. W. (1992). The effect of ocean sounds on sleep after coronary bypass graft surgery. *American Journal of Critical Care, 1,* 91–97.

Wilson, V. S. (1987). Identifications of stressors related to patients' psychologic responses to the surgical intensive care unit. *Heart & Lung, 16*(3), 267–273.

Wolpe, J. (1969). *The practice of behavioral therapy.* New York: Pergamon.

Woods, N. F. (1972). Patterns of sleep in postcardiotomy patients. *Nursing Research, 21*(4), 347–352.

Young, S. H., Muir-Nash, J., & Ninos, M. (1988). Managing nocturnal wandering behavior. *Journal of Gerontological Nursing, 14*(5), 6–12.

Zarcone, V. P., Jr. (1994). Sleep hygiene. In M. H. Kryger, T. Roth, & W. C. Dement (Eds.), *Principles and practice of sleep medicine* (2nd ed., pp. 542–546). Philadelphia: Saunders.

Zimmerman, L., Nieveen, J., Barnason, S., & Schmaderer, M. (1996). The effects of music interventions on postoperative pain and sleep in coronary artery bypass graft (CABG) patients. *Scholarly Inquiry for Nursing Practice: An International Journal, 10*(2), 153–174.

Chapter 3

Guided Imagery Interventions for Symptom Management

LUCILLE SANZERO ELLER

ABSTRACT

For the past several decades, papers in the nursing literature have advocated the use of cognitive interventions in clinical practice. Increasing consumer use of complementary therapies, a cost-driven health care system, and the need for evidence-based practice all lend urgency to the validation of the efficacy of these interventions. This review focuses specifically on guided imagery intervention studies identified in the nursing, medical and psychological literature published between 1966 and 1998. Included were 46 studies of the use of guided imagery for management of psychological and physiological symptoms. There is preliminary evidence for the effectiveness of guided imagery in the management of stress, anxiety and depression, and for the reduction of blood pressure, pain and the side effects of chemotherapy. Overall, results of this review demonstrated a need for systematic, well-designed studies, which explore several unanswered questions regarding the use of guided imagery. These include the effects of different imagery language, symptoms for which guided imagery is effective, appropriate and sensitive outcome measures, method of delivery of the intervention and optimum dose and duration of the intervention, and individual factors that influence its effectiveness.

Keywords: Guided Imagery, Visualization, Cognitive-Behavioral Techniques, Interventions, Symptom Management

Computerized searches of the literature included several databases: Medline (for 1966 through December, 1997), the Cumulative Index of Nursing and

Allied Health Literature (CINAHL) (from 1982 through November, 1997) and the psychological literature (PsycInfo) (for 1967 through November, 1997). The keywords "imagery," "guided imagery," and "visualization" were used. All searches were limited to the English language. PsycInfo searches were also limited to those addressing treatment and prevention. A total of 857 abstracts were retrieved, including 225 from CINAHL, 151 from Medline and 481 from PsycInfo. Article titles and abstracts were screened for keywords and phrases and included in the review as appropriate. Reference lists in articles examined were used to identify additional studies that met inclusion criteria. Case studies, laboratory studies, and dissertations were excluded. Also excluded were studies that included multiple interventions which could confound results. Therefore, excluded were studies combining guided imagery with music, use of journals for daily events, biofeedback, support groups, cognitive restructuring, and other stress management techniques.

Guided imagery has been studied for its effects on academic and athletic performance, and immune and neuroendocrine modulation. It has been used for mental rehearsal to enhance motor performance in rehabilitation and has been applied to the treatment of sexual dysfunction and post-traumatic stress disorder. Examination of these applications of guided imagery are beyond the scope of this chapter and were not included. Included from all sources were 46 studies of other-guided imagery, either pleasant or specific for desired change. The focus of this review is on research studies exploring the use of guided imagery, with or without relaxation, for therapeutic goals on psychological and physiological symptoms in adult subjects. Due to lack of semantic clarity in the use of the term "guided imagery," other studies utilizing this technique may inadvertently been omitted.

A considered decision was made to include studies that combined relaxation with guided imagery. It is suggested that a relaxation induction is necessary to produce an altered state of awareness and focused concentration, to control thought processes, and to intensify the image (Leuner, 1977), and the vast majority of studies of guided imagery include a relaxation induction.

DEFINITION OF TERMS

Imagery consists of the mental representation of all sensory, perceptual events. It includes visual, olfactory, proprioceptive, tactile, auditory and gustatory properties and occurs in the absence of external stimuli (Achterberg & Lawlis, 1982; Moye, Richardson, Post-White, & Justice, 1995; Sodergren, 1992). The images generate physiological and psychological responses that would occur as a result of the imagined external stimulus if it was actually present. Imagery creates a bridge between mind and body, linking perception, emotion and psychological, physiological, and behavioral responses (Achterberg, 1982, 1985; Klinger, 1980; Mast, Meyers, & Urbanski, 1987).

Guided imagery has been categorized as behavioral training or a cognitive technique in which the individual exerts active control over the focus of attention (Fawzy & Fawzy, 1994; Fishman & Loscalzo, 1987). It is a therapeutic process in which participants use an image to communicate with physiological processes outside conscious awareness to achieve specific health goals (Sodergren, 1992; Vines, 1988). Guided imagery includes synthesis of information, formation of cognitive strategies, and development of individual coping behaviors (Schandler & Dana, 1983).

CONTENT AND PROCESS OF GUIDED IMAGERY

Two types of imagery have been described: active imagery, in which the subject is guided through suggestion to evoke specific images, and receptive imagery, in which the subject's spontaneous images are the focus. Guided imagery is active imagery.

Both the content and process of guided imagery interventions must be considered. Content may include pleasant imagery or specific imagery. Pleasant imagery includes the mental construction or recall of a pleasant or relaxing experience (Daake & Gueldner, 1989). Pleasant imagery includes suggestions for visualization of peaceful or pleasant scenes, which may be selected by the subject, or may be a standardized pleasant image, such as a beach or mountain scene. Some authors have suggested that the most effective images are generated by the subjects themselves, and are related to their perceptions and experiences (Turkoski & Lance, 1996).

Specific imagery can be process-oriented, outcome-oriented, or both. Process- or task-oriented images describe the mechanism by which the desired outcome is to be achieved. For example, the image may be one of increasing blood flow to the heart. Outcome or end-result images describe the final desired result and often include emotional responses to the desired result (Achterberg, 1985; Dossey, 1995; Korn & Johnson, 1983). For example, an outcome image may include visualizing oneself in a healed state with feelings of vigor and joy.

Both process and end-result imagery language includes suggestions for the desired physiological, psychological, or behavioral change. The specific language may be symbolic or physiologically correct. Physiologically correct imagery language usually begins with instruction and graphic presentations of the relevant anatomy and/or physiology to the participant.

Metaphorical images are those in which symbolic, subject-selected imagery occurs in response to suggestions for specific physiological, psychological, or behavioral processes or end-states. The meaning of symbols and selection of metaphors is individually determined and based on beliefs, values, attitudes, and experiences which vary across individuals. Some researchers have suggested that the use of specific imagery, for example, symbolic images of destruction of cancer cells, may result in feelings of failure and helplessness if the imagined scenario does not occur (Bridge, Benson, Pietroni, & Priest, 1988).

One of the earliest and most-cited studies that explored the effects of guided imagery on survival in cancer patients used metaphorical process imagery for the destruction of cancer cells (Simonton, Matthews-Simonton, & Creighton, 1978). Subjects using guided imagery had significantly longer survival compared to statistical norms. However, there were several methodological problems in this study, including lack of a control group, self-selected sample bias, and inclusion of other potentially confounding interventions, such as psychotherapy, assertiveness training, and an exercise program.

Since published studies do not typically report the specific imagery language used, it is not possible to determine in how many cases the language employed may have resulted in the lack of significant results. In one study, Eller (1995) reported that two HIV-positive subjects dropped out of a guided imagery intervention because they found mention of "the virus" in the imagery script too stressful. Activation of the stress response may negate the potentially beneficial psychological and physiological effects of guided imagery. Little is known about optimum imagery language. Further studies of specificity of imagery language and use of subject-selected process and outcome images and language are warranted.

Lang's (1979) bioinformational theory of imagery posits that the therapeutic effectiveness of imagery is directly related to the subject's physiological response to images specific for desired change. The critical property of an effective imagery script is its elicitation of specific somatomotor, verbal, sense-organ, and visceral responses. Sensory qualities such as physical details are called stimulus imagery and create a visual context, but are passive and not critical to therapeutic outcomes. On the other hand, language which describes active responses is called response imagery, and include somatomotor events, visceral events, processor characteristics, and sense-organ adjustments. Use of response imagery has been related to autonomic nervous system responses such as pupil size, lacrimation, salivation, heart rate, blood pressure, bronchial constriction, and gastric motility and secretion. The critical properties of the therapeutic image are thought to be generated by active response language that elicits an active physiological response.

Studies supporting the theory that response-based imagery scripts are more effective in eliciting physiologic change measured autonomic response outcomes. Experiments were conducted in which the language of the imagery script was varied (Lang et al., 1980; Lichstein & Lipshitz, 1982). Stimulus scripts used vivid descriptions of surroundings, placing the subject in one scene of kite-flying on the beach and another of being trapped in a car with a yellowjacket. An example of stimulus language used is the phrase "You are flying a kite on the beach on a bright summer day" (Lang et al., 1980, p. 183). Response scripts used the same contextual elements, but instead used response language rather than visual descriptors. For example, "You breathe deeply as you run along the beach flying a kite" (Lang et al., 1980, p. 183). A neutral script, or control condition, was designed to elicit low or no physiological activation. The neutral scene began with the phrase "You are sitting in your living room reading on a Sunday afternoon" (Lang et al., 1980, p. 183). Only response script subjects demonstrated significant differences in heart rate, muscle tension, and respiration cycle length.

RELAXATION INDUCTION

It is unclear if a relaxation induction is necessary prior to the use of guided imagery or whether it confounds results. Most investigators initiated guided imagery with a relaxation technique. Guided imagery, a cognitive process, is thought to be facilitated by physiological relaxation procedures, which can enhance the focus of attention on physiological feedback (Rees, 1993; Schandler & Dana, 1983; Singer, 1974; Turkowski & Lance, 1996). However, in most studies, specific details of the relaxation induction were not reported. It is possible that some may have included lengthy relaxation techniques that, in and of themselves, qualify as interventions.

Five of the studies reviewed examined the effects of guided imagery alone without a relaxation induction. In a comparison of three types of imagery, neutral, positive and subject-selected, Jarvinien and Gold (1981) found that all three types of imagery significantly reduced depression when compared to a control group. Similarly, Eller (1995), in comparing imagery, relaxation, and a control condition, found that both imagery alone and relaxation alone reduced depression in persons with HIV. In the same study, fatigue was significantly reduced only in the imagery group. Two studies examined the effects of imagery alone on anxiety. Stephens (1992) reported that both imagery and progressive muscle relaxation attenuated increases in anxiety seen in the control group. Pickett and Clum (1982) reported that reductions in anxiety were greater in the imagery group when compared to relaxation and control groups. Finally, Wells (1989) found no effects on pain in a comparison of pleasant imagery, specific imagery, relaxation, and a control group. Taken together, these few studies suggest that imagery alone may have a differential effect on psychological and physiological outcomes. They lend support to the premise that imagery is different from, or more than, relaxation. Additional research is needed to study the effects of relaxation and guided imagery both separately and combined in order to determine the differential and synergistic effects of these interventions.

THEORETICAL FRAMEWORKS AND MECHANISMS OF ACTION OF GUIDED IMAGERY

In general, studies of guided imagery do not clearly link the intervention or outcome measures to theoretical frameworks. Theoretical frameworks or putative mechanisms of action for effects of guided imagery guided approximately one-third of studies reviewed. Theoretical frameworks included stress and coping (Collins & Rice, 1997; Manyande et al., 1995; Rees, 1995; Stephens, 1992; Tsai & Crockett, 1993); Psychoneuroimmunology (Andrews & Hall, 1990; Eller, 1995); Gate control theory (Daake & Gueldner, 1989; Wells, 1989); Orem's self-care deficit theory of nursing (Sloman, Brown, Aldana, & Chee, 1994; Troesch, Rodehaver, Delaney, & Yanes, 1993); cognitive theory (Turner & Jensen, 1993); Psychosynthetic theory (Ilacqua, 1994); Rogers' science of unitary human beings (Thompson & Coppens, 1994); Neuman health care systems model (Leja, 1989) and Selye's general adaptation syndrome (Holden-Lund, 1988). Several alternative psychological and physiological mechanisms of action for the effects of guided imagery have been suggested. These include cognitive restructuring, active coping, cognitive distraction, reduction of autonomic activity, and biochemical mediation of physiological and psychological processes.

Guided imagery may exert its effect as a cognitive method through the modification of maladaptive cognitive patterns with subsequent reduction of autonomic arousal and decrease in muscle tension (Fishman & Loscalzo, 1987; Tan, 1982; Zahourek, 1988). Negative cognitions or appraisals result in exacerbation of mood disturbances and pain. Alteration of meanings, assumptions and internal dialog surrounding specific images, and substitution of adaptive cognitions can attenuate negative experience (Lang, 1977; Meichenbaum, 1978). In the case of anxiety or depression, imagery can serve to replace negative internal processes with images of positive outcomes and realistic appraisal and more adaptive coping (Jarvinien & Gold, 1981). Turner and Jensen (1993) reported a significant decrease in maladaptive thoughts in a chronic pain population following a 6-week guided imagery intervention. Guided imagery may be an active coping skill, increasing the subject's sense of control, and decreasing feelings of helplessness and hopelessness (Kiecolt-Glaser et al., 1985; Lyles, Burish, Krozely, & Oldham, 1982). Mental rehearsal using relevant images can lead to increased control of maladaptive behaviors (Meichenbaum, 1978). Several studies explored the effects of guided imagery on control and coping. In persons with cancer (Baider, Uziely, & DeNour, 1994; Troesch et al., 1993), multiple sclerosis (Maguire, 1996), migraine headache (Ilacqua, 1993) and abdominal surgery (Manyande et al., 1995), guided imagery interventions significantly improved perceived control and coping related to medical treatment (Troesch et al., 1993), pain (Ilacqua, 1993; Manyande et al., 1995) and the impact of illness (Baider et al., 1994). All of these studies employed imagery specific for control and coping. In a study by Maguire (1996), declines in health-related locus of control observed in the control group were attenuated in the treatment group. In another study, specific imagery increased participants' ability to cope with cancer; however, effects on locus of control in this study were difficult to explain. Attribution of control to chance or powerful others, or external control, was reduced, which would suggest subjects' increased perceptions of personal control. However, internal locus of control was also significantly lower after the intervention (Baider et al., 1994). Investigators had no explanation for this observation.

Specific imagery was not effective in increasing subject sense of "mastery" in one study of persons with chronic emphysema and bronchitis (Moody, Fraser, & Yarandi, 1993). That study did not have a control group, therefore, without control comparisons, it is not possible to know whether comparative differences would have occurred. In another study, there was also no effect on perceived control in an independently living geriatric population. The type of imagery used was not described in this study. The authors noted a high functional level in the sample, so lack of change may be attributed to a ceiling effect (Kiecolt-Glaser et al., 1985).

It may be that the use of specific imagery or measurement of specific areas of control and coping related to illness resulted in differing results in these studies. Support for this is provided by findings in the Manyande et al. (1995) study that although specific coping with pain was significantly improved, overall coping was not.

It has been suggested that imagery influences the experience of pain by acting as a cognitive distraction. This is based on models of attention that posit that in the presence of competing stimuli, attention becomes selective and filters out nociceptive information (Turk & Meichenbaum, 1989). In addition, it may be that activity of higher brain centers during imagery inhibit the transmission of pain signals (Melzack & Wall, 1965). There is some evidence that pleasant imagery acts as a cognitive distraction technique. In a comparison of relaxing imagery and cognitive distraction, Vasterling, Jenkins, Tope, and Burish (1993) found both interventions equally effective in controlling anticipatory nausea and vomiting prior to chemotherapy. However, in another study, Pickett and Clum (1982) used specific surgical imagery followed by pleasant imagery as a "cognitive distraction" technique to reduce postsurgical pain and anxiety. Anxiety, and recalled "pain at its worst" scores were lower for the imagery group when compared to relaxation alone and a control condition. However, overall pain scores were not lower in the imagery group. This may have been due to a floor effect, since pain was measured 5 days post-surgery, when pain would have already subsided.

Imagery may function as one of many relaxation techniques (Smith, 1990). The relaxation effect results in reduction of autonomic activity and the concomitant physiological responses to catecholamine production (Benson, Beary, & Carol, 1974). In addition, relaxation may facilitate the release of endorphins which bind to opioid receptor sites in the central nervous system and block the transmission of painful impulses (Bloom, 1981).

Finally, some authors suggest that the mind does not distinguish between external and internal events, and responds identically to both (Cautela, 1977; Maltz, 1966; Naparstek, 1994; Siegel, 1986; Troesch et al., 1993). Thoughts and emotions elicit specific biochemical responses, creating a communication network between body and mind (Achterberg, 1985; Achterberg & Lawlis, 1982; Pert, 1985). Imagery directs the central and peripheral nervous systems to achieve specific outcomes through the elicitation of neurochemicals. In fact, there is support for this in studies that show that the same areas of the brain are activated by imagery or actual perceived events (Farah, 1984).

Psychological Symptoms

Stress. The effects of imagery on stress or psychological distress were explored in nine studies which included work populations (Lewis, 1987; Tsai & Crockett, 1993), postoperative patients (Holden-Lund, 1988; Manyande et al., 1995), cardiac patients (Collins & Rice, 1997), persons with cancer (Baider et al., 1994) subjects with self-reported symptoms of stress (Green et al., 1988; Schandler & Dana, 1983) and recent ex-smokers (Wynd, 1992). Stress was measured either by self-report (Baider et al., 1994; Green et al., 1988; Tsai & Crockett, 1993; Wynd, 1992) or physiological measures (Holden-Lund, 1988; Lewis, 1987; Manyande et al., 1995; Schandler & Dana, 1983). In all but one of the nine studies (Collins & Rice, 1997), symptoms were significantly reduced in persons in the guided imagery interventions.

In studies reporting significant results, two employed pleasant imagery (Tsai & Crockett, 1993; Wynd, 1992) while the others were specific for wound healing and recovery (Holden-Lund, 1988), pain reduction and coping (Manyande et al., 1995) a healthy body (Green et al., 1988) and reduction of tension or distress (Baider et al., 1994; Schandler & Dana, 1983). Instruction was provided in live format (Baider et al., 1994; Green et al., 1988; Tsai & Crockett, 1993; Wynd, 1992) or via audiotape (Holden-Lund, 1988; Manyande et al., 1995; Schandler & Dana, 1983) and to both individuals (Holden-Lund, 1988; Schandler & Dana, 1983; Manyande et al., 1995) and groups (Baider et al., 1994; Green et al., 1988; Wynd, 1992). Interventions were conducted between one (Baider et al., 1994; Green et al., 1988; Manyande et al., 1995) and seven times (Tsai & Crockett, 1993), with opportunity for participant practice noted in four studies (Green et al., 1988; Manyande et al., 1995; Tsai & Crockett, 1993; Wynd, 1992). However, frequency of practice was not included in analyses. Type of imagery, length of intervention, and method of delivery were not described in one study (Lewis, 1987).

The guided imagery groups reported significantly lower subjectively perceived stress than controls (Baider et al., 1994; Green et al., 1988; Tsai & Crockett, 1993; Wynd, 1992) and reductions in physiological indicators of stress including urinary cortisol levels (Manyande et al., 1995), palmar sweat (Lewis, 1987) and frontalis muscle tension (Schandler & Dana, 1983). One study reported a trend for decreased urinary cortisol (Holden-Lund, 1988).

In the one study that reported no effect, psychological distress related to cardiac disease was not reduced (Collins & Rice, 1997). The intervention was conducted once, live, with individuals, and followed by home practice over 6 weeks. Frequency-of-practice data were not included in analyses. The sample consisted of 20 intervention and 23 control subjects. Specific imagery referred to visualization of a "well healed and strong" heart, which may have been a reminder of disease and increased subjects' stress and could explain the lack of significant findings.

Mood. In seven studies where mood or affect were measured, three reported no significant effects of guided imagery, and four reported that outcomes were significantly improved following guided imagery interventions. In three of the four studies in which imagery significantly improved mood, subjects were persons with cancer (Bridge et al., 1988; Lyles et al., 1982; Vasterling et al., 1993). Subject-selected pleasant imagery interventions were delivered between three to six times in all three studies. The fourth studied a geriatric population and did not report the type of imagery (Kiecolt-Glaser et al., 1985). In that study, all psychological symptoms except depression improved significantly in response to the intervention which was delivered twelve times. All four studies ranged from 1 to 6 weeks in length, and the interventions were delivered live in an individual format.

In the studies where guided imagery had no effect, study samples included persons with multiple sclerosis (Maguire, 1996), burn patients (Achterberg, Kenner, & Lawlis, 1988) and women with breast cancer (Arathuzik, 1994). Imagery specific for physiological change was employed in all of the studies. Interventions were delivered once in a one-day pre-posttest (Arathuzik, 1994). The other two studies delivered the intervention six times, but did not provide sufficient information to ascertain length of the study (Achterberg et al., 1988; Maguire, 1996).

As in other studies of psychological states, the few studies examining mood used different populations, sample sizes, and frequency and length of the interventions, as well as different interventions themselves. Based on an evaluation of these few studies, it may be that self-selected pleasant imagery is more effective in improving mood than any specific process or outcome imagery. Specific imagery may serve as a reminder of health problems and, as such, be less effective in moderating affective states. Additional research is needed to validate the effects of guided imagery on global mood or psychological stress and distress.

Anxiety.   Twenty studies examined anxiety related to treatments, procedures, or health states. Of those, twelve reported significant reductions in anxiety, and seven reported no differences in anxiety in guided imagery intervention groups.

In the thirteen studies in which anxiety was significantly reduced, five examined guided imagery in chronically ill populations, including those with cancer (Burish, Carey, Krozely, & Greco, 1987; Carey & Burish, 1987; Lyles et al., 1982), multiple sclerosis (Maguire, 1996), and burns (Achterberg et al., 1988). Three studies included participants undergoing surgery or medical tests (Holden-Lund, 1988; Pickett & Clum, 1982; Thompson & Coppens, 1994), and five included persons involved in stressful life situations (King, 1988; Rees, 1993, 1995; Schandler & Dana, 1983; Stephens, 1992). Pleasant imagery of the participant's own choosing was used in five studies (Burish et al., 1987; Carey & Burish, 1987; King, 1988; Lyles et al., 1982; Thompson & Coppens, 1994), while the remainder used specific process or outcome imagery. For example, images were specific for wound healing (Holden-Lund, 1988), myelin repair (Maguire, 1996), and positive surgical outcomes (Pickett & Clum, 1982). The intervention was delivered live over one to six sessions (Burish et al., 1987; King, 1988; Lyles et al., 1982; Maguire, 1996; Pickett & Clum,

1982) or by audiotape over two to six sessions (Achterberg et al., 1988; Holden-Lund, 1988; Schandler & Dana, 1983; Stephens, 1992; Thompson & Coppens, 1994). One study compared live and audiotaped instruction (Carey & Burish, 1987). Two studies using audiotaped instruction did not report the number of times the intervention was delivered by investigators (Rees, 1993, 1995). In some cases, subjects practiced the intervention after initial instruction, however, frequency of practice data were not included in statistical analyses (Burish et al., 1987; Rees, 1993, 1995; Stephens, 1992). The length of studies ranged from one day to approximately 60 days, with most occurring over 2 to 4 weeks. In the study that lasted approximately 60 days, investigators stated that "the average length of time between [five chemotherapy] treatments was approximately 15 days;" however, no further information was given (Burish et al., 1987, p. 43). Seven studies had 11 to 18 subjects per cell (Burish et al., 1987; Carey & Burish, 1987; Holden-Lund, 1988; Lyles et al., 1982; Maguire, 1996; Pickett & Clum, 1982; Schandler & Dana, 1983), while the remainder had 20 to 50 subjects per cell. One study did not provide statistical comparisons, but did report larger mean decreases in anxiety in the intervention group compared to controls (Rees, 1993).

In the seven studies where guided imagery had no effect on anxiety, five tested guided imagery in persons with chronic illnesses, including cancer (Rapkin, Straubing, & Holroyd, 1991; Vasterling et al., 1993), cardiac illnesses (Collins & Rice, 1997) glaucoma (Kaluza & Stremple, 1995) and bronchitis and emphysema (Moody et al., 1993). The remaining two were in postoperative subjects (Manyande et al., 1995) or those with self-identified psychological symptoms (Green et al., 1988). Three of the studies did not include control groups (Green et al., 1988; Moody et al., 1993; Rapkin et al, 1991). One study employed the participant's own pleasant imagery (Vasterling, 1993), and one used a "standard guided imagery script," so it is not known whether this was specific or pleasant imagery (Moody et al., 1993). The other five used imagery specific for desired results, such as a "healed, strong heart." In five of the studies, the intervention was delivered only once (Collins & Rice, 1997; Green et al., 1988; Manyande et al., 1995; Moody et al., 1993; Rapkin et al., 1991), and in one of the five, the intervention was delivered via audiotape rather than live (Manyande et al., 1995). The remaining two studies included four (Moody et al., 1993) or sixteen (Kaluza & Stremple, 1995) sessions, and all were delivered live. In four studies, participants practiced the intervention following instruction; however, data on frequency and its relationship to outcomes were not provided (Collins & Rice, 1997; Manyande et al., 1995; Moody et al., 1993; Rapkin et al. 1991). The length of studies, where reported, ranged from 4 days (Manyande et al., 1995) to 16 weeks (Kaluza & Stremple, 1995). Most were from 3 to 6 weeks (Collins & Rice, 1997; Green et al.,

1988; Moody et al., 1993). Six studies had 9 to 15 subjects per cell (Green et al., 1988; Kaluza & Stremple, 1995; Moody et al., 1993; Rapkin et al., 1991; Vasterling et al., 1993), and the others had 20 to 26 subjects per cell (Collins & Rice, 1997; Manyande et al., 1995). Vasterling and colleagues did not provide pre- or posttest data for anxiety scores, but divided subjects by high and low anxiety at prechemotherapy, and reported no interaction between anxiety and the effects of guided imagery (Vasterling et al., 1993).

It appears that state anxiety may be amenable to modification with imagery techniques. In studies in which guided imagery was effective in reducing anxiety, type of imagery, methods of delivery, and length of the intervention varied. The interventions were delivered more than one time in 12 of 13 of these studies. Most studies that found no difference in anxiety used specific imagery and delivered the intervention only once. Populations and sample sizes were not considerably different across studies where significant and nonsignificant results were reported. Additional research is needed to determine whether frequency of delivery of the intervention or type of imagery language are the critical variables in determining the efficacy of guided imagery for reducing anxiety.

Depression. Fifteen studies explored the effects of guided imagery on depression. In eleven studies where the intervention was effective, clinical populations included cardiac, cancer, or postoperative patients (Burish et al., 1987; Collins & Rice, 1997; Leja, 1989; Lyles et al., 1982) or persons with chronic low back pain (Turner & Jensen, 1993) or HIV/AIDS (Eller, 1995). Primiparas (Rees, 1993, 1995) and depressed college students (Jarvinien & Gold, 1981; Propst, 1980; Schandler & Dana, 1983) made up the remaining study populations. In two studies, type of imagery included pleasant imagery chosen by the participant (Burish et al., 1987; Lyles et al., 1982), one study did not provide information about type of imagery (Turner & Jensen, 1993) and the remaining eight studies used specific imagery. These included images of a healed heart (Collins & Rice, 1997), accomplishment of specific tasks (Jarvinien, 1981; Leja, 1989; Rees, 1993, 1995) or reduction in tension or negative feelings (Eller, 1995; Schandler & Dana, 1983). One study with subjects who scored high on religiosity compared the effects of religious and nonreligious imagery (Propst, 1980). Across studies, the interventions were delivered in one to six sessions followed, in some cases, by home practice. In studies in which home practice of the intervention was performed, data were not included in analyses (Burish et al., 1987; Collins & Rice, 1997; Eller, 1995; Rees, 1993, 1995). The interventions were presented live in all but one study, in which guided imagery was delivered by audiotape (Eller, 1995). The intervention was presented in a group format in two studies (Propst,

1980; Turner & Jensen, 1993) and two gave no information (Rees, 1993, 1995) while the remaining seven used individual training. Length of studies ranged from 1 week (Leja, 1989) to more than 2 months (Burish et al., 1987). The majority of studies were from four to six weeks (Collins & Rice, 1997; Eller, 1995; Jarvinien, 1981; Propst, 1980; Rees, 1993, 1995). Four studies had between 9 and 15 subjects per cell (Burish et al., 1987; Jarvinien, 1981; Propst, 1980), and six studies had from 16 to 30 per cell (Collins & Rice, 1997; Eller, 1995; Lyles et al., 1982; Rees, 1993, 1995; Turner & Jensen, 1993). One study with five subjects in each cell (Leja, 1989) reported significant within-group, but not between-group, decreases in depression. Finally, the study which compared religious and nonreligious imagery reported a trend for reduced depression only in the religious imagery group (Propst, 1980).

Four studies reported no effects on depression of guided imagery interventions. Two clinical populations included persons with open angle glaucoma (Kaluza & Stemple, 1995), and chronic bronchitis and emphysema (Moody et al., 1993). The other two studied depressed college students (Gold, Jarvinien, & Teague, 1982) and geriatric nursing home residents (Abraham, Neundorfer, & Currie, 1992). All presented the intervention live in a group format. Studies included as few as two or four (Gold et al., 1982; Moody et al., 1993) and as many as 16 or 24 training sessions (Abraham et al., 1992; Kaluza & Stremple, 1995), and lasted from 3 to 28 weeks. The type of imagery used was specific for success (Gold et al., 1982), or desired physical or psychological changes (Abraham et al., 1992; Kaluza & Stremple, 1995). One study did not describe the type or content of imagery used, and also did not include a control group (Moody et al., 1993). Across studies, the number of subjects per cell ranged from 8 to 19.

Other psychological variables.   Other psychological outcome variables were examined in very few studies. Interpersonal sensitivity in subjects undergoing cardiac rehabilitation was improved in response to one session of instruction in specific guided imagery followed by home practice over 6 weeks (Collins & Rice, 1997). Hostility was reduced in cancer patients (Burish et al., 1987) and subjects who screened high on hostility (Schandler & Dana, 1983). Either the subject's own pleasant imagery (Burish et al., 1987) or imagery specific for tension reduction (Schandler & Dana, 1983) were employed. Interventions were conducted with individuals either three times in an audiotaped format (Schandler & Dana, 1983) or six times through live instruction with additional home practice (Burish et al., 1987).

One investigator replicated a study with primiparas that indicated improvements in self-esteem in response to the intervention (Rees, 1993, 1995). The imagery used was specific for successful conduct of daily tasks and home practice was employed. No information was provided regarding method of delivery or frequency of the intervention.

Loneliness (Kiecolt-Glaser et at., 1985), hopelessness (Abraham et al., 1992) and life satisfaction (Abraham et al., 1992; Kiecolt-Glaser et al., 1985) in geriatric populations, and pessimism in postsurgical head and neck cancer patients (Rapkin et al., 1991) were not significantly reduced in response to live, individual guided imagery instruction. Imagery was specific in two studies (Abraham et al., 1992; Rapkin et al., 1991) and not described in the other (Kiecolt-Glaser et al., 1985).

Physiological Symptoms

Blood pressure and heart rate.   Nine studies explored the effects of guided imagery on blood pressure and heart rate. In the seven studies where the interventions were effective, populations included individuals with essential hypertension (Crowther, 1983; Henry & Sanacore, 1987; Taylor, Farquhar, Nelson, & Agras, 1977) persons undergoing cancer chemotherapy (Burish et al., 1987; Lyles et al., 1982; Vasterling et al., 1993) or cardiac patients (Collins & Rice, 1997). In this last group, significant effects were reported only for heart rate. However, the control group had greater increases in cardiac medications, and this may explain the lack of difference in blood pressure between the control and intervention groups.

Participant-selected pleasant imagery was used in six studies, and, in addition, one study included specific imagery for a strong heart (Collins & Rice, 1997). In one case, "general imagery" which was not described was used (Henry & Sanacore, 1987). Interventions were conducted from one to eight times, and home practice was used in all studies except one (Vasterling et al., 1993). In all cases, interventions were delivered live on an individual basis. Studies ranged from one week to approximately 60 days in length. Sample sizes ranged from 10 to 23 subjects per cell.

In two studies in which guided imagery did not affect blood pressure or heart rate, subjects included postoperative (Manyande et al., 1995) or burn patients (Achterberg et al., 1988). In the Manyande et al. (1995) study, specific imagery for pain and coping was used. Interventions were conducted once, individually, by audiotape and followed by individual practice over 4 days. The study included 25 or 26 subjects per cell. In the Achterberg et al. (1988) study, specific imagery for wound care was used. The interventions were conducted individually, by audiotape, six times over an unspecified period of time, with no individual practice. There were 34 to 50 subjects per cell in the study. In both studies, patients were experiencing pain, and although guided imagery was reported to significantly reduce subjective indicators of pain, it did not decrease autonomic arousal secondary to pain.

Effects of chemotherapy. A series of studies compared the effects of guided imagery, attention-placebo, and no-treatment control in patients receiving chemotherapy (Burish et al., 1987; Burish & Lyles, 1981; Lyles et al., 1982). Live instruction with a guided image of a pleasant scene was delivered four to six times and followed by home practice with written instructions or an audiotape. The imagery was individually tailored to the preferences of the subject. Investigators reported reductions in negative affect and autonomic arousal, nausea, and anxiety during chemotherapy. There was no difference in postchemotherapy frequency of vomiting.

In a later study comparing guided imagery to cognitive distraction in 60 patients, after three live sessions, both were found equally effective in reducing the distress of chemotherapy (Vasterling et al., 1993). Pleasant imagery was specifically selected by the subject and the intervention was delivered in person. Redd, Rosenberger, and Hendler (1982) also reported reductions in anticipatory nausea and vomiting in response to therapist-selected pleasant imagery and mental imagery rehearsal of chemotherapy administration delivered live. Conversely, there was no difference in nausea and vomiting observed post-chemotherapy in a sample of patients using a standardized audiotape of guided imagery. The guided imagery used specific language for "no side effects" and "actively treating the disease" (Troesch et al., 1993). The use of negative language, and the inclusion of disease-specific language, may have resulted in the lack of significant findings in this study. Taken together, these studies suggest that guided imagery, using pleasant but not specific imagery language, may be effective in reducing the aversive effects of chemotherapy at varying points of treatment. Based on these studies, live delivery of the intervention, over three to six sessions, with or without home practice was effective. Additional research is needed regarding timing of the intervention and its effect of chemotherapy-related side effects.

Pain. In a review, Herr and Mobily (1992) described interventions validated by expert nurses for the management of pain. Simple guided imagery was identified as a pain intervention that used imagination for achievement of relaxation or cognitive distraction. Defining activities included suggestions to induce relaxation and the use of pleasant imagery.

Eleven studies that examined the effects of guided imagery on pain in clinical populations were reviewed. These included postoperative patients (Daake & Gueldner, 1989; Manyande et al., 1995; Pickett & Clum, 1982; Rapkin et al., 1991), persons with cancer (Arathuzik, 1994; Sloman et al.,

1994; Syrjala, Donaldson, Davis, Kippes, & Carr, 1995), chronic low back pain (Turner & Jensen, 1993), burns (Achterberg et al., 1988) migraine headache (Ilacqua, 1994) or those undergoing abortion (Wells, 1989). Six studies reported significant reductions in reported pain in response to the interventions (Achterberg et al., 1988; Daake & Gueldner, 1989; Manyande et al., 1995; Sloman et al., 1994; Syrjala et al., 1995; Turner & Jensen, 1993). Among those, three used specific imagery for pain reduction (Achterberg et al., 1988; Manyande et al., 1995; Syrjala et al., 1995), two used pleasant imagery (Daake & Gueldner, 1989; Sloman et al., 1994), and one did not report on type of imagery used (Turner & Jensen, 1993). Interventions were conducted for either one (Daake & Gueldner, 1989; Manyande et al., 1995) four to six (Achterberg et al., 1988; Sloman et al., 1994; Turner & Jensen, 1993) or twelve sessions (Syrjala et al., 1995). These were delivered in an individual format in all but one case where a group format was used (Turner & Jensen, 1993). In three studies, audiotape was used to deliver the interventions (Achterberg et al., 1988; Daake & Gueldner, 1989; Manyande et al., 1995). One study compared live and audiotape delivery of guided imagery. Practice of the intervention was included in all but one study (Achterberg et al., 1988). The length of the studies was 4 to 6 days in the postoperative studies, and 2 to 6 weeks in the others. It was not possible to determine the length of time elapsed in the study of burn patients. Sample sizes ranged from 14 to 26 per cell in all but one study which included 34 to 50 subjects per cell (Achterberg et al., 1988).

In five studies, no significant differences in reported pain were observed in persons in the guided imagery intervention. These studies included postoperative patients (Pickett & Clum, 1982; Rapkin et al., 1991), persons with breast cancer (Arathuzik, 1994), migraine headache (Ilacqua, 1993) or those undergoing abortion (Wells, 1989). Specific imagery for pain reduction was used in all studies, and one compared specific analgesic imagery with pleasant imagery (Wells, 1989). The intervention was delivered six times in one study (Ilacqua, 1993), and once in the remaining four studies. In only one study, which did not include a control group, participants practiced the intervention (Rapkin et al., 1991). The majority of studies ranged from 1 to 9 days; one did not report length of time (Ilacqua, 1993). Sample sizes ranged from 8 to 15 subjects per cell. It may be that in the case of pain, by using specific imagery language, negative suggestions were introduced by using the word "pain." Wells' (1989) findings lend some support to this possibility in that, although not statistically significant, subjects receiving pleasant imagery had lower pain and distress ratings than those in the specific imagery and control groups.

In a meta-analysis of cognitive coping strategies for pain control, Fernandez and Turk (1989) reviewed studies published between 1960 and 1988.

Studies were grouped into categories of pain coping strategies identified in a taxonomy developed by Wack and Turk (1984). These categories were based on an analysis of strategies used by subjects coping with laboratory pain induction experiments. Imagery strategies were the most effective in attenuating pain. Two strategies, neutral imagery and pleasant imagery, were included. Seven studies of neutral imagery represented 160 subjects, while 20 studies used pleasant imagery in a total of 558 subjects. The two largest effect sizes seen across strategies were reported for imagery studies which employed neutral imaginings (d = 0.74) and pleasant imaginings (d = 0.64). One caveat, however, is that the majority of these studies were conducted in the laboratory with induced pain and may not be generalizable to clinical populations.

An interdisciplinary expert panel commissioned by the U.S. Agency for Health Care Policy and Research (AHCPR) carefully reviewed studies of the management of cancer pain. The resulting clinical practice guideline recommends pleasant imagery, particularly images tailored to individual patient preferences, for reduction in pain intensity and distress (AHCPR, 1994). In the similarly derived clinical practice guideline for management of acute pain, AHCPR recommends the use of simple relaxation imagery for reducing mild to moderate pain, and as an adjunct for severe pain. Complex imagery is recommended for use by skilled personnel in the reduction of mild to moderate pain (AHCPR, 1992).

Other physical symptoms.   Effects of guided imagery on a variety of physical symptoms were explored in nine studies. In four studies, researchers reported improvements in symptoms or physical function. Significant improvements were reported in apthous ulcer recurrence (Andrews & Hall, 1990), fatigue in persons with HIV/AIDS (Eller, 1995) and intraocular pressure in persons with open angle glaucoma (Kaluza & Stremple, 1995) In addition, trends for improved physical function were observed in nutritionally at-risk persons with cancer (Dixon, 1984). Three studies employed specific imagery interventions, delivered individually either once (Eller, 1995) or 12 times (Andrews & Hall, 1990), or in a group format, 8 times (Kaluza & Stremple, 1995). One study did not report on method of delivery of the intervention. In all but one case (Kaluza & Stremple, 1995), home practice of the intervention was reported. Studies were either 6 (Eller, 1995), 16 (Dixon, 1984; Kaluza & Stremple, 1995) or 20 weeks in length (Andrews & Hall, 1990). Sample sizes per cell ranged from 7 subjects (Andrews & Hall, 1990) to 24 subjects (Eller, 1995).

In five studies, guided imagery interventions had no effect on somatic symptoms (Kaluza & Stremple, 1995), symptoms of multiple sclerosis (Maguire, 1996), frequency of migraine headache (Ilacqua, 1993) and functional status (Moody et al., 1993; Turner & Jensen, 1993). In a sixth study that examined the effects of imagery on wound healing, results were equivocal. Two indicators of healing, edema and exudate, were not significantly affected, while one, erythema, was significantly reduced in response to the intervention (Holden-Lund, 1988). In four of the six studies, specific imagery was employed. Two studies provided no information regarding the contents of the imagery (Moody et al., 1993; Turner & Jensen, 1993). One study did not include a control group (Moody et al., 1993). Frequency of the interventions ranged from four to eight times delivered over 4 days to 16 weeks. In four studies, the intervention was delivered live in a group format (Kaluza & Stremple, 1995; Maguire, 1996; Moody et al., 1993; Turner & Jensen, 1993). The other two studies used audiotaped interventions individually. All but one study (Ilacqua, 1993) included home practice of the intervention. Sample sizes ranged from 9 to 21 subjects per cell. No clear distinctions emerged in comparing studies reporting significant and nonsignificant results.

CONCLUSIONS AND FUTURE DIRECTIONS FOR RESEARCH

Of the 46 studies reviewed for this chapter, 40, or 87%, reported that guided imagery, with or without relaxation, resulted in improvements in the psychological or physiological outcomes examined. This may be an indication of the efficacy of the intervention. However, it may, instead, reflect a systematic bias in the publication of studies reporting significant findings.

There were multiple methodological differences across studies of guided imagery. These included type of imagery (specific or nonspecific); delivery of the intervention, including method (live or audiotaped; individual or group format) and frequency; frequency of practice of the intervention; and individual subject characteristics. Although several authors noted that relaxation was part of the imagery exercise, the effects of this intervention alone was not addressed.

Type of Imagery

Of the 40 studies which reported significant findings, 11 used participant-selected pleasant imagery (Bridge et al. 1988; Burish et al., 1987; Carey & Burish, 1987; Crowther, 1983; Daake & Gueldner, 1989; King, 1988; Lyles et al., 1982; Taylor et al., 1977; Thompson & Coppens, 1994; Vasterling et al., 1993; Wells, 1989); five used standardized or therapist-selected pleasant imagery (Henry & Sanacore, 1987; Kiecolt-Glaser et al., 1985; Moody et al., 1993; Redd et al., 1982; Turner & Jensen, 1993) and the remainder used imagery for specific psychological or physiological change. In studies where no differences in psychological or physiological symptoms were observed, studies employed specific imagery (Abraham et al., 1992; Arathuzik, 1994; Gold et al., 1982; Rapkin et al., 1991) or both participant-selected pleasant and specific imagery (Wells, 1989). One study provided no information regarding type of imagery used (Moody et al., 1983).

Method of Delivery of the Intervention

Live versus audiotape.   Where reported, the interventions were delivered live in 62% of the studies reviewed, and by audiotape in 27%. Audiotaped interventions are less labor-intensive, less costly, and more flexible than face-to-face interventions. However, there is insufficient evidence to support their use over live instruction.

Audiotaped and live methods of delivery of the same intervention were compared in two studies of persons with cancer. Carey and Burish (1987) examined effects of guided imagery on anxiety, nausea, blood pressure, and respiration. They reported no significant differences in outcomes of interventions delivered live by professionals when compared to audiotaped interventions. However, when compared to controls, only the live intervention significantly reduced postchemotherapy physiological arousal and anxiety. Sloman et al. (1994) also compared audiotaped and live instruction of relaxation with pleasant imagery. While both treatment groups differed significantly from controls in pain sensation, intensity, severity and non-opiate analgesic use, the two methods of delivery did not differ from each other. More evidence is needed to assess the equivalence of live or audiotaped delivery of guided imagery interventions.

Individual versus group instruction.   Sixty-five percent of studies reviewed conducted the interventions in an individual format, while 20% used group training. The remaining studies did not provide information regarding training sessions. No studies were found which compared delivery of the intervention in a group versus an individual format. As with audiotaped interventions, group delivery of the intervention is more cost-effective than individual instruction. However, it is possible that social support provided in a group would constitute a confounding variable. Additional research is needed to evaluate the use of group versus individual delivery of guided imagery.

Frequency of the Intervention

Frequency of the intervention data was provided in 32 of the studies that reported significant findings. Frequency ranged from one to three sessions in 41%, four to six sessions in 31%, and seven to twelve sessions in 22%. This differs from the findings of Borkovec and Sides (1979) who reported significant results only in studies using progressive muscle relaxation that included at least four teaching sessions. Six studies did not provide information regarding one or more features of the intervention, including method of delivery, format, or frequency (Dixon, 1984; Lewis, 1987; Rees, 1993, 1995; Stephens, 1992; Troesch et al., 1993).

Frequency of Practice

Individual participant practice of guided imagery following delivery of the intervention was reported in 17, or 45%, of the studies which reported significant differences and in four of the six studies which found no effect for the guided imagery intervention. In several studies, subjects were asked to practice the intervention at home, and in some cases were asked to log frequency of home practice. However, in most cases, the data were not systematically collected during the study or, if collected, were not included in analyses.

There were wide variations in frequency of practice in the seven studies that reported this data. It was reported that subjects practiced the intervention an average of seven times a day (Jarvinien & Gold, 1981); 5.46 (*SD* 1.92) times per week (Collins & Rice, 1997); 6.55 (*SD* 0.52) times per week (Crowther, 1983); 4.7 times per week (range 0–9 times) (Tsai & Crockett, 1993); 6 to 8 times per week (Dixon, 1984); approximately 29 times over 5 weeks (Henry & Sanacore, 1987); or 36.5 times (*SD* 15.89) over 6 weeks (Eller, 1995).

Only four studies examined relationships between frequency of practice and study outcomes. In two separate studies, researchers reported lack of significant correlations between frequency of practice and observed reductions in blood pressure (Crowther, 1983; Henry & Sanacore, 1987). Similarly, Jarvinien and Gold (1981) reported no relationship between frequency of practice and depression scores. In a study of the aversiveness of chemotherapy in cancer patients, Lyles et al. (1982) reported that subjects failed to keep accurate records of their home practice, and further stated that frequency of practice was not related to study outcomes. They did not explain this conclusion in view of their comment regarding inaccuracy in record keeping.

Several investigators suggest that skill in techniques is acquired with practice (Benson, 1975; Sims, 1987; Smith, 1990). For example, Collins and Rice (1997) reported significant reductions in subject reported tension levels pre- and post-practice across the 6 weeks of their study. However, it has not been established that reduction in tension is an appropriate indicator of skill acquisition in the use of guided imagery. In addition, frequency of practice alone may be necessary, but not sufficient, for development of skill in the use of guided imagery. Additional research is needed to identify indicators of skill development in the use of guided imagery, optimum frequency of practice, and the role of skill development in determining effectiveness of the intervention.

Individual Characteristics

It has been suggested that the effectiveness of guided imagery interventions is affected by several individual characteristics. These include expectancy of treatment effect, vividness or clarity of imagery, and hypnotizability. Although there has been much debate as to the importance of these individual factors, only eight intervention studies systematically explored them. Three studies (Crowther, 1983; Propst, 1980; Turner & Jensen, 1993) explored expectancy. In two studies, expectancy of treatment effect was used at pretreatment to assess equivalence of groups. However, the effects of expectancy were not included in posttreatment analyses. Only Propst (1980) included pretreatment expectancy of success of treatment in analyses and reported that expectancy was not significantly related to outcome measures.

In the two studies that measured hypnotizability, differing findings were reported. Andrews and Hall (1990) observed that hypnotizability of study participants was not significantly related to improvement in persons with recurrent apthous ulcers. However, Rapkin et al. (1991) found that hypnotizability was negatively correlated with anxiety scores as well as postsurgical complications and blood loss during surgery.

Image vividness or clarity is another factor that has been suggested to influence the outcomes of guided imagery interventions. Gold et al. (1982) reported that image clarity was significantly related to observed reductions in depression. Wynd (1992) reported that practice increased subjects' ability to image and that effective imagery reduced smoking recidivism in ex-smokers. Conversely, vividness of imagery was not related to effects of guided imagery on pain, distress, and coping in postoperative patients (Manyande et al., 1995). Some individuals are auditory while others are visual processors, with individual differences in ability to generate visual or auditory images (Kunzendorf,

1981). Therefore, visual vividness or clarity may not be relevant to the effects of guided imagery for all individuals.

Differing findings in these few studies may be at least partially related to the use of various measures for expectancy, vividness or clarity, and hypnotizability. There is insufficient evidence to support the premise that specific individual factors are related to the effectiveness of guided imagery interventions. Additional research, with methodological consistency, is needed to prove or disprove the role of these factors in the application of guided imagery for psychological and physiological symptom management.

Despite the lack of consistency in methods of research using cognitive interventions, the nursing literature is replete with theoretical papers encouraging the application of these strategies in clinical practice (Achterberg, 1982; Donovan, 1980; Dossey, 1995; Stephens, 1993). As long ago as 1977, Armstrong encouraged nurses to apply techniques utilizing altered states of consciousness to effect physiologic and behavioral change in their patients. The use of imagery in particular has been encouraged by several authors. Achterberg and Lawlis (1982) espoused the use of active receptive imagery to provide patients with insight into their illness, and active process imagery to alter the patient's perceptions and improve response. In addition, they encouraged the use of relaxation followed by imagery as mental rehearsal to reduce stress and anxiety. Vines (1988) discussed the potential for the use of guided imagery in nursing for behavior change, improved surgical outcomes, increased rest, easier childbirth, potentiation of medication effects, and faster healing. Houldin, McCorkle, and Lowrey (1993) and Birney (1991) described the research from other disciplines supporting the effect of psychological state on immune function. Despite the encouragement for cognitive techniques in nursing practice, the application of these techniques can only be based on empirical evidence of their effects. In addition, as this evidence is gathered through research, intervention protocols must be more clearly described and systematically executed to insure consistency in their application (Egan, Snyder, & Burns, 1992).

Comparability of outcomes across studies of guided imagery is difficult due to variations in sample populations, protocols, outcome variables, and instruments. There is a need for replication of studies; however, protocols were not reported in sufficient detail to permit adequate replication. Despite flaws in methodology, there is preliminary evidence for the effectiveness of guided imagery, particularly for the management of stress, anxiety and depression, and the reduction of blood pressure, pain, and the side effects of chemotherapy.

Increasing consumer interest in and use of complementary therapies, the current cost-driven health care system, and the need for evidence-based practice all support the need for research in the development and delivery of guided imagery interventions. Randomized controlled clinical studies with separation of interventions and clarification of protocols with specification of imagery language are needed. Rigor in the execution of interventions should be assessed thorough the inclusion of process evaluations during the course of the intervention. Consistency in the use of sensitive, reliable, valid outcome measures is also necessary. Once the methodology is clarified, well-designed studies that compare methods of delivery of interventions, variations in methods of instruction, frequency of delivery of the intervention, frequency of practice, and relevant personality variables are needed. Optimum dose and duration of interventions are unknown, as are those physical and psychological symptoms most amenable to treatment with guided imagery. These questions remain to be explored.

REFERENCES

Abraham, I. L., Neundorfer, M. M., & Currie, L. J. (1992). The effects of cognitive group interventions on cognitive functioning and depressive symptomatology among nursing home residents. *Nursing Research, 41*, 196–202.

Achterberg, J. (1985). *Imagery in healing*. Boston: New Science Library.

Achterberg, J., Kenner, C., & Lawlis, G. F. (1988). Severe burn injury: A comparison of relaxation, imagery and biofeedback for pain management. *Journal of Mental Imagery, 12*(1), 71–88.

Achterberg, J., & Lawlis, F. (1982). Imagery and health intervention. *Topics in Clinical Nursing, 3*(4), 55–60.

Agency for Health Care Policy and Research (AHCPR). (1992). *Acute pain management: Operative or medical procedures and trauma* (AHCPR Publication No. 92-0032). Rockville, MD: Author.

Agency for Health Care Policy and Research (AHCPR). (1994). *Management of cancer pain* (AHCPR Publication No. 94-0592). Rockville, MD: Author.

Andrews, V. H., & Hall, H. R. (1990). The effects of relaxation/imagery training on recurrent apthous stomatitis: A preliminary study. *Psychosomatic Medicine, 52*, 526–535.

Arathuzik, D. (1994). Effects of cognitive-behavioral strategies on pain in cancer patients. *Cancer Nursing, 17*(3), 207–214.

Armstrong, M. E. (1977). Use of altered states of awareness in nursing practice. *AORN Journal, 25*(1), 49–53.

Baider, L., Uziely, B., & De Nour, A. K. (1994). Progressive muscle relaxation and guided imagery in cancer patients. *General Hospital Psychiatry, 16*, 340–347.

Benson, H. (1975). *The relaxation response*. New York: William Morrow.

Benson, H., Beary, J., & Carol, M. (1974). The relaxation response. *Psychiatry, 37*, 37–46.

Birney, M. H. (1991). Psychoneuroimmunology: A holistic framework for the study of stress and illness. *Holistic Nursing Practice, 5*(4), 32–38.

Bloom, F. E. (1981). Neuropeptides. *Scientific American, 245*(4), 148–168.

Borkovec, T. D., & Sides, J. K. (1979). Critical procedural variables related to the physiological effects of progressive relaxation: A review. *Behavior Research and Therapy, 17,* 119–125.

Bridge, L. R., Benson, P., Pietroni, P. C., & Priest, R. G. (1988). Relaxation and imagery in the treatment of breast cancer. *British Medical Journal, 297,* 1169–1172.

Burish, T. G., Carey, M. P., Krozely, M. G., & Greco, A. (1987). Conditioned side-effects induced by cancer chemotherapy: Prevention through behavioral treatment. *Journal of Consulting and Clinical Psychology, 55*(1), 42–48.

Burish, T. G., & Lyles, J. N. (1981). Effectiveness of relaxation training in reducing the adverse reactions to cancer chemotherapy. *Journal of Behavioral Medicine, 4,* 65–78.

Carey, M. P., & Burish, T. G. (1987). Providing relaxation training to cancer chemotherapy patients: A comparison of three delivery techniques. *Journal of Consulting and Clinical Psychology, 55*(5), 732–737.

Cautela, J. R. (1977). Covert conditioning: Assumptions and procedures. *Journal of Mental Imagery, 1,* 53–65.

Collins, J. A., & Rice, V. H. (1997). Effects of relaxation intervention in phase II cardiac rehabilitation: Replication and extension. *Heart and Lung, 26*(1), 31–44.

Crowther, J. H. (1983). Stress management training and relaxation imagery in the treatment of essential hypertension. *Journal of Behavioral Medicine, 6*(2), 169–187.

Daake, D. R., & Gueldner, S. H. (1989). Imagery instruction in the control of postsurgical pain. *Applied Nursing Research, 2*(3), 114–120.

Dixon, J. (1984). Effect of nursing interventions on nutritional and performance status in cancer patients. *Nursing Research, 33*(6), 330–335.

Donovan, M. I. (1980). Relaxation with guided imagery: A useful technique. *Cancer Nursing, 3*(1), 127–132.

Dossey. B. (1995). Using imagery to help your patient heal. *American Journal of Nursing, 95,* 41–47.

Egan, E. C., Snyder, M., & Burns, K. R. (1992). Intervention studies in nursing: Is the effect due to the independent variable? *Nursing Outlook, 40*(4), 187–190.

Eller, L. S. (1995). Effects of two cognitive-behavioral interventions on immunity and symptoms in persons with HIV. *Annals of Behavioral Medicine, 17*(4), 339–347.

Farah, M. (1984). The neurological basis of mental imagery: A componential analysis. *Cognition, 18,* 245–272.

Fawzy, F. I., & Fawzy, N. W. (1994). A structured psychoeducational intervention for cancer patients. *General Hospital Psychiatry, 16,* 149–192.

Fernandez, E., & Turk, D. C. (1989). The utility of cognitive coping strategies for altering pain perception: A meta-analysis. *Pain, 38,* 123–135.

Fishman, B., & Loscalzo, M. (1987). Cognitive-behavioral interventions in management of cancer pain: Principles and application. *Medical Clinics of North America, 71*(2), 271–287.

Gold, S. R., Jarvinien, P. J., & Teague, R. G. (1982). Imagery elaboration and clarity in modifying college students' depression. *Journal of Clinical Psychology, 38*(2), 312–314.

Green, M. L., Green, R. G., & Santoro, W. (1988). Daily relaxation modifies serum and salivary immunoglobulins and psychophysiologic symptom severity. *Biofeedback and Self-regulation, 13*(3), 187–199.

Henry, P. E., & Sanacore, K. A. (1987). Relaxation methods in the control of essential hypertension. *Journal of the New York State Nurses Association, 18*(2), 19–32.

Herr, K. A., & Mobily, P. R. (1992). Interventions related to pain. *Nursing Clinics of North America, 27*(2), 347–369.

Holden-Lund, C. (1988). Effects of relaxation with guided imagery on surgical stress and wound healing. *Research in Nursing and Health, 11*(4), 235–244.

Houldin, A. D., McCorkle, R., & Lowrey, B. J. (1993). Relaxation training and psychoimmunological status of bereaved spouses. *Cancer Nursing, 16*(1), 47–52.

Ilacqua, G. E. (1994). Migraine headaches: Coping efficacy of guided imagery training. *Headache*, 99–102.

Jarvinien, P. J., & Gold, S. R. (1981). Imagery as an aid in reducing depression. *Journal of Clinical Psychology, 37*(3), 523–529.

Kaluza, G., & Stremple, I. (1995). Training and relaxation and visual imagery with patients who have open-angle glaucoma. *International Journal of Rehabilitation and Health, 1*(4), 261–273.

Kiecolt-Glaser, J. K., Glaser, R., Willinger, D., Stout, J., Messick, G., Sheppard, S., Ricker, D., Romisher, S. C., Briner, W., Bonnell, G., & Donnerberg, R. (1985). Psychosocial enhancement of immunocompetence in a geriatric population. *Health Psychology, 4*(1), 25–41.

King, J. V. (1988). A holistic technique to lower anxiety: Relaxation with guided imagery. *Journal of Holistic Nursing, 6*(1), 16–20.

Klinger, E. (1980). Therapy and the flow of thought. In J. E. Shorr, G. E. Sobel, P. Robin, & J. A. Connella (Eds.), *Imagery* (pp. 3–20). New York: McGraw-Hill.

Korn, E. R., & Johnson, K. (1983). *Visualization: The uses of imagery in the health professions.* Homewood, IL: Dow Jones Irwin.

Kunzendorf, R. G. (1981). Individual differences in imagery and autonomic control. *Journal of Mental Imagery, 5*, 47–60.

Lang, P. J. (1977). Imagery in therapy: An information processing analysis of fear. *Behavior Therapy, 8*, 862–886.

Lang, P. J. (1979). A bio-informational theory of emotional imagery. *Psychophysiology, 16*(6), 495–512.

Lang, P. J., Kozak, M. J., Miller, G. A., Levin, D. N., & McLean, A. (1980). Emotional imagery: Conceptual structure and pattern of somato-visceral response. *Psychophysiology, 17*(2), 179–192.

Leja, A. M. (1989). Using guided imagery to combat postsurgical depression. *Journal of Gerontological Nursing, 15*(4), 7–11.

Leuner, H. (1977). Guided affective imagery: An account of its development. *Journal of Mental Imagery, 1*(1), 73–91.

Lewis, H. (1987). An investigation into the effects of imagery compared with biofeedback in the management of stress in nurses. *Curatonis: South African Journal of Nursing, 10*(4), 11–12.

Lichstein, K. L., & Lipshitz, E. (1982). Psychophysiological effects of noxious imagery: Prevalence and prediction. *Behavioral Research and Therapy, 20,* 339–345.

Lyles, J. N., Burish, T. G., Krozely, M. G., & Oldham, R. K. (1982). Efficacy of relaxation training and guided imagery in reducing the aversiveness of cancer chemotherapy. *Journal of Consulting and Clinical Psychology, 50*(4), 509–524.

Maguire, B. I. (1996). The effects of imagery on attitudes and moods in multiple sclerosis patients. *Alternative Therapies in Health and Medicine, 2*(5), 75–79.

Maltz, M. (1966). *Psychocybernetics.* New York: Pocket.

Manyande, A., Berg, S., Gettins, D., Stanford, S. C., Mazhero, S., Marks, D. F., & Salmon, P. (1995). Preoperative rehearsal of active coping imagery influences subjective and hormonal responses to abdominal surgery. *Psychosomatic Medicine, 57,* 177–182.

Mast, D., Meyers, J., & Urbanski, A. (1987). Relaxation techniques: A self-learning module for nurses. *Cancer Nursing, 10*(4), 217–225.

Meichenbaum, D. (1978). Why does using imagery in psychotherapy lead to change? In J. L. Singer & K. S. Pope (Eds.), *The power of human imagination* (pp. 381–394). New York: Plenum.

Melzack, R., & Wall, P. D. (1965). Pain mechanisms: A new theory. *Science, 150,* 971–979.

Moody, L. M., Fraser, M., & Yarandi, H. (1993). Effects of guided imagery in patients with chronic bronchitis and emphysema. *Clinical Nursing Research, 2*(4), 478–486.

Moye, L. A., Richardson, M. A., Post-White, J., & Justice, B. (1995). Research methodology in psychoneuroimmunology: Rationale and design of the IMAGES-P clinical trial. *Alternative Therapies, 1*(2), 34–39.

Naparstek, B. (1994). *Staying well with guided imagery.* New York: Warner.

Pert, C. (1985). Neuropeptides and their receptors: A psychosomatic network. *Journal of Immunology, 135*(2 Suppl), 820S–826S.

Pickett, C., & Clum, G. A. (1982). Comparative treatment strategies and their interaction with locus of control in the reduction of postsurgical pain and anxiety. *Journal of Consulting and Clinical Psychology, 50*(3), 439–441.

Propst, L. R. (1980). The comparative efficacy of religious and nonreligious imagery for the treatment of mild depression in religious individuals. *Cognitive Therapy and Research, 4*(2), 167–178.

Rapkin, D. A., Straubing, M., & Holroyd, J. C. (1991). Guided imagery, hypnosis and recovery from head and neck cancer surgery: An exploratory study. *The International Journal of Clinical and Experimental Hypnosis, 39*(4), 215–226.

Redd, W. H., Rosenberger, P. H., & Hendler, C. S. (1982). Controlling chemotherapy side effects. *American Journal of Clinical Hypnosis, 25,* 161–172.

Rees, B. L. (1993). An exploratory study of the effectiveness of a relaxation with guided imagery protocol. *Journal of Holistic Nursing, 11*(3), 271–276.

Rees, B. L. (1995). Effect of relaxation with guided imagery on anxiety, depression and self-esteem in primiparas. *Journal of Holistic Nursing, 13*(3), 255–267.

Schandler, S. L., & Dana, E. R. (1983). Cognitive imagery and physiological feedback relaxation protocols applied to clinically tense young adults: A comparison on state, trait and physiological effects. *Journal of Clinical Psychology, 39*(5), 672–681.

Siegel, B. (1986). *Love, medicine and miracles.* New York: Harper & Row.

Simonton, O. C., Mathews-Simonton, S., & Creighton, J. (1978). *Getting well again.* New York: Bantam Books.

Sims, E. R. (1987). Relaxation training as a technique for helping patients cope with the experience of cancer: A selective review of the literature. *Journal of Advanced Nursing, 12*, 583–591.

Singer, J. L. (1974). *Imagery and daydream methods in psychotherapy and behavior modification.* New York: Academic Press.

Sloman, R., Brown, P., Aldana, E., & Chee, E. (1994). The use of relaxation for the promotion of comfort and pain relief in persons with advanced cancer. *Contemporary Nurse, 3*(1), 6–12.

Smith, J. C. (1990). *Cognitive-behavioral relaxation training.* New York: Springer.

Sodergren, K. M. (1992). Guided imagery. In M. Snyder (Ed.), *Independent nursing interventions* (pp. 103–124). New York: Wiley.

Stephens, R. L. (1992). Imagery: A treatment for nursing student anxiety. *Journal of Nursing Education, 31*(7), 314–320.

Stephens, R. L. (1993). Imagery: A strategic intervention to empower clients: Part II. A practical guide. *Clinical Nurse Specialist, 7*(5), 235–240.

Syrjala, K. L., Donaldson, G. W., Davis, M. W., Kippes, M. E., & Carr, J. E. (1995). Relaxation and imagery and cognitive-behavioral training to reduce pain during cancer treatment: A controlled clinical trial. *Pain, 63*(2), 189–198.

Tan, S. Y. (1982). Cognitive and cognitive-behavioral methods for pain control: A selective review. *Pain, 12*, 201–228.

Taylor, C. B., Farquhar, J. W., Nelson, E., & Agras, S. (1977). Relaxation therapy and high blood pressure. *Archives of General Psychiatry, 34*, 339–342.

Thompson, M. B., & Coppens, N. M. (1994). The effects of guided imagery on anxiety levels and movement of clients undergoing magnetic resonance imaging. *Holistic Nursing Practice, 8*(2), 59–69.

Troesch, L. M., Rodehaver, C. B., Delaney, E. A., & Yanes, B. (1993). The influence of guided imagery on chemotherapy-related nausea and vomiting. *Oncology Nursing Forum, 20*, 1179–1185.

Tsai, S. L., & Crockett, M. S. (1993). Effects of relaxation training combining imagery and meditation on the stress level of Chinese nurses working in modern hospitals in Taiwan. *Issues in Mental Health Nursing, 14*, 51–66.

Turk, D. C., & Meichenbaum, D. H. (1989). A cognitive-behavioral approach to pain management. In P. D. Wall & R. Melzack (Eds.), *Textbook of pain* (pp. 1001–1009). New York: Churchill Livingstone.

Turkoski, B., & Lance, B. (1996). The use of guided imagery with anticipatory grief. *Home Healthcare Nurse, 14*(199), 878–888.

Turner, J. A., & Jensen, M. P. (1993). Efficacy of cognitive therapy for chronic low back pain. *Pain, 52,* 169–177.

Vasterling, J., Jenkins, R. A., Tope, D. M., & Burish, T. G. (1993). Cognitive distraction and relaxation training for the control of side effects due to cancer chemotherapy. *Journal of Behavioral Medicine, 16*(1), 65–80.

Vines, S. W. (1988). The therapeutics of guided imagery. *Holistic Nursing Practice,* 2(3), 34–44.

Wack, J. T., & Turk, D. C. (1984). Latent structure of strategies used to cope with nociceptive stimulation. *Health Psychology, 3*(1), 27–43.

Wells, N. (1989). Management of pain during abortion. *Journal of Advanced Nursing, 14,* 56–62.

Wynd, C. A. (1992). Relaxation imagery used for stress reduction in the prevention of smoking relapse. *Journal of Advanced Nursing, 17,* 294–302.

Zahourek, R. P. (1988). Imagery. In R. P. Zahourek (Ed.), *Relaxation and imagery: Tools for therapeutic communication and intervention* (pp. 3–27). Philadelphia: W. B. Saunders.

Chapter 4

Patient-Centered Communication

SARAH JO BROWN

Abstract

The term patient-centered communication (PCC) has been used to describe a group of communication strategies and behaviors that promote mutuality, shared understandings, and shared decision making in health care encounters. There is evidence to suggest that advanced practice nurse and patients use these strategies to co-produce highly individualized clinical discourse. Although the communication behaviors associated with PCC have been studied separately, their impact as an integrated communications strategy has not been studied. Suggestions for developing PCC as a mid-range theory of health care communication encompassing other more specific communication concepts are offered.

Keywords: Patient-Centered Communication, Patient-Centredness, Health Care Discourse

Nurses have always been person-centered; they have considered patients' preferences, backgrounds, and the contexts of their lives while managing health problems. However, advanced practice nurses (APNs) assume expanded responsibilities for diagnosing, monitoring, and treating disease and illness states. The additional responsibilities can make it difficult for APNs to pay attention to the full meaning of what the patient is saying and think clearly about the processes underlying the problems the patient presents. Focusing on the meanings of what a patient is saying and responding in supportive ways to subtle messages are demanding tasks in and of themselves, as is the task of sorting through the content of what is being said for information that will enable one to determine the underlying nature of the person's problems and to recommend treatment. This dual set of goals is shared by patients who want to be respected as unique persons, yet also receive substantive assistance with their health problems. It is not clear how patients and providers strategically conduct themselves to achieve both goals within the context of their health care relationship.

Over the years providers have been admonished to be patient-centered in the way they talk with patients. When the concept was first introduced, the goal of patient-centered communication was to understand the patient's experiences from his or her point of view (Mathews, 1962; Stewart, 1984); however, the usage of the term has undergone change over the 35 years since the term was first introduced into the health care literature. Toward the objective of summarizing the state of knowledge regarding patient-centered communication (PCC), a review of the health care communication research follows. Special attention has been given to associations between the components of PCC and patient outcomes, and to the ways in which patient-centered communication is brought into relationship with clinical problem solving by advanced practice nurses. The terms "patient-centered communication" and "person-centered communication" will be used interchangeably in this paper, since they are interchanged throughout the clinical literature on the topic; the abbreviation PCC can be read as either.

ORIGINS OF THE TERM

Most likely, the term patient-centered communication was a derivation from Carl Rogers' term "client-centered therapy," which he used in his 1951 book to describe a non-directive approach to counseling (Rogers, 1951). Client-centered therapy was aimed at understanding the client as the client seems to himself. The counselor's deep understanding and acceptance of the patient were viewed as leading to the client seeing himself objectively and eventually to an integrated acceptance of self (Rogers, 1951).

In 1962 a nurse-researcher first used the term "patient-centeredness" in the nursing literature to describe communication in which the nurse "makes interpersonal responses that encourage the patient to disclose how he sees his world, what he is experiencing, and the meanings the experiences have for his daily life and for his feeling about himself" (Mathews, 1962, p. 155). The term "patient-centred [*sic*] medicine" was introduced into the medical literature in 1970 by Balint, Hunt, and Joyce, who contrasted it with "illness-centred medicine." Interestingly, a similar term, "person-centered speech" was used in the British speech communication literature in the early 1970s to describe a sociolinguistic mode of speaking that creates social solidarity between speakers with different social backgrounds (Applegate & Delia, 1980). It is not clear whether this term was derived from the health care literature or had an independent origin.

EVOLVING DEFINITION

In the early research on PCC, the operational definitions used consisted of discrete speech actions that encourage patients to disclose how they see their worlds and to express concerns, thoughts, and feelings (Byrne & Long, 1976; Kasch & Lisnek, 1984; Mathews, 1962; Stewart, 1984; Wallston, Cohen, Smith, & DeVellis, 1978). Speech actions that were viewed as serving this end included open-ended questions, prompts acknowledging that the provider is attentive and wants to hear more, and acknowledgment of nonverbal, emotional cues.

Over time, PCC came to viewed more broadly as communication strategies that take place across the discourse, rather at the level of the isolated statement. Foremost among these strategies is centering clinical discourse around the patient's story instead of around the clinical reasoning of the provider as traditionally had been done (Mishler, 1984; Smith, 1996). This view of PCC precludes reframing the patient's story into clinical language and sequence; instead, it requires leaving the patient's story intact as a personal account located in the patient's time and place. When the provider asks questions, they should relate to the chronology and meanings of what the patient has previously said—much like the flow by which a person in a social conversation acknowledges what the other person has just said, but goes on to ask for more details, or for clarification to understand it better (Shuy, 1983). The goal of the clinical encounter is to reach shared understandings of both the clinical and personal aspects of the patient's problems. To achieve shared understandings, the patient helps the provider see the personal meanings and implications of what he is experiencing, while the provider helps the patient see the technical (i.e., bioscientific) meanings of those experiences (Marshall, 1988; Tuckett, Boulton, Olson, & Williams, 1986). Perhaps, PCC is best now called an orientation to provider-patient discourse by which patient and provider co-produce mutual understandings and decisions (Tresolini and the Pew-Fetzer Task Force, 1994). The orientation inspires communication behaviors that give life to the orientation.

The following list of provider communication behaviors and strategies are those most frequently associated with the PCC orientation; studies describing each behavioral element are in parentheses.

- Allowing patients to give their accounts in their own language and chronology (Cecil & Killeen, 1997; Joos, Hickam, Gordon, & Baker, 1996; Kristjanson & Chalmers, 1990; Law & Britten, 1995; Mishler, 1984; Rowland-Morin & Carroll, 1990)
- A conversational style of interviewing (Brown, 1994; Hall, Roter, & Katz, 1987; Marshall, 1988; Morten, Kohl, O'Mahoney, & Pelosi, 1991)
- Eliciting patients' thoughts, perspectives, expectations, values, and goals (Henbest & Stewart, 1990; Mishler, Clark, Ingelfinger, & Simon, 1989; Roter & Hall, 1987; Stewart, 1984)
- Asking about the context of patients' lives (Bertakis, Roter, & Putnam, 1991; Brown, 1994; Price, 1989; Woolliscroft et al., 1989)
- Responding to patients' indirect and nonverbal clues regarding emotions and problems (Brykcznski, 1989; Kaplan, Greenfield, & Ware, 1989; Suchman, Markakis, Beckman, & Frankel, 1997)
- Providing patients with information for self-care and participation in health care decisions (Blanchard, Ruckdeschel, Fletcher, & Blanchard, 1986; Brykcznski, 1989; Daley, 1993; Johnson, 1993; Morten et al., 1991; Robbins et al., 1993; Rost, Carter, & Inui, 1989)
- Creating shared understandings with patients (Arborelius & Bremberg, 1992; Kristjanson & Chalmers, 1990)
- Collaboratively developing health care plans with patients (Allshouse, 1993; Johnson, 1993; Kaplan et al., 1989; Thom & Campbell, 1997)
- Expressing concern for the patient's well-being (Brown, 1994; Morten et al., 1991; Thom & Campbell, 1997)
- Creating social connectedness with patients by humor, touch, and modest personal sharing (Brown, 1994; Morten et al., 1991)

THE SAMPLE OF STUDIES

Even though there is clinical essay literature regarding PCC, particularly in the family medicine literature, searches of CINAHL, Medline, and LLBA from 1984 to 1997 using the term "patient-centered communication" produced no empirical studies. However, using the term "patient-centredness" (the British spelling) located five empirical studies (Henbest & Fehrsen, 1992; Henbest & Stewart, 1989, 1990; Law & Britten, 1995, Stewart, 1984). Two additional studies were found in which the learning of the trait of patient-centredness by student nurses was examined (French, 1994; Rolfe, 1994). In these empirical studies, patient-centeredness was conceptualized as the provider responding to the patient in ways that allow the patient to express all of the reasons for coming to a health care visit, including symptoms, thoughts, feelings, and expectations. This usage is consistent with the way in which the term was originally used, but does not comprehensively reflect its contemporary, North American usage (Gerteis, Edgman-Levitan, Daley, & Delbanco, 1993; Putnam & Lipkin, 1995; Smith, 1996).

Although PCC is defined as a multifaceted approach to communication in the essay literature, it has not been empirically studied as such. Instead, the communication behaviors that comprise PCC have been studied separately. In the reports of some of these studies of a particular communication behavior, the researcher invoked PCC as an explanatory framework for the behavior or set of behaviors. As a result, this review consists of health care communication studies with connections to PCC, rather than studies about PCC per se. The starting points were studies in which the behaviors studied were associated with PCC in either the introduction or conclusion section of the report; others studies addressing those behaviors were also included. Other communication behaviors became associated with PCC in the essay literature; for example, Kasch and Lisnek (1984) suggested several specific behaviors by which nurses strategically enact person-centered speech. Finally, five descriptive studies of advanced practice nurse communication were included, because their overall descriptions reveal that APNs do focus on the patient as a person as well as on disease and illness management and encourage patients to be co-producers of clinical discourse and decisions (Brown, 1994; Brykczynski, 1989; Johnson, 1993; Morten et al., 1991; Taylor, Pickens, & Geden, 1989). In summary, the studies included in this review are those that examined a behavior that has been conceptually associated with PCC or a set of behaviors that as an aggregate have been characterized by a researcher as "patient-centered."

The majority of studies in this review are of patient-physician communication, a distribution that reflects the makeup of health care communication research claiming a PCC framework. In recent years, social scientists and physician-researchers have studied patient-physician communication extensively, but nurse-patient communication has not received much attention from social scientists, nor has it received much attention from nurse-researchers. The unfortunate consequences of the under-representation of patient-nurse communication is that we do not know as much about patient-nurse communication as we do about patient-physician communication, and there are reasons to suspect that nurses, particularly advanced practice nurses, are highly patient-centered in their communication. In contrast, studies of physicians indicate that they have difficulty balancing patient-centeredness with a clinical task focus (Hall et al., 1987; Mishler, 1984), although a recent study of 50 family practice residents showed that many were willing to let patients take control of conversations (Cecil & Killeen, 1997). There are no studies reporting the prevalence of person-centered communication vis-a-vis problem-focused communication in either nursing or medicine.

RESEARCH METHODS OF THE STUDIES

The behavioral elements of PCC have been studied using interactional analysis systems, rating scales, interpretive methods, content analysis, and the constant comparison technique of analysis from grounded theory. The interactional analysis systems used content categories and/or speech act categories to count and profile what occurred (Bertakis et al., 1991; Cecil & Killeen, 1997; Hall et al., 1987; Morten et al., 1991; Roter & Hall, 1987; Stewart, 1984). Rating scales have been used mainly to characterize the informativeness (Street, 1991), and the emotional tone of entire interviews (Hall et al., 1987; Street & Wiemann, 1987). The interpretive methods, also referred to as discourse analysis, involve a variety of methods from sociolinguistics, sociology, and speech communications. Generally, these methods (e.g., discourse analysis, conversational analysis) involve detailed examination of the meanings of exchanges between the patient and the provider to understand how the participants attempt to accomplish their goals, how the participants work together to produce shared understanding, or how they are constrained in their communication (Brown, 1994; Johnson, 1993; Marshall, 1988; Mishler, 1984; Shuy, 1983). Constant comparison has been used to identify patterns in certain kinds of communication exchanges (Suchman et al., 1997) and to characterize the clinical discourse being analyzed (Morten et al., 1991; Thom & Campbell, 1997).

The methods of studying communication have moved from early interactional analysis systems and rating scales to interpretive methods that capture meaning, context, conversational cooperation, interpersonal assertiveness, and control. This shift from studying discrete speech actions to examining the emergent coherence and overall structure of clinical discourse has produced a much richer portrayal of how skilled providers co-produce understandings with patients. Although many instruments have been created to evaluate medical interviewing skills (Kraan, Crijnen, van der Vleuten, & Imbos, 1995; Ong, deHaes, Hoos, & Lammes, 1995), only one (Henbest & Stewart, 1989) was designed specifically to measure patient-centredness, although it is based on a definition of PCC that is not consistent with the current, broader usage of the term. Other instruments capture several but not all of the dimensions of PCC; specifically, they fail to capture whether/how conversational cooperation and mutual understandings are achieved. The complexities involved in developing an instrument that measures PCC in the multidimensional manner in which it is currently defined are immense, as there are many possible empirical indicators for each dimension. Moreover, some of the indicators of the behavioral elements involve subtle content, oblique reference to prior discussions, nonverbal behaviors, and sequences of behaviors that take on person-centered meaning across time. Thus, the development of an instrument that captures the dynamic and comprehensive nature of PCC awaits future efforts. The theoretical and empirical pieces would seem to exist, but the unifying of them to produce a reliable and valid measure of PCC will be an arduous task.

OUTCOMES

There is considerable empirical support for the effectiveness of each of the behavioral elements of PCC (Ong et al., 1995; Putnam & Lipkin, 1995; Stewart, 1995). For example, several studies have found that the "information yield" of interviews in which the provider asked open-ended questions is superior to those in which the provider asked many very specific questions (Beckman & Frankel, 1984; Marshall, 1988; Roter & Hall, 1987). It follows then that comprehensive person-centered interviewing has the potential to produce more accurate diagnoses and more relevant plans of care. Other associations between provider behaviors and outcomes are displayed in Table 4.1. In a review of 21 randomized controlled trials of physician-patient communication in which patient health was an outcome variable, effective communication was found to be associated with improved patient health outcomes (Stewart, 1995).

Establishing causal linkage between PCC and patient outcomes will be limited until a valid and reliable measure of PCC has been developed, because confidence about the association between provider action and patient outcomes is built by conducting studies with large sample sizes that establish associations across a large number of cases. Although discourse analysis has contributed major understandings regarding how PCC is enacted, it will be of limited use in establishing the linkage to patient outcomes because its labor-intensive methods (sometimes referred to as micro-analysis), severely constrain the sample size of studies employing it.

STRATEGIES FOR ACHIEVING A DUAL FOCUS

Although there is a sizeable body of studies examining the specific speech actions involved in producing person-centered communication, no studies directly examine how person-centered communication, either in its original limited sense or as an orientation to clinical discourse, affects the accuracy of provider's diagnostic and therapeutic reasoning, and vice versa. Consequently, to theorize about how person-centered communication and problem-centered communication are brought together in clinical discourse, the clinical

TABLE 4.1   PCC Behaviors and Research-Supported Outcomes

PCC Behaviors	Associated Outcomes (and supporting studies)
1. Patient-centeredness (enables patients to express)	1. Increased patient compliance, feeling of being understood, resolution of patients' concerns (Henbest & Stewart, 1990; Henbest & Fehrsen, 1992; Stewart, 1984)
2. Asks open-ended questions	2. Greater information yield (Beckman & Frankel, 1984; Marshall, 1988; Roter & Hall, 1987; Stewart, 1984; Woolliscroft et al., 1989)
3. Exerts less conversational control	3a. Increase in patient compliance & satisfaction (Cecil & Killeen, 1997)
	3b. Better physiological outcomes (Kaplan et al., 1989)
4. Encourages patient to be more active in conversation and decisions	4a. Higher overall health rating—functional & subjective (Kaplan et al., 1989)
	4b. Commitment to treatment (Tuckett et al., 1986)
5. Facilitates bidirectional information flow and shared understandings	5a. Increased patient follow-through with recommendations (Joos, Hickam, Gordon, & Baker, 1996; Rost, Carter, & Inui, 1989)
	5b. More accurate and complete information (Marshall, 1988)
6. Is informative/provides health information	6. Increased satisfaction with care (Robbins et al., 1993; Street, 1991)
7. Allows or encourages talk about psychosocial issues	7. Increased patient satisfaction (Bertakis et al., 1991)
8. Instructs, uses humor, & asks for opinion or view	8. Predicts the malpractice claim status of primary care physicians and surgeons (Levinson, Roter, Mullooly, Dull, & Frankel, 1997)
9. Provider expression of caring, warmth, interest, respect	9a. Increased trust (Thom & Campbell, 1997)
	9b. Increased satisfaction (Hall & Dornan, 1988; Hauck, Zyzanski, Alemagno, & Medalie, 1990)

essay literature and the research literature must be pieced together. Three strategies for combining person-centered communication with clinical problem solving are supported by research findings: a phased approach, an integrated approach, and an opportunities approach.

A Phased Strategy of PCC

The first strategy, which is prominent in the medical essay literature, recognizes two phases of the PCC interview (Levenstein, McCracken, McWhinney, Stewart, & Brown, 1986; Smith, 1996). In the initial patient-centered phase, the patient takes the lead and presents his problems. This is followed by a provider-centered phase, in which the provider takes the lead to further define the symptoms the patient described and to obtain information needed to rule out and rule in the diagnostic possibilities suggested by the patient's story (Smith, 1996). Although the essay literature advocates a phased approach to addressing the two agendas, there is little research literature describing how the two phases are enacted and how transitions are made from one to another; most importantly, there is little research regarding how this phased approach affects patients' ability to give their accounts and effect their plan of care. A study of the discourse between nurse practitioners and women in a large medical clinic lends some support to the phased strategy of enacting PCC (Johnson, 1993). The researchers described the history-taking phase as a time when the personal experience of the patient was allowed and encouraged to emerge. Shared language was used, and the nurse practitioners used the history-taking to "help the patient define and problem solve the situation" (p. 150). Even though the traditional segments of the primary care visit were in place to some degree, and person-centered communication strategies were used, there was no indication that the nurse practitioners viewed the segments as patient-centered and provider-centered phases.

A Totally Integrated Strategy

The second person-centered strategy was explicated from descriptive studies of nurse practitioners (Brown, 1994; Johnson, 1993; Morten et al., 1991) and from a more demanding view of what is considered person-centered interviewing (Mishler, 1984). When this strategy is used, the patient's experiences, concerns, and ideas regarding the nature of his problem are the central feature of *all* discourse, rather than being featured in a particular phase of the discourse, and the provider's clinical reasoning takes place to a large degree in the background, or in-and-around the patient's story. The clinical reconstruction of the patient's story into clinical language and sequences takes place in the provider's head, and the traditional phase structure of the primary care interview is not imposed on the discourse. This approach does not preclude the provider's asking questions, but the frequency will be minimal, because most important clinical information will emerge as the patient gives his account.

The strategy of using person-centered discourse across the entire interview was evident in a study of a nurse practitioner and three pregnant patients (Brown, 1992, 1994). The discourse was described as having a very flexible format in that clinical issues and daily life issues were interspersed. The discourse was likened to two friends coming together in conversation wherein neither person controls the dialogue, and one thing leads to another and each shows interest in what the other is saying. Similarly, in another study of nurse practitioners and patients receiving postpartum care, the discourse was described as an "easy give-and-take" and characterized by an "interspersion of chatty conversation" (Morten et al., 1991, p. 278). One gets the sense from these two childbearing care studies that there was an emergent flow of person-centered issues and clinical management issues, but there was also a sense of coherence resulting from discussing issues at length followed by either participant making a transition to another topic (Brown, 1994). The emergent format, bilateral introduction of topics, and easy flow from one topic to another resembled social conversation more than it did the traditional medical interview, and yet in the process clinical issues were raised and addressed.

It must be recognized, however, that the clinical management required in the clinical settings of both studies (Brown, 1994; Morten et al., 1991) was fairly straightforward, and this may have allowed the social conversation format to be used. There is some indication in Brown's study that the presence of a troubling symptom lessened the use of the conversational format. Also, the patients in both studies had established relationships with the nurse practitioners, which may have contributed to the social tone that was observed. Another explanation is that since all these studies involved women providers and women patients, the format may be one with which women are particularly skilled and comfortable (Kasch, Kasch, & Lisnek, 1987).

An exemplary medical interview in another study is of interest because it involved a male provider and a male patient (Mishler et al., 1989). The physician used explicit transitions, pauses, and acknowledgments to invite the patient to continue with his account. The content of the interview was centered almost entirely on topics introduced by the patient; the physician did introduce some topics, but did so by referring back to something the patient had said earlier. Importantly, recommendations were phrased in ways that recognized the patient as a competent person who ultimately would make his own deci-sions. At the end of the interview, the physician referred back to the event or circumstances that had brought the patient to the visit, which the researchers interpreted as "relocating the patient's problems within his real world of work rather than within a medical framework of symptoms, pains and medication" (p. 333). Although the content in Mishler et al. was not quite as "chatty" as the dialogue between the women in the nursing studies, it clearly was conversational in nature, and the patient's life world experiences were the central feature of the dialogue. The three studies together constitute evidence that some providers do not impose the traditional segments of the primary care interview on the discourse, but instead enact a format that is conversational, organized around the patient's story, and person-centered across the entire interview.

An Opportunities Strategy

A third approach to making clinical interviews more person-centered is called the "Windows of Opportunities" approach (Branch & Malik, 1993). These researchers described how in four of the 20 interviews they videotaped "highly experienced practitioners" recognized patients' comments indicating that the patient wanted to talk about personal, emotional, or family issues. The expert physicians responded by providing a "brief but intense" opportunity (lasting from 1 to 7 minutes) to explore these issues. In essence, these opportunities were viewed as breakouts from physician-centered communication that allow patients to discuss concerns and psychosocial issues; thus the overall structure is built around the "health problem," but the provider remains sensitive to patients' desires to introduce psychosocial information they feel is relevant.

The actual use of such opportunities was not supported in a study of how physicians respond to patients' expressions of emotion, in that most physicians allowed the opportunities for empathy to pass without acknowledgment (Cam-pion, Butler, & Cox, 1992; Suchman et al., 1997). The studies of advanced practice nurses (Brown, 1994; Brykcznski, 1989; Morten et al., 1991) reveal that these providers are apt to take note of patients' psychosocial and emotion-laden cues, and make inquiry about them.

Other Possible Strategies

Two other possible strategies for combining person-centered communication with disease-focused communication can be theorized, even though the research literature has not documented them. They are: (a) combining person-centered discourse with disease and illness discourse to different degrees in encounters occurring over time and (b) using a patient-centered assessment framework, such as functional health status, as a guide to a comprehensive clinical conversation (Brown, 1996). The lack of research evidence related to these two strategies may be due to the fact that provider-patient communication has not been studied in encounters taking place across time, nor has APN communication been studied much since functional health patterns became more prominent in the nursing literature.

There are fragments of evidence suggesting that person-centered communication is more prevalent in dialogue between patients and providers who have had previous encounters. In a study comparing differences between new versus established clinical relationships in a family practice clinic, established patient encounters were shorter and involved more chatting and less structuring of the encounter by the physicians (Bertakis & Callahan, 1992); this description is similar to those offered by Brown (1994) and Morten et al. (1991) of encounters in which the patients and nurse practitioners also had established relationships. Over time, single encounters may be more or less patient-centered, depending on whether there are physical health problems to be addressed.

The use of functional health as an assessment format may give person-centered communication a very different look, because functional health sits conceptually between patients' experiences of daily life and clinical concepts of disease and illness. Eliciting information from a functional health perspective may make links in either direction easy to make.

FACTORS AFFECTING THE ENACTMENT OF PCC

The extent to which PCC is employed in patient-provider discourse undoubtedly depends on many factors, including the purpose of the visit, the setting, the time available, the patient's communications style, the nature of the health issue or problem, and how acquainted the provider and patient are with one another. In a study of 8300 visits to physicians' offices, the elderly, those with less education, minority patients, and male patients had the least participatory visits, as did those who saw male physicians rather than female physicians. Participatory decision-making also increased as the tenure of the patient-physician relationship increased (Kaplan, Gandek, Greenfield, Rogers, & Ware, 1995). Similar personal characteristics plus patients' communications style were found to determine information-giving by physicians, leading the researcher to conclude that patients exert considerable control over the amount of information they receive (Street, 1991). A similar pattern emerged in a qualitative study of nurse-client interactions in community health practice: the tone, pace, and depth of the process of "creating common ground" was found to depend on care context, process skills of the nurse, and willingness of the client to engage (Kristjanson & Chalmers, 1990). Further support for the importance of the patient's role in producing patient-centered communication is found in a meta-analysis of patient characteristics that are predictive of physician and patient behavior in medical visits: the patient's health status was found to have considerable influence on communication (Hall, Roter, Milburn, & Daltroy, 1996). In summary, the patient plays a major role in determining the extent to which the discourse of his visit is patient-centered; however, some of the patient's characteristics undoubtedly constrain his ability to contribute to PCC.

The origins of the interpersonal ability to create shared understandings with another person are beyond the scope of this paper, but there may be gender-related differences in communication style that affect this ability. We know that female physicians engage in more social exchange, ask for and receive more psychosocial information, and provide more encouragement and reassurance than do male physicians (Bernzweig, Takayama, Phibbs, Lewis, & Pantell, 1997; Bertakis, Helms, Callahan, Azari, & Robbins, 1995; Law & Britten, 1995; Sprague-Zones, 1995; Street, 1991). These findings must be interpreted with caution, however, as it is not clear whether these differences by themselves are sufficient to produce changes in patient adherence to recommendations, in clinical outcomes, or in health care utilization. In a related matter, there is some evidence that modest educational effort can increase providers' abilities to elicit and respond to patients' concerns (French, 1994; Joos et al., 1996; Wallston et al., 1978). Thus, it would seem that PCC can viewed either as a complement to personal communication styles and caring human responses, or as a learned professional strategy for working with patients.

PRACTICALITY OF PCC

Even though the use of open-ended questions as a way of encouraging patients to talk about their concerns has been taught in nursing schools for years, there is evidence to suggest that they are not extensively used (Webster-Stratton, Glascock, & McCarthy, 1986). The pressures of tight appointment schedules and heavy case loads may influence practitioners to avoid using open-ended questions. However, in a study of 74 office visits the 17 patients (23%) who were given an uninterrupted opportunity to present their concerns took on average only 38 seconds to do so and never took more than two and a half minutes to complete their account (Beckman & Frankel, 1984). This study was conducted prior to the current era of short appointment times; the majority of patients today are undoubtedly well aware that providers do not have a lot of time, and make efforts to tell their stories in as brief a form as possible.

CONCLUSIONS

A small part of the health care communication research that has been conducted had conceptual origins within a communications paradigm, such as symbolic interactionism; another part was conducted within the context of a more specific conceptual framework, such as confirmation or empathy; but the largest part has been descriptive and/or interpretive in nature, that is, conducted apart from any a priori communication theory. These various approaches to studying health care communication have produced a multiplicity of isolated but partially overlapping characterizations of the health care communication process (e.g., empathetic communication, personal confirmation, mutuality, affective behavior, knowing the patient, and reassurance), and the commonality and connections between these interpersonal process concepts have not been explored or tested. As result, the research findings, concepts, and specific theories pertaining to health care communications lack coherency, which ultimately impedes understanding of how various interpersonal processes work in combination with one another.

As an orientation to health care communication that recognizes multiple interpersonal processes working together in the service of mutuality, shared understandings, and joint decision making, PCC could serve as a nascent framework for the development of a normative mid-range theory of health care communications encompassing the existing collection of more specific concepts and theories. The empirical evidence in support of the various concepts and variables that currently exist in health care communications theories and research would need to be appraised and the concepts and variables clustered on the basis of their similarity. The goals and collaborative interpersonal processes of PCC could provide a framework for this clustering.

The development of PCC as a comprehensive health care communication theory will require transforming its perspective from that of a provider strategy into a normative form of discourse by which patients and providers co-produce mutual understandings and decisions, thereby recognizing that the production of PCC as a shared responsibility, not solely the responsibility of the provider. There is a body of research findings regarding how patients' expectations, goals, and communication styles affect the discourse of clinical encounters that could be brought together with the PCC orientation to create a comprehensive co-production model. To be comprehensive, a co-production theory of health care communication should address the following aspects of health care communication:

1. illness, family, organizational, societal, and cultural contexts.
2. personal styles of communication (patient and provider).
3. types and purposes of health care discourse.
4. intentions, goals, and expectations (patient and provider).
5. relationship building.
6. conversational cooperation.
7. crafting mutual understandings.
8. patient outcomes.

Although the PCC orientation as it currently exists does not completely integrate all these aspects of health care communication, it does integrate many of them. For this reason it has the potential to serve as a unifying framework.

Ultimately we need to know if PCC as a multiple-process, integrated approach to health care communication has a positive effect on patients' health outcomes. Intermediate outcomes that would be of interest include: the patient's level of comfort in disclosing personal issues and information; the amount of information brought forth; the patient's views of the utility and acceptability of provider recommendations; the patient's adherence to providers' recommendations and utilization of health care services; and the provider's diagnostic and therapeutic accuracy.

Establishing the effects of PCC on end-point health outcomes such as clinical status, functional status, morbidity, and quality of life will be more difficult. To link PCC as it has been defined in this review to health outcomes, the following research will need to be undertaken:

1. Descriptive studies examining how the behavioral dimensions of PCC are used together.
2. Longitudinal studies of how PCC is enacted over time.
3. Examination of how PCC is enacted by expert, advance practice nurses.
4. Exploration of how patients' characteristics and communication styles interact with providers communication style to affect enactment of PCC
5. Examination of whether (and how) providers adjust their communication to patients' communication styles

6. Development of an instrument for measuring the dimensions on which a provider's communication is person-centered during an encounter
7. Exploration of how PCC and clinical reasoning affect one another.
8. Studies of communication situations other than the primary care visit; for example, encounters in which decisions regarding future clinical management are made or difficult information is imparted, or encounters taking place in the home or the workplace.

In defining, describing, specifying, and measuring PCC, it is imperative that its multi-dimensional, dyadic, and contextually embedded nature be respected. Although studying the interaction of the dyad is much more complicated than restricting the focus to the behaviors of one participant, future insights regarding how meaningful care is achieved will undoubtedly require consideration of how patients and providers work together to achieve their health care objectives (Jarrett & Payne, 1995). Clearly, the investigative skills and theoretical synthesis required to extend our understanding of PCC and its contributions to humanistic health care are demanding, but its conceptual and theoretical development could provide a valuable clinical and investigative tool.

REFERENCES

Allshouse, K. D. (1993). Treating patients as individuals. In M. Gerteis, S. Edgman-Levitan, J. Daley, & T. L. Delbanco (Eds.), *Through the patient's eyes: Understanding and promoting patient-centered care* (pp. 19–44). San Francisco: Jossey-Bass.

Applegate, J. L., & Delia, J. G. (1980). Person-centered speech, psychological development, and the contexts of language usage. In R. St. Clair & H. Giles (Eds.), *The social and psychological contexts of language* (pp. 245–282). Hillsdale, NJ: Erlbaum.

Arborelius, E., & Bremberg, S. (1992). What can doctors do to achieve a successful consultation? Videotaped interviews analysed by the "consultation map" method. *Family Practice, 9,* 61–66.

Balint, M., Hunt, J., & Joyce, D. (1970). *Treatment or diagnosis: A study of repeat prescriptions in general practice.* Toronto: Lippincott.

Beckman, H. B., & Frankel, R. M. (1984). The effect of physician behavior on the collection of data. *Annals of Internal Medicine, 91,* 692–696.

Bernzweig, J., Takayama, J. I., Phibbs, C., Lewis, C., & Pantell, R. H. (1997). Gender differences in physician-patient communication: Evidence from pediatric visits. *Archives of Pediatric Adolescent Medicine, 151,* 586–591.

Bertakis, K. D., & Callahan, E. J. (1992). A comparison of initial and established patient encounters using the Davis Observation Code. *Family Medicine, 24,* 307–311.

Bertakis, K. D., Helms, L. J., Callahan, E. J., Azari, R., & Robbins, J. A. (1995). The influence of gender on physician practice style. *Medical Care, 33,* 407–416.

Bertakis, K. D., Roter, D., & Putnam, S. M. (1991). The relationship of physician medical interview style to patient satisfaction. *Journal of Family Practice, 32,* 175–181.

Blanchard, C. G., Ruckdeschel, J. C., Fletcher, B. A., & Blanchard, E. B. (1986). The impact of oncologists' behaviors on patient satisfaction with morning rounds. *Cancer, 58,* 387–391.

Branch, W. T., & Malik, T. K. (1993). Using "windows of opportunities" in brief interviews to understand patients' concerns. *Journal of American Medical Association, 269,* 1667–1668.

Brown, S. J. (1992). Tailoring nursing care to the individual client: Empirical challenge of a theoretical concept. *Research in Nursing & Health, 15,* 39–46.

Brown, S. J. (1994). Communication strategies used by an expert nurse. *Clinical Nursing Research, 3,* 43–56.

Brown, S. J. (1996). Direct clinical practice. In A. B. Hamric, J. A. Spross, & C. M. Hanson (Eds.), *Advanced nursing practice: An integrative approach* (pp. 109–138). Philadelphia: Saunders.

Brykcznski, K. A. (1989). An interpretive study describing the clinical judgment of nurse practitioners. *Scholarly Inquiry for Nursing Practice: An International Journal, 3,* 75–104.

Byrne, P. S., & Long, B. E. L. (1976). *Doctors talking to patients.* London: Her Majesty's Stationery Office.

Campion, P. D., Butler, N. M., & Cox, A. (1992). Principle agendas of doctor and patients in general practice consultations. *Family Practice, 9,* 181–190.

Cecil, D. W., & Killeen, I. (1997). Control, compliance, and satisfaction in the family practice encounter. *Family Medicine, 29,* 653–657.

Daley, J. (1993). Overcoming the barrier of words. In M. Gerteis, S. Edgman-Levitan, J. Daley, & T. L. Delbanco (Eds.), *Through the patient's eyes: Understanding and promoting patient-centered care* (pp. 72–95). San Francisco: Jossey-Bass.

French, P. (1994). An experimental study of the effects of learning climate on patient-centred decision-making. *International Journal of Nursing Studies, 31,* 593–605.

Gerteis, M., Edgman-Levitan, S., Daley, J., & Delbanco, T. L. (Eds.). (1993). *Through the patient's eyes: Understanding and promoting patient-centered care.* San Francisco, CA: Jossey-Bass.

Hall, J. A., & Dornan, M. C. (1988). What patients like about their medical care and how often they are asked: A meta-analysis of the satisfaction literature. *Social Science and Medicine, 27,* 935–939.

Hall, J. A., Roter, D. L., & Katz, N. R. (1987). Task versus socioemotional behaviors in physicians. *Medical Care, 25,* 399–412.

Hall, J. A., Roter, D. L., Milburn, M. A., & Daltroy, L. H. (1996). Patients' health as a predictor of physician and patient behavior in medical visits: A synthesis of four studies. *Medical Care, 34,* 1205–1218.

Hauck, F. R., Zyanski, S. J., Alemango, S. A., & Medalie, J. H. (1990). Patient perceptions of humanism in physicians: Effects on positive health behaviors. *Family Medicine, 22,* 447–452.

Henbest, R. J., & Fehrsen, G. S. (1992). Patient-centredness: Is it applicable outside the West? Its measurement and effect on outcomes. *Family Practice, 9,* 311–317.

Henbest, R. J., & Stewart, M. A. (1989). Patient-centredness in the consultation: 1. A method for measurement. *Family Practice, 6,* 249–253.

Henbest, R. J., & Stewart, M. A. (1990). Patient-centredness in the consultation: 2. Does it really make a difference. *Family Practice, 7,* 28–33.

Jarrett, N., & Payne, S. (1995). A selective review of the literature on nurse-patient communication: Has the patient's contribution been neglected? *Journal of Advanced Nursing, 22,* 72–78.

Johnson, R. (1993). Nurse practitioner-patient discourse: Uncovering the voice of nursing in primary care practice. *Scholarly Inquiry for Nursing Practice: An International Journal, 7,* 143–157.

Joos, S. K., Hickam, D. H., Gordon, G. H., & Baker, L. H. (1996). Effects of a physician communication intervention on patient care outcomes. *Journal of General Internal Medicine, 11,* 147–155.

Kaplan, S. H., Gandek, B., Greenfield, S., Rogers, W., & Ware, J. E. (1995). Patient and visit characteristics related to physicians participatory decision-making style: Results from the Medical Outcomes Study. *Medical Care, 33,* 1176–1187.

Kaplan, S. H., Greenfield, S., & Ware, J. E. (1989). Assessing the effects of physician-patient interactions on the outcomes of chronic disease. *Medical Care, 27,* S110–S127.

Kasch, C. R., Kasch, J. B., & Lisnek, P. (1987). Women's talk and nurse-client encounters: Developing criteria for assessing interpersonal skill. *Scholarly Inquiry for Nursing Practice: An International Journal, 1,* 241–255.

Kasch, C. R., & Lisnek, P. M. (1984). Role of strategic communication in nursing theory and research. *Advances in Nursing Science, 7*(1), 56–71.

Kraan, H. F., Crijnen, A., van der Vleuten, C., & Imbos, T. (1995). Evaluation instruments for medical interviewing skills. In M. Lipkin, S. M. Putnam, & A. Lazare, *The medical interview: Clinical care, education, and research* (pp. 460–472). New York: Springer Verlag.

Kristjanson, L., & Chalmers, K. (1990). Nurse-client interactions in community-based practice: Creating common ground. *Public Health Nursing, 7,* 215–223.

Law, S. A., & Britten, N. (1995). Factors that influence the patient centredness of a consultation. *British Journal of General Practice, 45,* 520–524.

Levenstein, J. H., McCracken, E. C., McWhinney, I. R., Stewart, M. A., & Brown, J. B. (1986). The patient-centred clinical method: 1. A model for the doctor-patient interaction in family medicine. *Family Practice, 3,* 24–30.

Levinson, W., Roter, D. L., Mullooly, J. P., Dull, V. T., & Frankel, R. M. (1997). Physician-patient communication: The relationship with malpractice claims among primary care physicians and surgeons. *Journal of the American Medical Association, 277,* 553–559.

Marshall, R. S. (1988). Interpretation in doctor-patient interviews: A sociolinguistic analysis. *Culture, Medicine and Psychiatry, 12,* 201–218.

Mathews, B. P. (1962). Measurement of psychological aspects of the nurse-patient relationship. *Nursing Research, 11,* 154–162.

Mishler, E. G. (1984). *The discourse of medicine: Dialectics of medical interviews.* Norwood, NJ: Ablex.

Mishler, E. G., Clark, J. A., Ingelfinger, J., & Simon, M. P. (1989). The language of attentive patient care: A comparison of two medical interviews. *Journal of General Internal Medicine, 4,* 325–335.

Morten, A., Kohl, M., O'Mahoney, P., & Pelosi, K. (1991). Certified nurse midwifery care of the postpartum client: A descriptive study. *Journal of Nurse-Midwifery, 36,* 276–288.

Ong, L. M. L., de Haes, J. C. J. M., Hoos, A. M., & Lammes, F. B. (1995). Doctor-patient communication: A review of the literature. *Social Science & Medicine, 40,* 903–918.

Price, M. J. (1989). Qualitative analysis of the patient-provider interactions: The patient's perspective. *Diabetes Educator, 15,* 144–148.

Putnam, S. M., & Lipkin, M. (1995). The patient-centered interview: Research support. In M. Lipkin, S. M. Putnam, & A. Lazare (Eds.), *The medical interview: Clinical care, education, and research* (pp. 530–537). New York: Springer Verlag.

Robbins, J. A., Bertakis, K. D., Helms, L. J., Azaris, R., Callahand, E. J., & Creten, D. A. (1993). The influence of physicians practice behaviors on patient satisfaction. *Family Medicine, 25,* 17–20.

Rogers, C. R. (1951). *Client-centered therapy.* Boston: Houghton Mifflin.

Rolfe, G. (1994). Some factors associated with change in patient-centredness of student nurses during the Common Foundation Programme in nursing. *International Journal of Nursing Studies, 31,* 421–436.

Rost, K., Carter, W., & Inui, T. (1989). Introduction of information during the initial medical visit: Consequences for patient follow-through with physician recommendations for medication. *Social Science & Medicine, 28,* 315–321.

Roter, D. L., & Hall, J. A. (1987). Physicians' interviewing styles and medical information obtained from patients. *Journal of General Internal Medicine, 2,* 325–329.

Rowland-Morin, P. A., & Carroll, J. G. (1990). Verbal communication skills and patient satisfaction: A study of doctor-patient interviews. *Evaluation & the Health Professions, 13,* 168–185.

Shuy, R. W. (1983). Three types of interference to an effective exchange of information in the medical interview. In S. Fisher & A. D. Todd (Eds.), *The social organization of doctor-patient communication* (pp. 189–202). Washington, DC: Center for Applied Linguistics.

Smith, R. C. (1996). *The patient's story: Integrated patient-doctor interviewing.* Boston: Little, Brown.

Sprague-Zones, J. (1995). Gender effects in physician-patient interaction. In M. Lipkin, S. M. Putnam, & A. Lazare, *The medical interview: Clinical care, education, and research* (pp. 163–171). New York: Springer Verlag.

Stewart, M. A. (1984). What is a successful doctor-patient interview? A study of interactions and outcomes. *Social Science & Medicine, 19,* 167–175.

Stewart, M. A. (1995). Effective physician-patient communication and health outcomes: A review. *Canadian Medical Association Journal, 152,* 1423–1433.

Street, R. L. (1991). Physicians' communication and parents' evaluations of pediatric consultations. *Medical Care, 29,* 1146–1152.

Street, R. L., & Wiemann, J. M. (1987). Patients' satisfaction with physicians' interpersonal involvement, expressiveness, and dominance. In M. L. McLaughlin (Ed.), *Communication yearbook* (Vol. 10, pp. 592–612). Beverly Hills, CA: Sage.

Suchman, A. L., Markakis, K., Beckman, H. B., & Frankel, R. (1997). A model of empathetic communication in the medical interview. *Journal of the American Medical Association, 277,* 678–682.

Taylor, S. G., Pickens, J. M., & Geden, E. A. (1989). Interactional styles of nurse practitioners and physicians regarding patient decision making. *Nursing Research, 38,* 50–55.

Thom, D. H., & Campbell, B. (1997). Patient-physician trust: An exploratory study. *The Journal of Family Practice, 44,* 169–176.

Tresolini, C., & the Pew-Fetzer Task Force. (1994). *Health profession education and relationship-centered care: Report of the Pew-Fetzer Task Force on advancing psychosocial health education.* Triangle Park, NC: Pew Health Professions Commission.

Tuckett, D., Boulton, M., Olson, C., & Williams, A. (1986). *Meetings between experts.* New York: Tavistock.

Wallston, K. A., Cohen, B. S., Smith, R. A., & DeVellis, B. M. (1978). Increasing nurses' person-centeredness. *Nursing Research, 27,* 151–155.

Webster-Stratton, C., Glascock, J., & McCarthy, A. M. (1986). Nurse practitioner-patient interactional analyses during well child visits. *Nursing Research, 35,* 247–249.

Woolliscroft, J. O., Calhoun, J. G., Billiu, G. A., Stross, J. K., MacDonald, M., & Templeton, B. (1989). House Officer interviewing techniques: Impact on data elicitation and patient perceptions. *Journal of General Internal Medicine, 4,* 108–114.

PART II

Pain

Chapter 5

Acute Pain

MARION GOOD

ABSTRACT

The review of acute pain describes the problem of unresolved pain and its effects on the neural, autonomic, and immune systems. Conceptualizations and mechanisms of pain are reviewed as well as theories of pain management. Descriptive studies of patient and nurse factors that inhibit effective pain management are discussed, followed by studies of pharmacological and nonpharmacological interventions. Critical analysis reveals that most studies were atheoretical, and therefore, this proliferation of information lacked conceptual coherence and organization. Furthermore, the nature and extent of barriers to pain management were described, but few intervention studies have been devised, as yet, to modify the knowledge, beliefs, and attitudes of nurses and patients that are barriers to pain management. Although some of the complementary therapies have sufficient research support to be used in clinical pain management, the physiological mechanisms and outcomes need to be studied. It is critical at this time to design studies of interventions to improve assessment, decision making, attentive care, and patient teaching.

Keywords: Pain, Acute Pain, Postoperative Pain

Acute pain is a major health problem, and inadequate relief can result in adverse short and long-term psychological and physiological effects that are an ethical and economic burden on the health care system and society. The International Association for the Study of Pain (IASP) Subcommittee on Taxonomy defines pain as "an unpleasant sensory or emotional experience associated with actual or potential tissue damage or described in terms of such damage" (1979, p. 249). Acute pain usually signals injury, has a recent onset and brief duration, and subsides as healing of the injury occurs; it may be associated with increased autonomic activity and anxiety (Fields, 1987). Chronic pain persists beyond expected healing; often the specific injury is not known, and the pain may last for more than 1 to 6 months (Jurf & Nirschl, 1993).

This review focuses on advances in the empirical work on theories, mechanisms, and management of acute pain and on patient and nurse factors, from 1990 until early 1998. Other important reviews of acute pain have appeared since 1990: *Acute Pain Management: Operative or Medical Procedures and Trauma* (Acute Pain Management Guideline Panel, 1992); *Textbook of Pain* (3rd edition) (Wall & Melzack, 1994), and *Symptom Management: Acute Pain* (National Institute of Nursing Research Priority Expert Panel on Symptom Management: Acute Pain, 1994); these are excellent references. This chapter focuses on substantive advances in interdisciplinary knowledge of acute pain.

Published studies in English were obtained from computer searches of Medline, Cumulative Index to Nursing and Allied Health Literature (CINAHL), Healthstar, and Psychological Abstracts using the keywords pain, acute, surgical, post-operative, pain management, assessment, and pathophysiology. To access interventions, other key words were entered: pharmacology, music therapy, therapeutic touch, imagery, relaxation therapy, distraction, and massage. In addition, the author's file of articles were screened and acute pain researchers' names were used in retrieval. Between 1990 and January 1998, with the keywords of acute pain, there were 3,482 articles found in Medline, and 284 research articles found in CINAHL. The search was then limited by excluding the following topics: pain in children, labor, cancer, orthopedics, chronic conditions, and pain measurement. To further limit the sample, the following were prioritized for inclusion: review articles, recent research, and studies relevant to nursing.

PROBLEM

Although the undertreatment of pain in hospitals has been well established for over 20 years, studies continue to explore the nature and extent of the problem. For example, a recent telephone survey of adults in 500 U.S. households found that 57% of adults said their primary fear before surgery was pain, while 77% reported they had experienced pain after surgery and 80%

of these experienced moderate to severe pain (Warfield & Kahn, 1995). In a sample of intensive care unit (ICU) patients, 63% reported moderate to severe pain, with inadequate relief, and difficulty communicating pain (Puntillo, 1990). Yet in another study, ICU and postoperative patients were given only 30% to 37% of the maximum opioid ordered, with no documentation of the effects of analgesics (Tittle & McMillan, 1994).

The potential outcomes of unrelieved acute pain are serious: complications and delayed recovery from inhibition of respiration, peristalsis, ambulation, and immune function, and increased coagulation, fluid retention, and prolonged pain (Acute Pain Management Guideline Panel, 1992). For example, in human survivors of serious illness, over a third with moderate to severe pain still had it 2 and 6 months later (Desbiens et al., 1997). Sleep is also affected by pain, and analgesics are the most helpful in getting the patient back to sleep, but fewer analgesics are given at night because of assessment difficulties and patients' reluctance to report pain (Closs, 1992). These problems have spurred continued investigations of pain theories, assessment, and interventions in nursing and other health care disciplines.

THEORIES OF PAIN AND PAIN MANAGEMENT

Conceptual Approaches to Pain

In patients with life-threatening injuries or illnesses, qualitative themes of discomfort were found: pain was often set in the context of the disease and the body's responses; and having pain included vulnerable feelings, endurance, and thoughts of suicide and death. Investigators defined comfort as the relief of discomfort, understood only in relation to it (Morse, Bottorff, & Hutchinson, 1995).

Mahon's concept analysis of pain found that pain is tiring and interferes with relationships, but surprisingly, it gives meaning to life. She described pain as dominating, unpleasant, seemingly endless, preceded by a stimulus, and causing physical or mental damage (1994). Some pain, however, does not arise from a damaging stimulus; examples are contraction of viscera or light touch on hypersensitive skin near a wound. Thus, Cerverro and Merskey (1996) suggest that pain evoking stimuli be termed allogenic, rather than noxious. A survey of expert nurses resulted in defined characteristics of acute and chronic pain, and separate nursing diagnoses were recommended (Simon, Baumann, & Nolan, 1995).

Descriptive Theories

Lenz, Pugh, Milligan, Gift, and Suppe (1997) recently published a descriptive theory of unpleasant symptoms including dyspnea, nausea, fatigue, and pain and suggested that there are sufficient commonalities among the symptoms to warrant the generalized theory. Further, the symptoms are often experienced simultaneously, with synergistic patient effects. For example, seriously ill patients who have nausea and/or dyspnea have more pain than those who do not have these additional symptoms; thus treating nausea and dyspnea may help to relieve pain (Desbiens, Mueller-Rizner, Connors, & Wenger, 1997). The first issue of *Pain Forum* in 1996 celebrated the 30th anniversary of publication of the gate control theory of pain; the original Melzack and Wall (1965) article that appeared in *Science* was republished. Melzack (1996) traced the theory through the years in terms of paradigm shifts, and proposed a new neuromatrix theory of pain to take into account current knowledge about the brain and the mystery of phantom limb pain.

Mechanisms of Pain

Knowledge of acute pain mechanisms has increased recently (Cousins, 1994). We now know that the injury response involves primary hyperalgesia or increased peripheral sensitization at the area of injury (inhibited by nonsteroidal anti-inflammatory drugs [NSAIDS]) and secondary hyperalgesia or increased tenderness in adjacent areas due to central sensitization, that is, central nervous system (CNS) changes. Genetic and biochemical changes in the CNS at the spinal and supra-spinal level can develop into persistent post injury states. These changes include second messengers that trigger the prolonged "wind-up," "after discharge," and sprouting that occur in spinal neurons from repetitive peripheral stimulation. In addition, there is recruitment of "third messengers" such as c-fos, permitting genetic encoding of increased responsiveness of dorsal horn neurons. (Several other recent reviews of the mechanisms of pain expand on this information [Hopkin, 1997; Paice, 1991; Puntillo, 1988]).

The discovery of these mechanisms has led to animal studies of pain prevention in which investigators found that the hyper excitability of spinal neurons could be prevented, and c-fos decreased, with small doses of analgesics given before the noxious stimulation (Cousins, 1994). In a clinical study, S. M. Gordon, Dionne, Brahim, Jabir, and Dubner (1997) found that intrathecal long-acting local anesthetics decreased central hyperexcitability and pain. These studies provide empirical evidence that pain pathways can be interrupted by preventive management with opioids, local anesthetics, and NSAIDS

(Goldstein, 1995); however, more research is needed to determine the treatment dose and duration (Dahl & Kehlet, 1993).

Cousins (1994) noted that risk factors for development of persistent postoperative pain include genetic predisposition; degree and duration of pain prior to surgery; surgical factors, such as incision type, percentage of trauma and stretching, delayed or inadequate analgesia; and middle to old age. Further, the stress response to tissue injury and to acute pain activates the sympathetically mediated fight-or-flight responses of increased heart rate, peripheral resistance, blood pressure, cardiac output, and coagulation, and decreased immunocompetence. Kehlet (1989) showed that 48- to 72-hour maintenance of a combined local anesthetic and opioid neural blockade produced a powerful modification of the stress response to surgical injury. This finding has been the basis of study and increased use of this combination epidural analgesia in postoperative patients.

Others investigated physiological responses to pain and surgery as powerful stressors which result in neuroendocrine activity and suppressed immune response and metastasis of cancer cells. They have found that in rats, surgery enhances metastasis, while it suppresses the natural killer (NK) cells needed to control metastasis. These reactions, however, were blocked by an analgesic dose of morphine (Page & Ben-Eliyahu, 1997a). Unrelieved acute pain is more than an issue of temporary suffering; it has long-term ethical implications of cost in terms of health and resources.

In addition to pathological effects of pain, there are mechanisms than modulate pain. These include descending neurons from the brain to the dorsal horn of spinal cord that release inhibitory substances such as substance P, serotonin, norepinephrine, and endogenous opioids (Puntillo, 1988).

Theories of Pain Management

Several theories of pain management have recently been published in nursing journals. Kolcaba (1994) who defined comfort as the satisfaction of basic human needs for relief, ease, or transcendence that arise from stressful health care situations, suggested that comfort is related to interventions that enhance it and to desirable outcomes of care. Comfort is state specific and an immediate goal of patient care. Comfort care has been described as a nursing art (Kolcaba, 1995), and is linked to patient care through assessment, intervention, patient evaluation, and engagement in health-seeking behavior. This theory of comfort care is described relative to terminal illness (Kolcaba & Fisher, 1996; Vendlinski & Kolcaba, 1997). In a qualitative study, Zalon (1997) found that frail, elderly women dealing with pain after surgery reported pain as immediate, but comfort and trust gave them security. Pain required endurance, control, and the ability to discover strategies to relieve it.

Good and Moore (1996) conceptualized an acute pain management theory from national guidelines (Acute Pain Management Guideline Panel, 1992). The theory prescribes multimodal intervention, attentive care, and patient participation to achieve a balance between analgesics and side effects. This theory is supported by studies cited in the guidelines and by several subsequent studies (Good, 1998).

In Greipp's (1992) model, pain is described as an ethical problem with potential to dehumanize victims who are dependent on nurses for knowledgeable, timely, compassionate, and effective care. The model describes factors that affect the quality of pain care: patient and nurse biological essences, such as gender and age, and inhibitors to nurse-patient interactions, such as personal experiences, culture, and belief systems.

A theory of chronotherapeutic or time-dependent approaches to pain assessment and intervention was inductively derived from chronobiologic literature and validated in three investigations. This theory postulates that analgesic therapy delivered in synchrony with the patient's pain rhythms will improve postoperative outcomes (Auvil-Novak, 1997).

Dalton and Blau (1996) have examined the learning process involved in changing the practice of pain management using theories of cognitive learning, adult learning, problem solving, self-efficacy, self-protection, attitude theory, value conflict, reasoned action, and persuasion. They recommend that agencies use these theories to influence the motivation, attitudes, education, and sense of empowerment of nurses.

ASSESSMENT

Patient Factors

Studies continue to explore patient and nurse factors that contribute to the problem of undertreatment of pain. Greipp's model (1992) indicates that patients' biological essences, including gender and age, are related to their experience and communication of pain.

Gender.   Fillingim and Maixner (1995) speculate that the lack of consensus on gender differences in pain response is due to the absence of a model. Therefore, they review the literature from the position that females exhibit greater sensitivity to pain. They conclude that studies are needed on the nature and physiology of gender differences, including menstrual cycle and childbirth effects. This is especially important in light of findings that surgery reduced NK cell immunity to metastasis more in female rats than in males (Page & Ben-Eliyahu, 1997b).

A laboratory study found no sex differences in response to thermal stimulation, but women had lower thresholds and tolerance to electrical pain (Lautenbacher & Rollman, 1993). Faucett, Gordon, and Levine (1994) found that 242 men reported significantly less postoperative dental pain than 301 women. However, a study of three large clusters of patients experiencing clinical pain showed no difference between males and females (Lander, Fowler-Kerry, & Hill, 1990), nor did a large study of hospitalized adults (Desbiens et al., 1996).

Other studies have shown that females and males respond differently to analgesics. In dental surgery patients, two k-opioid analgesics, nalbuphine (Nubain) and Butorphanol (Stadol), produced greater analgesia in women than in men (Gear et al. 1996). A review by Vallerand (1995) found that being female was a significant predictor of inadequate pain management. This may be related to gender differences in pain and analgesic response, or to gender stereotyping. In the emergency department, female patients were perceived to have more pain, and they received more medications and stronger analgesics than males; however, pain, rather than gender stereotyping, was related to pain management practices (Raftery, Smith-Coggins, & Chen, 1995).

Age. Interviews with 5,176 seriously ill hospitalized adults in a prospective cohort study revealed that nearly 50% reported pain; older patients reported less pain (Desbiens et al., 1997). Unfortunately, pain in older adults has often been dismissed as expected, and is therefore tolerated rather than managed. A review of age-related differences in pain perception and report (Gibson & Helme, 1995) has shown that pain in older adults is due to pathology rather than age. Age does result in decreased transmission of pain impulses and increased pain threshold, but reduced endogenous opiate modulation may counteract the effect.

There are changes in the incidence of pain in several body locations as aging occurs: joint pain increases, while headache, chest, abdominal, and facial pain decrease. The belief of elderly adults that pain is a normal part of the aging process could potentially alter patients' inclination to report pain. Older adults have a higher pain threshold and under-report pain, but this does not mean it hurts less. It is recommended that older adults be asked regularly about their pain, and if they report any, it should be considered in exactly the same manner as that of a younger person (Gibson & Helme, 1995).

Closs, Fairtlough, Tierney, and Currie (1993) found that the majority of orthopedic patients over the age of 70 had significant pain, but none received more than half the maximum prescribed amount of opiate. This may have been because of a greater analgesic effect from opioids in elders, or it may have been that beliefs and lack of knowledge about pain management were barriers to adequate pain control (Brockopp, Warden, Colclough, & Brockopp, 1996).

Assessment of pain in the confused elderly population is especially problematic. Standards of self-report are insufficient because of patient difficulties with processing and speech. Nurses do not understand confusion among the elderly in relation to pain assessment (Brockopp, Warden, Colclough, & Brockopp, 1993), and do not routinely try to manage discomfort during turning and mobilization (Miller, Moore, Schofield, & Ng'andu, 1996). Nurses need to rely on family and other long-term care givers to provide specific behaviors that can be used to identify pain in elders (Miller, Neelon, et al., 1996).

Beliefs.   Greipp's ethical model of pain describes patient beliefs as potential inhibitors of a beneficial management decision (1992). Such beliefs include the notion that one should not mention when one is in pain, or that pain is a result of wrong doing and is necessary for recovery (Brydon & Asbury, 1996). Beliefs that postoperative pain is unavoidable, that analgesics are bad for one's health, and a fear of addiction cause some patients to rarely express pain or ask for analgesia. Lack of assertiveness, insecurity, and suboptimal interactions with nurses contribute (Francke & Theeuwen, 1994; Winefield, Katsikitis, Hart, & Rounsefell, 1990).

A large multicenter study found that 15% of patients were dissatisfied with pain control, especially those with more severe pain, greater anxiety, depression, alteration of mental status, and lower income (Desbiens et al., 1996). Some investigators have found that patients reported satisfaction with pain management despite having moderate to severe pain and waiting for analgesics. The reasons for the incongruence were not clear, and the authors recommend exploring them with patients (Miaskowski, Nichols, Brody, & Synold, 1994; Ward & Gordon, 1994). Others found that it is the perception of having control over pain that relates most to satisfaction (Pellino & Ward, 1998), or the perception of relief following "as needed" doses (Ward & Gordon, 1996).

Cultural background.   Pain beliefs and responses common to various races, nationalities, and cultures can inhibit effective pain management, especially when the nurse does not understand these perspectives. Villarruel and de Montellano (1992) found there were six themes in ancient Mesoamerica that were related to the cultural meaning of pain in contemporary Mexican-Americans. These six themes were acceptance of pain, endurance, stoicism, predetermination, punishment, and person-environment balance. Faucett et al. (1994) found that subjects of European descent reported significantly less pain than Black Americans or Latinos. McDonald (1994) found that White patients received significantly more total opioids than ethnic minority patients.

In their review, Calvillo and Flaskerud (1991) found that nurses underestimated patients' pain, regardless of cultural background; however, the ethnicity and culture of the patient influenced the extent of the differences between patient and nurse assessment. In a subsequent study, Calvillo and Flaskerud (1993) found no significant differences between Mexican-American and Anglo-American women in pain and amount of analgesia, but nurses judged the two ethnic groups' pain response differently, assigning more pain to Anglo-Americans. Nurses' pain ratings were significantly correlated with patients' education, place of birth, language, and religion. Nurses in hospitals with large populations of minorities may be more understanding of cultural factors than nurses in other hospitals; one study found that Hispanics in the emergency department were not undermedicated compared to Whites (Karpman, Del Mar, & Bay, 1997). Knowing cultural differences should lead to sensitive care, but not to stereotyping.

In the preceding studies of patient factors there were five research reviews (Calvillo & Flaskerud, 1991; Fillingim & Maixner, 1995; Gibson & Helme, 1995; Vallerand, 1995; Villarruel & de Montellano, 1992). Of the individual studies, most were surveys and descriptive studies with a few random or total samples. The mean sample size in this section was 126 excluding two large studies from a sample of 5,176 subjects. Measures included: patient knowledge, attitudes, beliefs, comfort, emotional status, functional status, ethnicity, satisfaction, and confusion. Although one-third of the articles included no recommendations for future research, the others gave suggestions for studying the meaning of pain across cultures, gender differences in pain response, pain assessment in confused elders, and type of illness in relation to expression of pain.

Nursing Factors

According to Greipp (1992), nurses' biological essences, beliefs, education, personal, and professional experiences affect their pain management decisions. In a review, Sullivan (1994) found that the age of the nurse, educational preparation, years of experience, personal pain experience, religion, and clinical subspecialty influenced pain management decisions.

Nursing education.   Incorrect nursing decisions are preceded by inadequate education—4 hours or less spent on pain content in many baccalaureate nursing programs, requiring nurses to acquire knowledge, skills and appropriate attitudes through clinical work after graduation. Faculty have revealed that their knowledge and beliefs about pain and their curriculum pain content are less than optimal (Ferrell, McGuire, & Donovan, 1993). A survey of 351 baccalaureate and associate degree programs found that 8 hours of pain instruction were allotted, with little instruction in nonpharmacological methods for relief (Zalon, 1995).

Inadequate knowledge and inaccurate beliefs, such as overconcern with addiction and respiratory depression, also contribute to poorer pain management. Many nurses also lack knowledge about the likelihood of addiction when giving opioid analgesics. When Ferrell, McCaffery, and Rhiner (1992) reviewed nursing textbooks, they found that nearly all used confusing terminology, and some actually promoted nurses' fear of patient addiction. Until textbooks are revised, educators can use two recent pain publications (Acute Pain Management Guideline Panel, 1992; American Pain Society, 1992).

Wakefield (1995) engaged nurses in a series of in-depth unstructured interviews and found that they tended to categorize patients according to symptoms or overt pain behaviors, and this resulted in patients not being believed when they reported pain. Gujol (1994) found that nurses' assessment and management of pain was affected by length of time after surgery and patient ventilator status. Patient complaints of pain in the early postoperative period and patients on ventilators were more likely to be believed and treated with larger narcotic doses than were complaints of pain from patients in the later postoperative period or those not on a ventilator. Patients whose pain endures for several days may be at particularly high risk of undermedication.

Using hypothetical patients, students attributed more pain to depressed patients, and both student and registered nurses attributed more pain when test results of physical pathology were positive (Halfens, Evers, & Abu-Saad, 1990). Clearly, nurses believe patients' pain more when they think there is a reason for it. McCaffery and Ferrell (1997) suggested teaching nurses to be more empathetic with patients and providing them pain management materials.

Decision making.   Guyton-Simmons and Ehrmin (1994) observed 61 ICU expert nurses as they interacted with ICU ventilator patients and interviewed the nurses immediately afterward. In patients who were not able to verbalize pain, nurses assessed pain based on observations of increased restlessness, anxiety, guarded movement, and change in facial expressions; they also monitored physiological changes as signs of pain and evidence of relief after medication. The nurse tried to distinguish typical from atypical pain based on type of surgery, days since surgery, and other factors. If atypical, further assessment was done. Prevention of pain and ability to move freely and breathe deeply were important.

Puntillo et al. (1997) tested a pain assessment and intervention notation algorithm consisting of lists of behavioral and physiological indicators for making inferences about the pain intensity of critical care patients. They found moderate to strong correlations between behavioral and physiological indicators and nurses' ratings of pain, which were not significantly lower than those of the patients.

When 53 nurses were asked about potential inhibitors of effective pain management, they listed physician and patient/family knowledge and cooperation, along with nursing knowledge and time. The ethical dilemmas they noted were overmedication or undermedication, conflicts with physicians or patients, and concern about opioid side-effects (Ferrell, Eberts, McCaffery, & Grant, 1997).

Wallace, Reed, Pasero, and Olsson (1995) surveyed nurses in 24 hospitals randomly sampled and stratified on the basis of size and found that practitioners did not recognize their own inadequacies and did not see the need for change. They recommended finding ways to develop awareness of deficiencies in knowledge and practice.

In the preceding section on nurse factors, there were two research reviews (Ferrell et al., 1992; Sullivan, 1984). Of the individual studies, 93% were survey or descriptive designs. The mean sample size was 142. Measures included nurses' knowledge, attitudes, beliefs, and decisions, patients' behavioral expressions of pain, and hospitals' acute pain programs. Two-thirds of the authors made no recommendations for further study, but others suggested studies of expert nurses in various sized agencies, intervention studies, and how agencies support or inhibit the use of new knowledge.

INTERVENTIONS

Good and Moore (1996) propose that nurses (a) administer pharmacological and nonpharmacological interventions; (b) assess pain and side effects regularly and intervene, reassess, and reintervene until relief is obtained; and (c) teach patients to participate in pain management and to set goals for relief.

Pharmacological Interventions

Analgesic administration.   Intravenous (IV) patient-controlled analgesia (PCA) and epidural analgesia (EA) have largely replaced traditional intermittent methods of intramuscular (IM) or intravenous (IV) bolus (Woolf & Chong, 1993). A review by Thomas and Rose (1993) concluded that IV/PCA is generally more effective than IM, and studies have also found that IV/PCA increases patient satisfaction (Snell, Fothergill-Bourbonnais, & Durocher-Hendriks, 1997), and is effective and safe for hospitalized patients (Sidebotham, Monique, Dijkhuizen, & Schug, 1997), and mentally intact chronically ill older adults when carefully titrated and monitored (Egbert, Parks, Short, & Burnett, 1990; Maxwell, 1996). However, few studies have looked at structured preoperative PCA teaching (Williams, 1996). Persons with high anxiety and less social support have been found to make more frequent PCA demands and have higher postoperative pain (Gill, Ginsberg, Muir, Sykes, & Williams, 1990). Chronotherapeutic administration of opioid to match diurnal pain variation resulted in greater postoperative pain relief and decreased toxicity (Auvil-Novak, 1997).

Conflicting results were found for pain relief with the addition of a continuous infusion (Cokefair, Smith, & Gries, 1996; Dawson et al., 1995). One large survey concluded that nurses should monitor closely when continuous infusion is added to demand PCA, and be alert to possible drug interactions or activation of the pump by someone other than the patient (Fleming & Coombs, 1992).

Epidural analgesia (EA) has been shown to provide greater pain control and patient satisfaction than that of PCA opioids (Eriksson-Mjöberg, Svensson, Almkvist, Ölund, & Gustafsson, 1997; Schug & Fry, 1994), it can be managed on a postoperative unit with appropriate monitoring (Scott, Beilby, & McClymont, 1995), and results in greater patient satisfaction, and increased pulmonary function (Simpson, Wahl, DeTraglia, Speck, & Taylor, 1992). Further, the combination of epidural anesthetic and analgesic management has been shown to minimize physiological stress responses to surgery and pain, and prevent the complications of acute pain (Brown & Mackey, 1993). Patient-controlled epidural anesthesia (PCEA) offers immediate patient control and even analgesia levels.

Analgesic combinations. A review by Hopf and Weitz (1994) indicates that new combinations of drugs can improve pain relief and reduce the opioid requirement. Ketorolac, an injectable NSAID, has been found to potentiate the effect of morphine after orthopedic surgery at rest and during movement (Picard, Bazin, Conio, Ruiz, & Schoeffler, 1997), and is also effective with fentanyl PECA (Grass et al., 1993).

A nurse researcher reviewed the mechanism of action of four new neurotransmitters that may eventually contribute to pain modulation (Miaskowski, 1997). Her research group found analgesic synergy in rats with intrathecal combinations of the μ-opioid agonist with δ or κ-selective opioid agonists (Miaskowski, Sutters, Taiwo, & Levine, 1992). In a clinical study, morphine analgesia was enhanced by adding Baclofen, a Gamma-amino butyric acid (GABA) agonist, thereby activating both opioid and $GABA_A$ receptors (Gordon et al., 1995).

In the pharmacological section there were eight research reviews (Brown & Mackey, 1993; Cokefair et al., 1996; Hopf & Weitz, 1994; Miaskowski, 1997; Simpson et al., 1992; Thomas & Rose, 1993; Williams, 1996; Woolf & Chong, 1993). Of the 14 individual studies, eight (57%) were randomly assigned, with six of these experimental and two comparative. The remainder were retrospective, comparative, or survey designs, which are appropriate for some research questions, but less prescriptive than prospective trials of interventions. Most of the pharmacological studies did not use a formal theory, but were based on concepts such as preemptive analgesia, combination therapy, and personal control.

In this section the mean group size was 27. Measures included frequent pain VAS, cognitive function, oxygen saturation, pain after coughing or moving, and side effects, complications, recovery, satisfaction, and locus of control. Authors recommended that the following be studied in the future: combined opioid and nonopioid PCA, synergic medication effects, opioid adjuncts to decrease side effects, preoperative pain education, and nursing care of patients with epidural analgesia.

Nonpharmacological Interventions

Complementary nursing therapies.   A review of psychological and physical complementary therapies by Stevenson (1995) lists the following as having sound support: preoperative information, relaxation, guided imagery, breathing training, cognitive reframing, distraction, music, massage, acupuncture, and Transcutaneous Electrical Nerve Stimulation (TENS). The evidence on the effects of hypnosis, humor therapy, biofeedback, aroma therapy, reflex zone therapy, acupressure (shiatsu), and Therapeutic Touch is inconclusive. Blankfield (1991) reviewed clinical trials which employed hypnosis, suggestion, or relaxation and found that these techniques reduced analgesic intake or pain in 13 of 15 studies. Other positive outcomes were decreased hospital stay, and improved postoperative emotional response and recovery.

Although Sindhu's meta-analysis of 49 studies of nonpharmacological interventions found evidence that relaxation and patient teaching were effective in reducing pain, results were mixed because the studies were small. There were large standard errors, and Sindhu concluded that larger randomized controlled trials were needed to decrease variability (1996). A meta-analysis of 191 studies of the effects of psychoeducational care of adult surgical patients supported reliable, small to moderate beneficial effects for pain and distress (Devine, 1992).

Three intervention validation studies have been conducted using two-round Delphi surveys. The first included interventions related to pain (Herr & Mobily, 1992). The second included relaxation, distraction, and guided imagery for pain (Mobily, Herr, & Kelley, 1993). The third was designed to validate cutaneous stimulation interventions such as heat and cold for pain (Mobily, Herr, & Nicholson, 1994). Experts said that although these are not widely used in clinical settings, they are important interventions for pain. The authors suggest that the activities be used to standardize interventions in research, practice, and education.

Relaxation.   Relaxation is the most widely evaluated nonpharmacological method of postoperative pain management (Acute Pain Management Guideline Panel, 1992); however, until recently, small sample sizes, lack of randomization, and lack of pretest controls were common, perhaps contributing to the varying results. An integrated review found that most of the 16 studies in which relaxation was tested reduced at least the affective component of pain, and sometimes the sensory component. However, the mean of 18 subjects per treatment group was inadequate (Good, 1996). A larger study with 125 subjects per group has found that jaw relaxation reduces both the sensory and affective components of postoperative pain on ambulation and rest on postoperative days 1 and 2 (Good, Stanton-Hicks, Grass, Anderson, & Schoolmeesters, In revision).

Music.   In the laboratory, Whipple and Glynn (1992) found that listening to soothing and stimulating music elevated pain detection and tolerance of both mechanical and thermal pain stimulation. Good (1996) reviewed six studies that used music for postoperative pain and found that most reduced pain; but only two were randomized, and the sample sizes were small for the large standard deviations of pain. Henry (1995) reviewed six studies on the effect of music on patients in ICU, with similar findings. Mengazzi, Paris, Kersteen, Flynn, and Trautman (1991) found that music was an effective adjuvant for management of pain during laceration repair in the emergency department. Good and Chin (1998) used Western music for postoperative pain in Taiwan with mixed effectiveness due to either the small music group (n = 16) or to patient preferences for Taiwanese popular songs and Buddhist hymns. Interestingly, music was effective without medication. None of these patients happened to have analgesics in effect at the time of testing.

Other investigators have found no effect on pain among patients receiving 30 minutes of music on Days 2 and 3 following coronary artery bypass graft. These results, however, may have been due to the mild intensity and low variability of pain in these patients (Zimmerman, Nieveen, Barnason, & Schmaderer, 1996). Two small studies in the postanesthesia recovery unit (PACU) found no effect for music, but patients perceived the experience as relaxing and pleasant (Heiser, Chiles, Fudge, & Gray, 1997; Heitz, Symreng, & Scamman, 1992).

Imagery.   In a recent review of guided imagery, Giedt (1997) described the principles of guided imagery, and said that a placebo effect is very likely to account in part for the efficacy of the strategy. (This review is a notable resource on the concepts of psychoneuroimmunology in relation to guided imagery.) For colorectal surgical patients, a guided imagery tape with healing suggestions was used along with background music for 3 days preoperatively to calm and focus patients. During induction, surgery, and recovery, the same music was used without the narrative, and the imagery tape was used for 6 days postoperatively. The outcomes included decreased postoperative anxiety, worst pain, and opioid requirements, and increased patient satisfaction (Tusek, Church, Strong, Grass, & Fazio, 1997). However, patient adherence to use of the tape was not reported.

Therapeutic touch.   In a qualitative study of 6 postoperative patients, Barrington (1994) found substantial evidence that therapeutic touch (TT) reduced or eliminated postoperative pain, and produced perceived relaxation, soothing, calming, and an overall feeling of well-being. However, in a experimental comparison of TT, placebo, and standard opioid analgesic intervention in 108 patients, TT did not decrease abdominal surgical pain more than the placebo; however, TT increased the time before requesting further analgesic medication compared to the placebo (Meehan, 1993).

Massage.   Based on practice articles and preliminary studies of massage for relaxation and cancer pain, Nixon, Teschendorff, Finney, and Karnilowicz (1997) found that controlling for age, massage produced significantly lower 24-hour perceptions of pain in 16 subjects compared to matched controls. Patients aged 41 to 60 years benefitted more from massage and tolerated a longer massage time than younger and older patients. This study matched the subjects in the two groups. It should be replicated with a larger and randomized sample using a computerized minimization program so that confounding factors are balanced across groups (Zeller, Good, Anderson, & Zeller, 1997).

Patient teaching.   Good and Moore (1996) recommend patient teaching about attitudes and expectations, reporting pain, obtaining medication, and using pharmacological and nonpharmacological adjuvants such as NSAIDS and complementary therapies. Gammon and Mulholland (1996) found that 41 patients who were given preoperative procedural, sensory, and coping information used significantly less IM analgesics, mobilized sooner, coped more effectively, and went home 2 days earlier than the controls. However, Hawkins and Price (1993) found no significant difference in postoperative pain between groups with a preoperative patient education video on pain management, although the video was valued by the 20 patients and reduced analgesic intake during mild pain. Differences in results between these two studies may have been due to sample size, measurement differences, and none to mild pain in 45% of subjects in the Hawkins and Price study.

Goal-setting and attentive care.   Good and Moore (1996) suggest that goal-setting for relief, along with frequent assessment, intervention, and reassessment for effect, is important to manage pain. The American Pain Society Quality of Care Committee (1995) developed quality improvement guidelines for institutional coordination of responsive analgesic care and prompt action to relieve pain. A survey by Beck and Larrabee (1996) found that patients' reports of achievement of their goals were related to patient-perceived quality of nursing care. Voigt, Paice, and Pouliot (1995) found that a flowsheet requiring frequent documentation of pain and analgesics for moderate or severe pain helped reduce pain. Scott (1994) demonstrated patient participation in pain assessment with a Pain Assessment Chart (PAC) given to experimental patients to be used every 2 hours postoperatively. Subjects recorded pain scores every 2 hours and set a goal for relief. Nurses recorded analgesics and possible side effects on the bedside PAC. Although there was no difference in satisfaction scores in this pilot study, it is an innovative way to encourage patient participation in pain management.

In the nonpharmacological studies there were two meta-analyses (Devine, 1992; Sindhu, 1996) and five research reviews (Blankfield, 1991; Gammon & Mulholland, 1996; Giedt, 1997; Good, 1996; Henry, 1995; Stevenson, 1995). Of the 18 individual studies, seven (39%) used a middle-range theory and two (11%) used a nursing conceptual model. There were nine (50%) randomized and seven (39%) quasi-experiments. Three used the Delphi method to validate interventions.

The mean treatment group size of 28 in the nonpharmacological studies is comparable to that of the pharmacological studies ($n = 27$), but should be larger because of only moderate effects on pain. The nonpharmacological studies included various VAS measures of pain: sensation, distress, worst, least, average, now pain (current pain), and pain during coughing and deep breathing. Outcomes included anxiety, sleep, and mobilization. Authors suggested that future studies identify onset and duration of effects, and determine the effect of complementary therapies on sleep, anxiety, and immune function. Most studies in this review did not use either a conceptual framework or a middle-range theory. To communicate results efficiently, findings need to be related to middle-range theories by the investigator, thereby organizing them conceptually. Specific pain theories may eventually merge into more general theories of unpleasant symptoms and comfort, but the specific goal is to relieve pain. The intervention section included a higher percentage of review articles and meta-analyses (29%) than the patient/nurse articles in the assessment section (16%), demonstrating the need for more review articles discussing patient and nurse factors. In addition, studies of patients and nurses included only 1 (3%) that was randomly assigned and 1 (3%) that was blinded; while in studies of pharmacological and nonpharmacological methods, 17 (53%) were randomly assigned, 8 (25%) were single- or double-blinded, and 4 (13%) were placebo-controlled. Half of the investigators made no recommendations for further research. Most assessment studies used descriptive designs: the paucity of intervention studies highlights the need for more to solve the problems of beliefs and attitudes in patients and nurses. These will contribute improving the nursing assessment, attentive care, and patient education.

RECOMMENDATIONS

Unrelieved pain is not only unpleasant, but can also cause neural, immune, and genetic changes that can result in chronic pain. Prevention and effective relief of acute pain may reduce these outcomes, improve sleep and immune function, and reduce complications and metastasis. This review has examined acute pain studies published since 1990 in the disciplines of nursing, medicine, psychology, and neuroscience. It has synthesized theoretical and empirical information about patient and nurse factors as well as pharmacological and nonpharmacological interventions. A limitation is that studies were not retrieved from the citations of the included articles. Analysis indicated that there need to be intervention studies for modifying the patient and nurse factors that inhibit effective pain management. Further, although complementary therapies are important, it is crucial that nurses study ways of improving the primary nursing functions that these therapies complement: accurate assessment, ethical decision making, attentive care, and effective patient teaching for participation.

There continues to be a need for studies of opiate combinations and interactions of gender and receptor types. There must be a greater understanding of genetic, cultural, early experiences, and age in relation to pain. Human studies are needed on the effect of pain management on immune factors, the spread of cancer, and increased nervous system sensitivity (Stein & Yassouridis, 1997).

More indirect measures of pain need to be devised; examples include supplemental analgesic intake, PCA attempts, pulmonary function, and time to next analgesic requirement. In addition, biological markers such as positron emission tomography (PET) are being used to demonstrate brain structures that increase activity with noxious stimulation (Derbyshire et al., 1997). Researchers also need to identify the role of plasma measures of stress such as adrenocorticotrophic hormone, cortisol, and β-endorphin in the pain experience (McKinney, Tims, Kumar, & Kumar, 1997). Study designs should avoid pre- and intra-operative treatments with effects that continue postoperatively. To detect differences between groups, pain should be measured during high pain times and activities (Stein & Yassouridis, 1997).

With increased patient, physician, nurse, and federal interest in research on nonpharmacological therapies, more attention should be paid to the capacity of designs to rule out placebo and other nonspecific effects. Independent evaluation to establish the effects of treatments beyond nonspecific effects is difficult in pain studies because the subjective measures and therapies cannot always be blind to the patient. Use of an inert placebo condition, blind data collectors, and adding indirect and more covert measures of pain can counter threats to the validity of these studies (Jonas, 1993; Turner, Deyo, Loeser, Von Korff, & Fordyce, 1994).

Although acute pain continues to be a problem, an increasing body of research findings is directed at its relief; recommendations for future study have been made. Utilization of research findings will help reduce acute pain.

ACKNOWLEDGMENTS

The author gratefully acknowledges the contributions of doctoral students Sandra Siedlecki, Catherine Stiller, Laree Schoolmeesters, Suzanne Vendlinski, Saffa Salem, and Gannon Johnson, who played important roles in searching the literature, organizing and screening the research articles, and preparing the references.

REFERENCES

Acute Pain Management Guideline Panel. (1992). *Clinical Practice Guideline: Acute pain management operative or medical procedures and trauma* (AHCPR Pub. No. 920032). Rockville, MD: Agency for Health Care Policy and Research.

American Pain Society. (1992). *Principles of analgesic use in the treatment of acute pain and chronic cancer pain* (3rd ed.). Skokie, IL: Author.

American Pain Society Quality of Care Committee. (1995). Quality improvement guidelines for the treatment of acute pain and cancer pain. *JAMA, 274*(23), 1874–1880.

Auvil-Novak, S. E. (1997). A middle-range theory of chronotherapeutic intervention for postsurgical pain. *Nursing Research, 46*(2), 66–71.

Barrington, R. (1994). A naturalistic inquiry of post-operative pain after therapeutic touch. *NLN-Pub.* No. 14-2607, 199–213.

Beck, K. L., & Larrabee, J. H. (1996). Measuring patients' perceptions of nursing care. *Nursing Management, 27*(9), 32B–32D.

Blankfield, R. P. (1991). Suggestion, relaxation, and hypnosis as adjuncts in the care of surgery patients: A review of the literature. *American Journal of Clinical Hypnosis, 33*(3), 172–186.

Brockopp, D., Warden, S., Colclough, G., & Brockopp, G. (1996). Elderly people's knowledge of and attitudes to pain management. *British Journal of Nursing, 5*(9), 556–558, 560–562.

Brockopp, D. Y., Warden, S., Colclough, G., & Brockopp, G. W. (1993). Nursing knowledge: Acute postoperative pain management in the elderly. *Journal of Gerontological Nursing, 19*(11), 31–37.

Brown, D. L., & Mackey, D. C. (1993). Management of postoperative pain: Influence of anesthetic and analgesic choice. *Mayo Clinic Proceedings, 68*(8), 768–777.

Brydon, C. W., & Asbury, A. J. (1996). Attitudes to pain and pain relief in adult surgical patients. *Anaesthesia, 51*(3), 279–281.

Calvillo, E. R., & Flaskerud, J. H. (1991). Review of literature on culture and pain of adults with focus on Mexican-Americans. *Journal of Transcultural Nursing, 2*(2), 16–23.

Calvillo, E. R., & Flaskerud, J. H. (1993). Evaluation of the pain response by Mexican American and Anglo American women and their nurses. *Journal of Advanced Nursing, 18*, 451–459.

Cervero, F., & Merskey, H. (1996). What is a noxious stimulus? *Pain Forum, 5*(3), 157–161.

Closs, S. J. (1992). Patients' night-time pain, analgesic provision and sleep after surgery. *International Journal of Nursing Studies, 29*(4), 381–392.

Closs, S. J., Fairtlough, H. L., Tierney, A. J., & Currie, C. T. (1993). Pain in elderly orthopaedic patients. *Journal of Clinical Nursing, 2*, 41–45.

Cokefair, A., Smith, H. S., & Gries, C. A. (1996). An investigation of the current literature on the effectiveness of patient-controlled analgesia methods. *CRNA: The Clinical Forum for Nurse Anesthetists, 7*(3), 126–134.

Cousins, M. (1994). Acute and postoperative pain. In P. D. Wall & R. Melzack (Eds.), *Textbook of pain* (pp. 357–384). New York: Churchill Livingstone.

Dahl, J. B., & Kehlet, H. (1993). The value of pre-emptive analgesia in the treatment of postoperative pain. *British Journal of Anaesthesia, 70*, 434–439.

Dalton, J., & Blau, W. (1996). Changing the practice of pain management: An examination of the theoretical basis of change. *Pain Forum, 5*(4), 266–272.

Dawson, P. J., Libreri, F. C., Jones, D. J., Libreri, G., Bjorkstein, A. R., & Royse, C. F. (1995). The efficacy of adding a continuous intravenous morphine infusion to patient-controlled analgesia (PCA) in abdominal surgery. *Anaesthesia and Intensive care, 23*(4), 453–458.

Derbyshire, S., Jones, A., Gyulai, F., Clark, S., Townsend, D., & Firestone, L. (1997). Pain processing during three levels of noxious stimulation produces differential patterns of central activity. *Pain, 73*(3), 431–445.

Desbiens, N. A., Mueller-Rizner, N., Connors, A. F., & Wenger, N. (1997). The relationship of nausea and dyspnea to pain in seriously ill patients. *Pain, 71*(2), 149–156.

Desbiens, N. A., Wu, A. W., Alzola, C., Mueller-Rizner, N., Wenger, N. S., Connors, A. F. Jr., & Phillips, R. S. (1997). Pain during hospitalization is associated with continued pain six months later in survivors of serious illness. *American Journal of Medicine, 102*(3), 269–276.

Desbiens, N. A., Wu, A. W., Broste, S. K., Wenger, N. S., Connors, A. F. Jr., Lynn, J., Yasui, Y., Phillips, R. S., & Fulkerson, W. (1996). Pain and satisfaction with pain control in seriously ill hospitalized adults: Findings from the SUPPORT research investigations. *Critical Care Medicine, 24*(12), 1953–1961.

Devine, E. C. (1992). Effects of psychoeducational care for adult surgical patients: A meta-analysis of 191 studies. *Patient Education and Counseling, 19*, 129–142.

Egbert, A. M., Parks, L. H., Short, L. M., & Burnett, M. L. (1990). Randomized trial of postoperative patient-controlled analgesia vs. intramuscular narcotics in frail elderly men. *Archives on Internal Medicine, 150*(9), 1897–1903.

Eriksson-Mjöberg, M., Svensson, O., Almkvist, A., Ölund, A., & Gustafsson, L. L. (1997). Extradural morphine gives better pain relief than patient-controlled i.v. morphine after hysterectomy. *British Journal of Anaesthesia, 78*, 10–16.

Faucett, J., Gordon, N., & Levine, J. (1994). Differences in postoperative pain severity among four ethnic groups. *Journal of Pain and Symptom Management, 9*(6), 383–389.

Ferrell, B. R., Eberts, M. T., McCaffery, M., & Grant, M. (1997). Clinical decision making and pain. *Cancer Nursing, 14*(6), 289–297.

Ferrell, B. R., McCaffery, M., & Rhiner, M. (1992). Pain and addiction: An urgent need for change in nursing education. *Journal of Pain and Symptom Management, 7*(2), 117–123.

Ferrell, B. R., McGuire, D. B., & Donovan, M. I. (1993). Knowledge and beliefs regarding pain in a sample of nursing faculty. *Journal of Professional Nursing, 9*(2), 79–88.

Fields, H. L. (1987). *Pain.* New York: McGraw-Hill.

Fillingim, R. B., & Maixner, W. (1995). Gender differences in the responses to noxious stimuli. *Pain Forum, 4*(4), 209–221.

Fleming, B. M., & Coombs, D. W. (1992). A survey of complications documented in a quality-control analysis of patient-controlled analgesia in the postoperative patient. *Journal of Pain and Symptom Management, 7*(8), 463–469.

Francke, A. L., & Theeuwen, I. (1994). Inhibition in expressing pain: A qualitative study among Dutch surgical breast cancer patients. *Cancer Nursing, 17*(3), 193–199.

Gammon, J., & Mulholland, C. W. (1996). Effect of preparatory information prior to elective total hip replacement on post-operative physical coping outcomes. *International Journal of Nursing Studies, 33*(6), 589–604.

Gear, R. W., Miaskowski, C., Gordon, N. C., Paul, S. M., Heller, P. H., & Levine, J. D. (1996). Kappa-opioids produce significantly greater analgesia in women than in men. *Nature Medicine, 2*(11), 1248–1250.

Gibson, S. J., & Helme, R. D. (1995). Age differences in pain perception and report: A review of physiological, psychological, laboratory and clinical studies. *Pain Reviews, 2*(2), 111–137.

Giedt, J. (1997). Guided imagery: A psychoneuroimmunological intervention in holistic nursing practice. *Journal of Holistic Nursing, 15*(2), 112–127.

Gil, K. M., Ginsberg, B., Muir, M., Sykes, D., & Williams, D. A. (1990). Patient-controlled analgesia in postoperative pain: The relations of psychological factors to pain and analgesic use. *The Clinical Journal of Pain, 6*(2), 137–142.

Goldstein, F. J. (1995). Preemptive analgesia: A research review. *MEDSURG Nursing, 4*(4), 304–308.

Good, M. (1996). Effects of relaxation and music on post-operative pain: A review. *Journal of Advanced Nursing, 24*, 905–914.

Good, M. (1998). A middle range theory of acute pain management; Use in research. *Nursing Outlook, 46*(3), 120–124.

Good, M., & Chin, C. (1998). The effects of Western music on postoperative pain in Taiwan. *The Kaohsiung Journal of Medical Sciences, 14*(2), 94–103.

Good, M., & Moore, S. M. (1996). Clinical practice guidelines as a new source of middle-range theory: Focus on acute pain. *Nursing Outlook, 44*(2), 74–79.

Good, M., Stanton-Hicks, M., Grass, J. A., Anderson, G. C., Choi, C., & Schoolmeesters, L. J., & Salman, A. (In press). Relief of postoperative pain with jaw relaxation, music, and their combination, *Pain*.

Gordon, N. C., Gear, R. W., Heller, P. H., Paul, S., Miaskowski, C., & Levine, J. D. (1995). Enhancement of morphine analgesia by the $GABA_B$ agonist Baclofen. *Neuroscience, 69*(2), 345–349.

Gordon, S. M., Dionne, R. A., Brahim, J., Jabir, F., & Dubner, R. (1997). Blockade of peripheral neuronal barrage reduces postoperative pain. *Pain, 70*, 209–215.

Grass, J., Sakima, N. T., Valley, M., Fischer, K., Jackson, C., Walsh, P., & Bourke, D. L. (1993). Assessment of Ketorolac as an adjuvant to fentanyl patient-controlled analgesia after radical retropubic prostatectomy. *Anesthesiology, 78*(4), 642–647.

Greipp, M. E. (1992). Undermedication for pain: An ethical model. *Advances in Nursing Science, 15*(1), 44–53.

Gujol, M. C. (1994). A survey of pain assessment and management practices among critical care nurses. *American Journal of Critical Care, 3*(2), 123–128.

Guyton-Simmons, J., & Ehrmin J. T. (1994). Problem solving in pain management by expert intensive care nurses. *Critical Care Nurse, 14*, 37–44.

Halfens, R., Evers, G., & Abu-Saad, H. (1990). Determinants of pain assessment by nurses. *International Journal of Nursing Studies, 27*(1), 43–49.

Hawkins, R., & Price., K. (1993). The effects of an education video on patients' requests for postoperative pain relief. *The Australian Journal of Advanced Nursing, 10*(4), 32–40.

Heiser, R. M., Chiles, K. C., Fudge, M., & Gray, S. E. (1997). The use of music during the immediate post-operative recovery period. *AORN, 65*(4), 777–785.

Heitz, L., Symreng., T., & Scamman, F. L. (1992). Effect of music therapy in the postanesthesia care unit: A nursing intervention. *Journal of Postanesthesia Nursing, 7*(1), 22–31.

Henry, L. L. (1995). Music therapy: A nursing intervention for the control of pain and anxiety in the ICU: A review of the research literature. *Dimensions of Critical Care Nursing, 16*(6), 295–304.

Herr, K. A., & Mobily, P. R. (1992). Interventions related to pain. *Nursing Clinics of North America, 27*(2), 347–369.

Hopf, H. W., & Weitz, S. (1994). Postoperative pain management. *Archives of Surgery, 129*(2), 128–132.

Hopkin, K. (1997). Show me where it hurts: Tracing the pathways of pain. *The Journal of NIH Research, 9*(10), 37–43.

International Association for the Study of Pain Subcommittee on Taxonomy. (1979). Pain terms: A list with definitions and usage. *Pain, 6*, 249–252.

Jonas, W. B. (1993). Evaluating unconventional medical practices. *The Journal of NIH Research, 5*, 64–67.

Jurf, J. B., & Nirschl, A. L. (1993). Acute postoperative pain management: A comprehensive review and update. *Critical Care Nursing Quarterly, 16*(1), 8–25.

Karpman, R. R., Del Mar, N., & Bay, C. (1997). Analgesia for emergency centers' orthopaedic patients: Does an ethnic bias exist? *Clinical Orthopaedics & Related Research, 334*, 270–275.

Kehlet, H. (1989). Surgical stress: The role of pain and analgesia. *British Journal of Anesthesia, 63*, 189–195.

Kolcaba, K. (1995). Comfort as process and product, merged in holistic nursing art. *Journal of Holistic Nursing, 13*(2), 117–131.

Kolcaba, K. Y. (1994). A theory of holistic comfort for nursing. *Journal of Advanced Nursing, 19*, 1178–1184.

Kolcaba, K. Y., & Fisher, E. (1996). A holistic perspective on comfort care as an advance directive. *Critical Care Nursing Quarterly, 18*(4), 66–76.

Lander, J., Fowler-Kerry, S., & Hill, A. (1990). Comparison of pain perceptions among males and females. *The Canadian Journal of Nursing Research, 22*(1), 34–41.

Lautenbacher, S., & Rollman, G. B. (1993). Sex differences in responsiveness to painful and non-painful stimuli are dependent upon the stimulation method. *Pain, 33*, 255–264.

Lenz, E. R., Pugh, L. C., Milligan, R. A., Gift, A., & Suppe, F. (1997). The middle-range theory of unpleasant symptoms: An update. *Advances in Nursing Science, 19*(3), 14–27.

Mahon, S. M. (1994). Concept analysis of pain: Implications related to nursing diagnoses. *Nursing Diagnosis, 5*(1), 14–25.

Maxwell, L. E. (1996). Acute pain management: Evaluation of the effectiveness of intravenous patient-controlled analgesia with vascular patients. *Canadian Journal of Cardiovascular Nursing, 7*(1), 10–14.

McCaffery, M., & Ferrell, B. R. (1997). Influence of professional vs. personal role on pain assessment and use of opioids. *Journal of Continuing Education in Nursing, 28*(2), 69–77.

McDonald, D. D. (1994). Gender and ethnic stereotyping and narcotic analgesic administration. *Research in Nursing & Health, 17*, 45–49.

McKinney, C. H., Tims, F. C., Kumar, A. M., & Kumar, M. (1997). The effects of selected classical music and spontaneous imagery on plasma beta-endorphin. *Journal of Behavioral Medicine, 20*(1), 85–99.

Meehan, T. C. (1993). Therapeutic touch and postoperative pain: A Rogerian research study. *Nursing Science Quarterly, 6*(2), 69–78.

Melzack, R. (1996). Gate control theory. *Pain Forum, 5*(1), 128–138.

Melzack, R., & Wall, P. D. (1965). Pain mechanisms: A new theory. *Science, 150*(3699), 971–979.

Mengazzi, J. J., Paris, P. M., Kersteen, C. H., Flynn, B., & Trautman, D. E. (1991). A randomized, controlled trial of the use of music during laceration repair. *Annals of Emergency Medicine, 20*(4), 348–350.

Miaskowski, C. (1997). Innovations in pharmacologic therapies. *Seminars in Oncology Nursing, 13*(1), 30–35.

Miaskowski, C., Nichols, R., Brody, R., & Synold, T. (1994). Assessment of patient satisfaction utilizing the American Pain Society's quality assurance standards on acute and cancer-related pain. *Journal of Pain and Symptom Management, 9*(1), 5–11.

Miaskowski, C., Sutters, K. A., Taiwo, Y. O., & Levine, J. D. (1992). Antinociceptive and motor effects of delta/mu and kappa/mu combinations of intrathecal opioid agonists. *Pain, 49*, 137–144.

Miller, J., Moore, K., Schofield, A., & Ng'andu, N. (1996). A study of discomfort and confusion among elderly surgical patients. *Orthopaedic Nursing, 15*(6), 27–34.

Miller, J., Neelon, V., Dalton, J., Ng'andu, N., Bailey, D., Jr., Layman, E., & Hosfeld, A. (1996). The assessment of discomfort in elderly confused patients: A preliminary study. *Journal of Neuroscience Nursing, 28*(3), 175–182.

Mobily, P. R., Herr, K. A., & Kelley, L. S. (1993). Cognitive-behavioral techniques to reduce pain: A validation study. *International Journal of Nursing Studies, 30*(6), 537–548.

Mobily, P. R., Herr, K. A., & Nicholson, A. C. (1994). Validation of cutaneous stimulation interventions for pain measurement. *International Journal of Nursing Studies, 31*(6), 533–544.

Morse, J. M., Bottorff, J. L., & Hutchinson, S. (1995). The paradox of comfort. *Nursing Research, 44*(1), 14–19.

National Institute of Nursing Research Priority Expert Panel on Symptom Management: Acute Pain. (1994). *National Nursing Research Agenda. Volume 6: Symptom Management: Acute Pain* (NIH Publication No. 94-2421). Bethesda, MD: National Institutes of Health.

Nixon, M., Teschendorff, J., Finney, J., & Karnilowicz, W. (1997). Expanding the nursing repertoire: Effect of massage on post-operative pain. *American Journal of Advanced Nursing, 14*(3), 21–26.

Page, G. G., & Ben-Eliyahu, S. (1997a). The immune-suppressive nature of pain. *Seminars in Oncology Nursing, 13*(1), 10–15.

Page, G. G., & Ben-Eliyahu, S. (1997b). Increased surgery-induced metastasis and suppressed natural killer cell activity during proestrus/estrus in rats. *Breast Cancer Research and Treatment, 45*(2), 159–167.

Paice, J. A. (1991). Unraveling the mystery of pain. *ONF, 18*(5), 843–849.

Pellino, T. A., & Ward, S. E. (1998). Perceived control mediates the relationship between pain severity and patient satisfaction. *Journal of Pain and Symptom Management, 15*(2), 110–116.

Picard, P., Bazin, J. E., Conio, N., Ruiz, F., & Schoeffler, P. (1997). Ketorolac potentiates morphine in postoperative patient-controlled analgesia. *Pain, 73*(3), 401–406.

Puntillo, K. A. (1988). The phenomenon of pain and critical care nursing. *Heart & Lung, 17*(3), 262–271.

Puntillo, K. A. (1990). Pain experiences of intensive care unit patients. *Heart & Lung, 19*(5), 526–533.

Puntillo, K. A., Miaskowski, C., Kehrle, K., Stannard, D., Gleeson, S., & Nye, P. (1997). Relationship between behavioral and physiological indicators of pain, critical care patients' self-reports of pain and opioid administration. *Critical Care Medicine, 25*(7), 1159–1166.

Raftery, K. A., Smith-Coggins, R., & Chen, A. H. (1995). Gender-associated differences in emergency department pain management. *Annals of Emergency Medicine, 26*(4), 414–421.

Schug, S. S., & Fry, R. A. (1994). Continuous regional analgesia in comparison with intravenous opioid administration for routine postoperative pain control. *Anaesthesia, 49*(6), 528–532.

Scott, D. A., Beilby, D. S., & McClymont, C. (1995). Postoperative analgesia using epidural infusions of fentanyl with bupivacaine. A prospective analysis of 1,014 patients. *Anesthesiology, 83*(4), 727–737.

Scott, I. E. (1994). Effectiveness of documented assessment of postoperative pain. *British Journal of Nursing, 3*(10), 494–501.

Sidebotham, D., Monique, R. J., Dijkhuizen, R. J., & Schug, S. A. (1997). The safety and utilization of patient-controlled analgesia. *Journal of Pain and Symptom Management, 14*(4), 202–209.

Simon, J. M., Baumann, M. A., & Nolan, L. (1995). Differential diagnostic validation: Acute and chronic pain. *Nursing Diagnosis, 6*(2), 73–79.

Simpson, T., Wahl, G., DeTraglia, M., Speck, E., & Taylor, D. (1992). The effects of epidural versus parenteral opioid analgesia on postoperative pain and pulmonary function in adults who have undergone thoracic and abdominal surgery: A critique of research. *Heart & Lung, 21*(2), 125–138.

Sindhu, F. (1996). Are non-pharmacological nursing interventions for the management of pain effective? A meta-analysis. *Journal of Advanced Nursing, 24*, 1152–1159.

Snell, K. C., Fothergill-Bourbonnais, F., & Durocher-Hendriks, S. (1997). Patient-controlled analgesia and intramuscular injections: A comparison of patient pain experiences and postoperative outcomes. *Journal of Advanced Nursing, 25*, 681–690.

Stein, C., & Yassouridis, A. (1997). Peripheral morphine analgesia. *Pain, 71*(2), 119–121.

Stevenson, C. (1995). Non-pharmacological aspects of acute pain management. *Complementary Therapies in Nursing and Midwifery, 1*(3), 77–84.

Sullivan, L. M. (1994). Factors influencing pain management: A nursing perspective. *Journal of Post Anesthesia Nursing, 9*(2), 83–90.

Thomas, V. J., & Rose, F. D. (1993). Patient-controlled analgesia: A new method for old. *Journal of Advanced Nursing*(18), 1719–1726.

Tittle, M., & McMillan, S. C. (1994). Pain and pain-related side effects in an ICU and on a surgical unit: Nurses' management. *American Journal of Critical Care, 3*(1), 25–30.

Turner, J. A., Deyo, R. A., Loeser, J. D., Von Korff, M., & Fordyce, W. E. (1994). The importance of placebo effects in pain treatment and research. *JAMA, 271*(20), 1609–1614.

Tusek, D., Church, J. M., Strong, S. A., Grass, J. A., & Fazio, V. W. (1997). Guided imagery: A significant advance in the care of patients undergoing elective colorectal surgery. *Diseases of the Colon Rectum, 40*(2), 172–178.

Vallerand, A. H. (1995). Gender differences in pain. *Image: The Journal of Nursing Scholarship, 19*(3), 14–27.

Vendlinski, S., & Kolcaba, K. Y. (1997). Comfort care: A framework for hospice nursing. *The American Journal of Hospice and Palliative Care, 14*, 271–276.

Villarruel, A. M., & de Montellano, B. O. (1992). Culture and pain: A Mesoamerican perspective. *Advances in Nursing Science, 15*(1), 21–32.

Voigt, L., Paice, J. A., & Pouliot, J. (1995). Standardized pain flowsheet: Impact on patient-reported pain experiences after cardiovascular surgery. *American Journal of Critical Care, 4*(4), 308–313.

Wakefield, A. B. (1995). Pain: An account of nurses' talk. *Journal of Advanced Nursing*(21), 905–910.

Wall, P. D., & Melzack, R. (1994). *Textbook of pain* (3rd ed.). New York: Churchill Livingstone.

Wallace, K. G., Reed, B. A., Pasero, C., & Olsson, G. L. (1995). Staff nurses' perceptions of barriers to effective pain management. *Journal of Pain & Symptom Management, 10*(3), 204–213.

Ward, S. E., & Gordon, D. (1994). Application of the American Pain Society quality assurance standards. *Pain, 56*, 299–306.

Ward, S. E., & Gordon, D. B. (1996). Patient satisfaction and pain severity as outcomes in pain management: A longitudinal view of one setting's experience. *Journal of Pain and Symptom Management, 11*(4), 242–251.

Warfield, C. A., & Kahn, C. H. (1995). Acute pain management. Programs in U.S. hospitals and experiences and attitudes among U.S. adults. *Anesthesiology, 83*(5), 1090–1094.

Whipple, B., & Glynn, N. J. (1992). Quantification of the effects of listening to music as a noninvasive method of pain control. *Scholarly Inquiry for Nursing Practice, 6*(1), 43–62.

Williams, C. (1996). Patient-controlled analgesia: A review of the literature. *Journal of Clinical Nursing, 5*, 139–147.

Winefield, H. R., Katsikitis, M., Hart, L. M., & Rounsefell, B. F. (1990). Postoperative pain experiences: Relevant patient and staff attitudes. *Journal of Psychomatic Research, 34*(5), 543–552.

Woolf, C. J., & Chong, M. S. (1993). Preemptive analgesia: Treating postoperative pain by preventing the establishment of central sensitization. *Anesthesia and Analgesia, 77,* 362–379.

Zalon, M. L. (1995). Pain management instruction in nursing curricula. *Journal of Nursing Education, 34*(6), 262–267.

Zalon, M. L. (1997). Pain in frail, elderly women after surgery. *Image: Journal of Nursing Scholarship, 29*(1), 21–26.

Zeller, R., Good, M., Anderson, G. C., & Zeller, D. (1997). Strengthening experimental design by balancing confounding variables across eight treatment groups. *Nursing Research, 46*(6), 345–349.

Zimmerman, L., Nieveen, J., Barnason, S., & Schmaderer, M. (1996). The effects of music interventions on postoperative pain and sleep in coronary artery bypass graft (CABG) patients. *Scholarly Inquiry for Nursing Practice: An International Journal, 10*(2), 153–174.

Chapter 6

The Chronobiology, Chronopharmacology, and Chronotherapeutics of Pain

Susan E. Auvil-Novak

ABSTRACT

Data for this review of chronobiology, chronopharmacology, chronotherapeutics and pain were derived from electronic searches of the medical
literature (Medline) utilizing both Silver Platter and OVID search engines.
Further information was obtained from personal conversations with members of the International Society for Chronobiology involved in chronopharmacology and pain research and reviews of non-Medline-referenced
materials and journals such as Chronobiologia and the Annual Review of
Chronopharmacology. A variety of data from proceedings were available,
but was not utilized because of their nonrefereed status and the relative
unavailability of such sources; however, peer-reviewed, published proceedings have been included in this review.

A total of 62 studies were identified as relevant to this review of
biological rhythms and pain; of these, only 6 were conducted by nurses.
Studies were broadly categorized by purpose as experimental chronobiology
in humans (9), experimental chronobiology in animals (12), clinical chronobiology (25), chronopharmacology in animals (6), chronopharmacology
in humans (6), and chronotherapeutic interventions (4). All statistically
significant findings were reported at the $p < 0.05$ level.

Keywords: Pain, Circadian Rhythm, Chronobiology, Chronopharmacology, Chronotherapeutics

THE UBIQUITOUS NATURE OF PAIN

Millions of individuals throughout the world have the common experience of
pain each day. Despite the widespread availability of pharmacologic agents

and the advent of automatic drug delivery devices, pain is one of the most frequently encountered clinical problems. Recently, federal agencies published several guidelines regarding clinical practice policies for management of pain describing the severity of the problem. Both acute pain (Acute Pain Management Guideline Panel, 1992) and intractable cancer pain (Cancer Pain Management Guideline Panel, 1994) have been identified as areas of concern.

The undertreatment of both acute and chronic pain has been extensively documented over the past decade. Findings from previous research suggest that serious deficiencies exist in the establishment of analgesic dosage regimens for satisfactory relief of pain (Acute Pain Management Guideline Panel, 1992; Atwell et al., 1984; Austin, Stapleton, & Mather, 1980a, b; Cancer Pain Management Guideline Panel, 1994; Jacox, Ferrel, Heidrich, Hester, & Miakowski, 1992; Spetzler & Anderson, 1987).

Variability in the absorption rate of injections and delays in narcotic administration have been cited as factors resulting in inadequate analgesia. Further, several studies indicate that nurses and physicians have difficulty accurately assessing the patient's analgesic requirements, though only recently has the magnitude of this problem been recognized. A vicious cycle of pain anxiety, fear, helplessness, and sleep deprivation develops in patients experiencing acute pain (Acute Pain Management Guideline Panel, 1992) and chronic pain can exacerbate individual suffering by worsening common feelings of anxiety, helplessness, and depression (Cancer Pain Management Guideline Panel, 1994).

Historically, medical research has focused on either the development of more potent analgesics, slow release formulations, or automatic drug delivery devices in the search for improved pain relief. Advances in programmable pump technology and patient-controlled analgesia (PCA) have yielded significant decreases in the time required to deliver medication when compared to traditional analgesic delivery via either oral or intramuscular routes. Yet these strategies have failed to effectively alleviate suffering. Pain relief remains an elusive goal for many individuals.

Analgesic therapy has traditionally been administered based on the homeostatic assumption that the most effective way to maintain a constant level of medication in the blood is to give relatively constant doses of an agent over time. Thus, it is hypothesized that the body will maintain a steady state plasma concentration of drug. However, research has demonstrated that physiologic functions do not remain constant, but rather vary predictably over time.

The study of biological time structure is an emerging discipline known as "chronobiology." The evaluation of biological rhythms has provided important clues in determination of the efficacy of analgesic administration and the development of new therapies in the treatment of pain. A greater emphasis on rhythmicity may provide strategies for more effective pain relief.

During the last several decades numerous studies have demonstrated that pharmacologic properties and therapeutic effects vary with the time of administration. This evaluation of time-dependent differences in pharmacologic activity is often referred to as chronopharmacology. This rhythmicity has been only partially explored in relation to the effectiveness of analgesia and pain relief.

BIOLOGICAL RHYTHM RESEARCH

Biological rhythms are genetic in origin, persist without time clue or cue, can be characterized for a species with inter-individual differences, and are influenced by cyclic variations of environmental factors called "zeitgebers" or "synchronizers" (Reinberg & Smolensky, 1983). Inside the body, rhythms oscillate with different periods and represent statistically significant biological changes that occur in reproducible waveforms. These patterns may have periods from seconds to years, and the rhythms of many functions may overlap, producing elaborate changes in physiological function over time.

A rhythm may be characterized in terms of the duration of a cycle (τ or period); the time series average (M or mesor); the variability of the rhythm (A amplitude), and the crest time (ϕ or acrophase). Rhythms of various lengths may be studied, including: Ultradian ($<$ 1 to 20 hr), infradian (greater than 28 hr); circaceptan (rhythms of about a week); Circannual (seasonal, 12-month), and circatrigenitan or circamensal (30-day or monthly). Circadian (20–28 hr) rhythms are most frequently measured.

Chronobiologic research methods require that biological markers or processes be measured over several natural time cycles (seconds, minutes, hours, days, months, or years). These measurements are analyzed statistically using several different methods, and the characteristics of the resulting rhythm are defined (Reinberg, 1992).

The identification and description of the characteristics of a rhythm is often the initial phase of biological rhythm research. These descriptive studies are often referred to as "rhythm hunts." The majority of all chronobiologic studies currently published are of this type. Once the rhythm of interest has been identified, and characteristics defined, the second phase of biological rhythm research is to identify the mechanisms that drive the rhythmic nature of the phenomena of interest. These first two phases of research are typically performed in both animals and humans, and can be biological or pharmacological in nature. The third phase of clinical research in biological rhythms is the development of interventions and therapies that will improve the outcome or effectiveness of treatment.

CHRONOBIOLOGIC STUDIES IN EXPERIMENTAL POPULATIONS

Early efforts by researchers to define a pain signature in time measured responses to experimentally induced pain. The stimulus most often used was electric shock, although thermal gradients were also utilized. In these early studies, painful stimuli were applied to various anatomical sites in both humans and animals. Experimentally induced pain was used to mimic the effects of clinical disease. Differences in thresholds to pain and tolerance to noxious stimuli were commonly measured.

Experimental Pain Studies in Humans

The earliest documented chronobiologic studies of pain occurred just prior to the beginning of World War I and involved the experimental induction of painful stimuli to healthy humans. Two researchers (Grabfield & Martin, 1912) (Martin & Grabfield, 1914) detected circadian variations in the sensory threshold of electrically induced painful stimuli in humans. Greatest irritability (lowest tolerance) occurred at 1030 hrs, while lowest irritability was found to exist at two time periods, 2330–0100 and 0400–0500 hrs. In 1937, Jores and Frees applied electrical stimuli to teeth and discovered a circadian variation in dental pain, with peak pain threshold or minimum pain occurring at about 1600 hrs.

Procacci and others (Procacci, Della Corte, Zoppi, & Maresca, 1974), in a study of 19 men and 35 women, experimentally induced painful thermal stimuli to the skin during the subject's waking hours. The authors demonstrated the presence of diurnal changes in the cutaneous pain threshold in these subjects with an increase in pain sensitivity in the evening hours. This was the first study to demonstrate gender-related differences in peak pain threshold. Maximal pain intensity in male subjects peaked 1 to 3 hours earlier than female subjects, depending on the stage of the woman's menstrual cycle.

Davis, Buchsbaum, and Bunney (1978) discovered, using a group of 35 subjects, that those having somatosensory evoked potentials recorded in the morning were significantly less pain-sensitive for both response criterion and sensitivity measures when compared to those tested in the evening. In 136 male volunteers, thermal stimulus or electric shock was applied to the front teeth throughout the day (Pollmann & Harris, 1978). The authors found the pain threshold to be maximal in the early afternoon and minimal in the early morning. One subject was tested for 3 years and a circannual (annual) rhythm was discovered with maximum pain threshold in October and minimum in May.

In eleven subjects, Strian and co-workers (Strian, Lautenbacher, Galfe, & Holzl, 1989) found diurnal variations, specific to pain in some subjects when both hot and cold thermal stimuli were applied to the hand and foot at various times for 2 days. The authors discovered the existence of a period of time of increased pain sensitivity between 1500–2300 hrs. Although the researchers state that their findings were consistent with other studies, they believed their data to be inconclusive.

Gobel and Cordes (1990) applied painful stimuli to the cranial muscles in 12 healthy men using a modified pressure cuff. Intensity of pain was measured on a Likert-type scale. The authors found that pain sensitivity was lowest at 1400 hrs and reached a peak at 0200 hrs. No time-of-day difference in pain threshold was noted. However, a gender effect was identified, with women possessing twice the sensitivity of men.

Bourdalle-Badie and others (Bourdalle-Badie, Bruguerolle, Labreque, Robert, & Erny, 1990) used the nociceptive flexion reflex and a verbal scale to measure circadian variation in pain in five men. Electric stimuli were applied during 6 4-hour time periods throughout several days of testing. Reflex threshold was highest in the late afternoon (1700 hrs) and lowest in the early morning (0100 hrs) but pain intensity, as measured by the verbal scale, was highest in the early morning (0400 hrs).

Experimental Pain Studies in Animals

Beginning in the 1970s, experimental studies measuring the response and tolerance to painful stimuli were also performed in animal models. Results from some of the first studies suggested that a daily rhythmic change in the tolerance to noxious stimuli existed in healthy mice kept on a 12/12 light-dark cycle with lights on at 0600 hrs (Frederickson, Burgis, & Edwards, 1977; Wesche & Frederickson, 1978, 1981). Using the hot plate test, the optimum time of stimulus tolerance was found to be at the end of the normal rest and beginning of the normal activity period (evening), while minimum tolerance was found to exist during the beginning of the normal rest period (morning). It was found that hypophysectomy did not alter the time-dependent nature of either stimulus tolerance or brain levels of met-enkephelin.

Similar results have been discovered in other predominantly nocturnal rodent species and in the hamster (Bodnar, Kelly, Spiaggia, & Glussman, 1978; Buckett, 1981; Crockett, Bornschein, & Smith, 1977; Kavaliers & Hirst, 1983; Kavaliers, Hirst, & Tesky, 1983; Kavaliers & Ossenkopp, 1988; Pickard, 1987). Hamra and others (Hamra, Kamerling, Wolfsheimer, & Bagwell, 1993) measured pain sensitivity in horses on a normal summer photoperiod (10/14 light-dark). Responses to pain were best tolerated at 0900 hrs with a secondary peak at 1500 hrs. Levels of circulating endorphins were found to be highest during the early activity phase.

Both circadian (24-hour) and circamensal (estrus-related) changes in tolerance to pain have been studied in rats (Martinez-Gomez, Cruz, Salas, Hudson, & Pachero, 1994). Female rats on a 12/12 light-dark cycle were evaluated for response to noxious stimulus using the tail-flick method. Measurements were taken shortly after lights on (just before sleep) and 2 and 8 hours after lights off (activity period). It was determined that maximum threshold to pain occurred early in the activity period and that lower thresholds to pain were associated with estrus. It was further discovered that ovariectomy had no effect on circadian variation in pain threshold, but completely eliminated circamensal rhythms.

Factors Influencing Experimental Pain Study Outcomes

In animals, experimentally induced pain is generally found to be best tolerated near the beginning of the activity span and least tolerated near the beginning of the rest cycle, regardless of the nocturnal or diurnal nature of the species studied. In contrast, human experimental studies have reported conflicting results, with peak intensity of pain occurring either in the morning, afternoon or evening, but consistently most severe during the waking hours. These discrepancies may be related to several factors. The type of stimulus used for induction of experimental pain, and the part of the anatomy to which the stimulus was applied, was not consistent across these studies. Further, a variety of different stimuli of varying intensity was presented to diverse human populations, in contrast to the strict genetic control achieved with animal populations. In addition, although animal subjects were synchronized to a sleep-activity or light-dark schedule (generally 12 hours of light and 12 hours of dark), no such synchronization was reported in human experimental studies. This finding is relevant because the sleep-activity pattern is one of the most important synchronizers of human biological rhythms. Further, dietary intake is highly variable among human subjects. It is not known to what extent caffeine, alcohol, or medications may have impacted the sleep-wake patterns of these individuals. It has also rarely been reported whether or not any of the individuals participating in the study were shift workers. In contrast to the strictly controlled light and dietary patterns of laboratory animals, assumptions cannot be made about activity and dietary patterns of human volunteers.

CHRONOBIOLOGIC STUDIES IN CLINICAL POPULATIONS

Several studies have suggested that various circadian and other rhythms exist in a variety of diseases. Rhythms of pain severity differ with the type of disease and with health and degree of pain involved. The identification and characterization of pain rhythms in clinical populations is relatively new. Studies that identify rhythmicity in pain for a variety of populations began during the 1970s and may be of either prospective or retrospective design.

Chronic Pain

Folkard and others (Folkard, Glynn, & Lloyd, 1976) identified a temporal pattern in intensity of intractable pain experienced by 41 patients independent of the cause of pain or the use of analgesics. Clients in a hospital pain unit were asked to subjectively self-rate individual pain intensity and alertness using a visual analog scale, and to monitor oral temperature every 2 hours while awake, for a 7-day period. These same clients also completed the Eysenck Personality Inventory that provides scores on personality dimensions of extraversion, neuroticism, and social conformity. Results indicated that pain increased over the day, except for two peaks at 1200 and 1800, with the acrophase estimated to occur around 20.30 hours. Investigators also found that female subjects rated their pain as more intense than male subjects, and that clients who went outside of the home to work experienced less pain than those who stayed at home. No support for the relationship between pain sensitivity and temperature or pain and alertness was demonstrated.

Diurnal variation in pain has also been found in arthritic patients. Levi and others (Levi, Le Louarn, & Reinberg, 1985) found that osteoarthritis of the hip and knee had different peak times for pain in the 517 patients studied. Biological rhythmicity was discovered in 14 rheumatoid arthritis patients for symptoms of disease (pain and stiffness) when compared to age- and gender-matched controls (Bellamy, Sothern, Campbell, & Buchanan, 1991). It was discovered that peak pain and stiffness occurred in the morning upon rising, and troughs in these symptoms occurred in the afternoon. In general, research findings suggest that patients with osteoarthritis reported maximal pain at the end of the day, while patients with rheumatoid arthritis experienced an early morning peak in pain perception.

Several studies have been performed on pain related to cardiovascular disease. One of the first clinical research projects to study biological rhythms and cardiovascular pain was performed by Master (1960). A later study by Mattioli and others (Mattioli, Cioni, & Adreoli, 1986) validated the previous findings that a rhythm in angina existed, with peak episodes occurring between 0500–0800 hrs. In this same study, the addition of pharmacotherapy reduced the number of angina episodes in 187 patients who had not previously received medication, but did not change the peak time of the angina attack.

A peak in morning chest pain frequency related to myocardial ischemia has been reproduced with similar results in several studies involving hundreds of subjects (Beamer et al., 1987; Cannon et al., 1997; Hausmann, Licthlen, Nikutta, Wenzlaff, & Daniel, 1991; Thompson, Sutton, Jowett, & Pohl, 1991).

Circadian changes have also been recorded in severity and symptoms of headache in a few studies. Early work suggested a morning peak in migraine occurrence and pain with an evening trough (Ostfeld, 1963). Migraine head-aches were also studied by Solomon (1992) who studied 15 subjects with headache for 20 weeks. In the 215 episodes recorded, a significant rhythm was discovered with peak time at 1000 hrs and trough at 2400 hrs.

Despite large numbers of subjects, little research has been performed on chronic cancer pain. Bruera, Macmillan, Kuehn, and Miller (1992) found that in 61 cancer patients, extra doses of opioid analgesics were administered between 1000–2200 hrs. Another study (Sittl, Kamp, & Knoll, 1990) used a visual analog scale (VAS) on chronic patients and determined that peak pain occurred at 1800 hrs.

Two other studies evaluated cancer pain in patients using visual analogue and verbal scales. Vanier and others (Vanier, Labreque, & Lepage-Savary, 1992) studied 8 cancer patients and discovered the greatest demand for hydro-morphone delivered by PCA pump between 1800–2200 hrs. Pain scores at 2200 hrs were double the magnitude of those measured at 1400 hrs.

In a related study (Wilder-Smith, Schimke, & Bettiga, 1992) highest pain intensity in 20 patients as measured by a verbal scale was found during the waking hours (0800–2200 hrs.) when compared to pain during the night. Standard 16 mg.-doses of morphine were administered at 4-hour intervals around the clock.

Acute Pain

Circadian rhythms in pain have also been recorded in patients with sickle-cell disease. Auvil-Novak, Novak, and El Sanadi (1996) discovered a peak emergency room presentation time in the early evening for patients with sickle-cell vaso-occlusive pain crisis. A potential mechanism for this process has been suggested from a study of eight patients receiving meperidine for therapy (Ritschel, Bykadi, Ford, Bloomfield, & Levy, 1983). It was discovered that evening elimination half-life was 46% greater and serum levels were 70% lower when compared to morning values. Further, a significant correlation was found for blood drug level during the morning, but not during the evening.

In a group of dental patients, 5,706 demands for analgesics after dental surgery demonstrated significant circadian and weekly variation. During days 2 and 3 postoperatively, patients demonstrated a morning peak, reversing to an evening peak on day 6 and 7 resulting from post-dental surgery (Pollmann & Hildebrandt, 1987).

Graves and others (1983) used patient-controlled analgesia therapy to identify a circadian rhythm in the morphine requirements of 46 patients undergoing elective gastric bypass surgery. Pain and sedation status were evaluated every 2 hours. Data collected from the PCA pumps by residents were analyzed in 2-hour periods for a 36–72 hour duration when patients were allowed to use the pumps. The investigators identified that sedation rankings at 0300 were significantly higher than rankings at 0900, 1500, 2100, indicating a tendency towards lower sedation rankings in the daytime and higher sedation levels at night. Peak morphine utilization in these postsurgical patients was determined to occur at 0900 and was the lowest at 0300.

A study of 19 postsurgical gynecologic cancer patients examined retrospectively 24-hour patterns in self-administered boluses of morphine and hydromorphone achieved with a PCA pump (Auvil-Novak et al., 1988). For 9 patients receiving morphine and 10 receiving hydromorphone, peak demand occurred in the early morning and was lowest during the night. It was also discovered that this increased demand for analgesic during the morning was frequently unfulfilled because of the lockout interval utilized in the current regimen in PCA delivery. Patients apparently were unable to receive adequate quantities of analgesic for pain relief, despite the use of a concurrent, continuous basal dose of analgesic.

In a follow-up analysis (Auvil-Novak, Novak, Smolensky, Morris, & Kwan, 1990) a similar patient subset consisting of 45 gynecologic oncology patients was retrospectively studied at the same cancer center. All patients received only morphine sulfate following exploratory laparotomy with vertical midline incision for gynecologic malignancies without the use of a concurrent basal infusion. In this sample of patients, both 12- and 24-hour rhythms were confirmed, with the major peak in morphine sulfate delivery between 0800 and 1200 and a second minor peak occurring approximately 12 hours later. Results from both studies suggests that most of the patients were required to use the pump continuously throughout the 24 hour period, and were awake all night in an effort to maintain adequate analgesia, thus preventing normal sleep.

Similar results of sleep disturbance have been documented by Closs (1990, 1992) in 170 post-surgical patients who had their sleep disturbed by pain during their hospital stay, and a follow-up study that examined nurses' patterns of analgesic provision to 36 patients throughout the day. The author found that less analgesic was administered by the nurse during the night shift when compared to either day or evening shifts. The 24-hour pattern in administration of intramuscular opiates indicated lower provisions of analgesic during the night. Although the author speculated that circadian rhythms might provide the rationale for the findings, the explanation was quickly dismissed as unlikely, since the patients claimed they awoke during the night in pain.

In contrast, a double-blind study of 55 thoracic and abdominal surgical patients (Labreque, Lepage-Savary, & Poulin, 1988) demonstrated a rhythmic peak in pain, as measured by VAS, between 1830 hr and 1915 hr when morphine was delivered subcutaneously either continuously or every 4 hours by injection. A subsequent study by the authors conducted in 24 patients who had abdominal surgery demonstrated dual peaks of morphine requirements occurring between 0800 and 1200 hr and 1600 and 2000 hr (Dunn, Blouin, & Labreque, 1993).

Factors Influencing Clinical Study Outcomes

Research findings within clinical populations appear to be relatively congruent, and maximal pain was reported to occur either in the morning (rheumatoid arthritis, angina, migraine, dental, gastric bypass); evening (cancer, sickle cell, postsurgical thoracic and abdominal); or both morning and evening (postsurgical gynecologic oncology, general surgical, and postsurgical abdominal). It is unclear why this temporal variability in pain of various etiology occurs, and it is not known to what extent measurement issues may impact the findings.

Several different measures have been utilized to identify the timing of maximal pain in various clinical populations. Visual analog scales, verbal scales, analgesic utilization patterns, and time of emergency room presentation have all been used as measures of pain. Only two studies reported how visual analog and verbal rating scales were anchored in time, indicating whether or not they were measuring the perception of pain in the immediate present or over a specified period of time. A single pain measurement may be reflective of either a) the current pain level, b) the average pain occurring during the period, or c) the highest level of pain occurring during the period. This is in contrast to describing the frequency of data collection. When performing time-dependent research, anchoring the instrument in time is essential for accurate comparison of several cycles of data.

Only one study addressed the relationship between analgesic requirements and pain perception. In a study of 71 postsurgical gynecologic oncology patients, (Auvil-Novak, 1992) a significant relationship was demonstrated between patients' perception of pain as measured by VAS and attempts at analgesic administration for two postoperative days using the PCA pump. A positive relationship between pain intensity scores and requests for analgesic was supported in that study.

Further, the studies that utilized time of emergency room presentation made the assumption that maximal pain perception would result in the individual seeking treatment. This assumption has yet to be validated.

The results of these studies suggest that careful interpretation of the data must be made given the subtle differences in research methodologies. Further differences across clinical populations such as variations in hospital routines, individual unit activity patterns, dietary intake, and supplemental medications need to be addressed when comparing the reported results. Within populations factors such as type of surgery, analgesic agent used, drug delivery method favored, and even statistical analysis methods may impact study results.

Experimental Versus Clinical Studies

The results from studies of humans with clinically related pain must be reviewed separately from studies of experimental pain. Temporal responses to painful stimuli in healthy volunteers and in animal models without disease may be different than pain measured in humans with clinical disease. Healthy subjects may be better able to cope with intermittent stress and pain than individuals with a continuous disease process. Variations in the location and duration of clinical versus experimental pain would likely yield differences in study results. Painful stimuli are applied to experimental volunteers in epochs significantly lower in duration and intensity when compared to clinically related pain. External stimulation cannot adequately reflect clinical pain symptomology. The manifestation of clinical pain includes variables beyond simple pain stimulus and reception. For example, electric current applied to teeth may accurately mimic clinical dental pain, but not the pathophysiology. Researchers cannot reproduce the inflammatory response and the release of algogenic substances at the incision or injury site that is present with clinical pain.

All of the clinical research studies reviewed have identified a rhythm of a particular period for a specific disease. Further research is required to adequately identify and characterize pain rhythms in new populations and to validate previously identified rhythms.

CHRONOPHARMACOLOGIC STUDIES IN PAIN

Pharmacologic agents are administered to individuals to enhance the probability of a desired outcome. Chronopharmacology is, more precisely, the study of the influence of biological rhythms on the kinetics and pharmacodynamics of medications, including how pharmacologic agents and the timing of their administration affect biological rhythm structure (Reinberg & Smolensky, 1983). Chronopharmacologic research can further be classified into studies related to chronopharmacokinetics, chronesthesy, and chronergy. Chronopharmacokinetics refers to rhythmic influences in the bioavailability, metabolism, and excretion of medicines, while chronesthesy is defined as rhythmic changes in the susceptibility of target biosystems to medications or metabolites. Chronesthesy usually involves studies of periodic changes in receptors or membrane phenomena. Chronergy refers to the rhythmic changes in any effect of an agent, and involves both the desired effect, chronoeffectiveness, and the corresponding undesired effect, chronotoxicity (Reinberg, Smolensky, & Labreque, 1986). Several studies related to pain relief have been chronopharmacologic in nature. Chronopharmacologic studies in pain have been useful in understanding mechanisms of action of analgesics agents and the neurochemistry of pain.

Chronopharmacologic Studies in Animals

Endorphins are neurotransmitters located at most of the synaptic relay points of major pain pathways ranging from the sites in the dorsal horn of the spinal cord, periaqueductal gray, thalamus, and cortex. Endorphins appear to be neurotransmitters into interneurons, since they are located in regions critical to the relay or integration of somatosensory information. They appear to modulate transmission at multiple levels of the nervous system (Davis, 1983). Enkephalins appear to provide similar functions. Endorphins interact with several other pathways in which serotonin, substance P, norepinephrine, melatonin, and cholecystokinin are active. Endorphins are present in the brain and in the pituitary. Many effects of pituitary beta-endorphin (B-EP) have been associated with the actions of adrenocorticotropin (ACTH).

It has been demonstrated in 42 male albino rats (Kelly, 1979), exposed to stressful stimuli and then sacrificed 20 minutes after, that ACTH and beta-lipoprotein (B-LPH) are secreted concomitantly. Research suggests that basal levels of ACTH/B-LPH/B-EP in rat plasma are not constant, but manifest parallel circadian rhythmicity (Voulteenaho, Leppalouoto, & Mannisto, 1982). These circadian changes are ultimately coordinated by the suprachiasmatic nucleus (Moore-Ede, Czeisler, & Richardson, 1983; Suda, Hayaishi, & Nakagawa, 1979).

Other research (Davis, 1983) suggests pituitary beta-endorphin might mediate circadian changes in pain sensitivity, since 24-hour variation in pain appreciation follows circadian rhythmicity in adrenocorticotropin secretion. Voulteenaho and others (1982) demonstrated that basal levels of adrenocorticotropin, beta-lipoprotein, and beta-endorphin in the plasma of rats exhibit parallel circadian rhythms.

Wesche and Frederickson (Wesche & Frederickson, 1981) further demonstrated that hypophysectomy does not alter variation in the responsiveness of mice to pain. In addition, they further identified a similar 24-hour rhythm in pituitary and brain endorphins (Wesche & Frederickson, 1978, 1981).

These animal studies were performed primarily on rodents in a controlled laboratory setting. The rhythms discovered may not be applied directly to diurnally active species. Investigations in human subjects are difficult and costly to perform, but are requisite for affirmation of neurochemical rhythms.

Chronopharmacologic Studies in Man

Rhythmicity in circulating endorphin levels has also been detected in man. Ten healthy male volunteers, ages 20–32, were studied in a sleep laboratory where blood samples were obtained every 2 hours for a 24-hour period. Circadian variation of Beta-endorphin (B-EP) was established with the lowest levels between 2200 and 0330 hours and the highest levels between 0400 and 1000. There was also a correlation with cortisol levels suggesting a similar secretory pattern between B-EP and ACTH (Dent et al., 1981). Rhythmic alteration of neurotransmitters at the synaptic relay points of major pain pathways suggests that temporal variation in pain stimulus reception is probable.

Data suggest that individual differences in pain sensitivity are mediated by endorphins. In an early study (Buchsbaum, Davis, & Bunney, 1977) 21 healthy subjects were divided into pain-sensitive and pain-insensitive subgroups, and experimental electric shocks were administered. The insensitive subjects found electric shock significantly more painful after naloxone administration, while the sensitive group experienced the shocks as less painful. Evoked potentials demonstrated similar significant group differences.

Naber and others (1981) discovered circadian rhythms in cerebral spinal fluid (CSF) and plasma of an opioid substance in monkeys and humans when sampled every 2 hours. A peak in the morning at 1000 hrs and a trough at 2200 hrs was reported. These data have been confirmed by others, where a morning peak in plasma beta endorphin levels in 20 neonates and 10 adults was discovered (Hindmarsh, Tan, Sankaran, & Laxdahl, 1989).

The level of CSF endorphins and substance P in patients also appears to correlate with their need for narcotics in the postoperative state (Tamsen, Sakurada, & Wahlstrom, 1982). Basal levels of endorphin may be predictive of how much narcotic a patient will require to control pain in the post-operative period (Tamsen, Hartvig, & Dahlstrom, 1980).

Data obtained both from laboratory studies in animals and clinical studies in humans suggest that circadian variations exist for circulating levels of endorphins, enkephalins, and substance P, with peak levels occurring generally during the activity span. Results of these predictable fluctuations suggest mechanisms for discovered peaks and troughs in tolerance and sensitivity to either external or inherent painful stimuli. As such, these results give credence to the development of chronotherapeutic strategies in pain control.

CHRONOTHERAPEUTIC STUDIES IN PAIN

Once the chronopharmacology of a particular agent is understood, the final aim of performing chronopharmacologic research is the development of pharmacologic therapeutic interventions or chronotherapies. By manipulation of the timing of administration, medications are administered in synchrony with the individual's biological time structure in order to enhance the desired and reduce the undesired effects (Reinberg, 1992; Reinberg & Smolensky, 1983).

Unfortunately, very few researchers have integrated chronobiologic or chronopharmacologic data to develop chronotherapies and test interventions for improved treatment of pain. Development of chronotherapies may be as simple as the modification of routine dosing schedules of orally administered agents, or as complex as the development of analgesic regimens delivered intravenously or epidurally. The origin of these therapies is grounded in the evaluation of temporal changes in either symptomology or pharmacology. Currently, chronotherapies have been developed for arthritis and acute postsurgical pain.

Arthritis

Work in arthritis has produced several studies suggesting that modification of the dosing schedule of nonsteroidal anti-inflammatory agents and glucocorticoid improve pain relief. Clench and others (Clench, Reinberg, Dziewanowska,

Ghata, & Smolensky, 1981) evaluated time-varied single-dose ingestion of indomethacin in 9 subjects. It was discovered that evening ingestion of drug led to smallest peak serum concentration and longest time to peak concentration (longest plasma half-life).

In a study of 517 arthritis patients, Levi and others (Levi et al., 1985) discovered that different times of administration of indomethacin increased dosing tolerance by a factor of four and doubled analgesic effect. Individuals with high levels of pain in the morning had greater pain relief with evening dosing when compared to those with high levels of afternoon pain who benefited most from morning dosing. A later study of 26 rheumatoid arthritis patients (Arvidson, Gudbjornsson, Larsson, & Hallgren, 1997) demonstrated that early morning ingestion (0200 hrs) of a small dose of glucocorticoid improved pain and stiffness and reduced inflammatory modulators when compared to a normal dosing schedule.

Postsurgical Pain

In post-surgical pain Auvil-Novak and others (Auvil-Novak, 1992) developed a chronotherapeutic treatment regimen employing a sinusoidal basal infusion to compare the efficacy of chronotherapeutic versus constant basal and demand-only PCA therapy for postoperative pain relief. Seventy-one postoperative gynecologic oncology patients were randomly assigned to one of three experimental groups; VAS scores for pain intensity, pain relief, the number of unmet attempts, and the number of requests for analgesia were obtained at 4-hr intervals for a 72-hour period postoperatively. Pain intensity scores were significantly lower for chronotherapeutic and constant basal groups when compared to demand-only. Significantly greater pain relief was obtained only by the chronotherapeutic group, and 42% of the constant basal infusion group required at least one dosage reduction due to oversedation, while none of the individuals in either the demand-only or chronotherapeutic regimens required reductions in PCA dose. In addition, 46% of the constant basal group developed atelectasis, as compared to 27% in the demand-only and 10% in the chronotherapeutic group. Findings from these few studies suggest that significantly greater pain relief and decreased toxicity and side effects result from chronotherapeutic regimens.

CONCLUSIONS AND RECOMMENDATIONS FOR FUTURE RESEARCH

There is a paucity of literature investigating biological rhythms in pain perception, given the increased interest in acute and chronic pain relief (Acute Pain Management Guideline Panel, 1992; Cancer Pain Management Guideline

Panel, 1994). The cyclic changes of endogenous opioid compounds in both humans and animals suggest that temporal variation of analgesic administration would improve treatment effectiveness. However, alarmingly few studies have been performed to study time-dependent changes in the pharmacodynamics of analgesics. Even fewer studies utilized chronobiologic principles to develop chronotherapies for pain relief. Of the studies that were reviewed, chronobiologic studies in human populations frequently did not synchronize individuals prior to temporal evaluation, and did not discuss the potential effects of confounding medications. The majority of studies utilized small sample sizes and did not report statistical power. Only two studies referred to the use of a theoretical framework (Auvil-Novak, 1997).

The literature reviewed in this work suggests that the body of knowledge concerning biological rhythms and pain offers insight into the development of analgesic dosing regimens that could optimize pain relief; further research in this area is warranted. Evaluation of a pain signature in time for a variety of disease processes would eventually lead to the development of therapies based on principles of biological rhythm research. Scientific investigation in this area would enhance the effectiveness of current pain therapy regimens. A significant effort should be made to develop clinical studies to further identify and validate rhythms in both acute and chronic pain populations. Results of these studies could readily be used to develop improved analgesic therapies for the improved relief of pain, and reduction of undesired symptoms related to both short- and long-term use of analgesic agents.

Finally, very little of the work on biological rhythms and pain has been performed by nurse researchers. Since the traditional role of nurses has been to provide patient care around the clock, nurses in both clinical and research roles are in a unique position to develop and execute biological rhythm research related to pain and analgesia.

REFERENCES

Acute Pain Management Guideline Panel. (February 1992). *Acute pain management: Operative or medical procedures and trauma: Clinical Practice Guidelines* (AHCPR Publication No. 92-0032). Rockville, MD: Agency for Health Care Policy and Research.

Arvidson, N. G., Gudbjornsson, B., Larsson, A., & Hallgren, R. (1997). The timing of glucocorticoid administration in rheumatoid arthritis. *Annals of the Rheumatic Diseases, 56*, 27–31.

Atwell, R. J., Flanigan, R. C., Bennet, R. L., Allen, D. C., Lucas, B. A., & McRoberts, J. W. (1984). Efficacy of patient-controlled analgesia in patients recovering from flank incisions. *Journal of Urology, 132*, 701–703.

Austin, K. L., Stapleton, J. V., & Mather, L. E. (1980a). Multiple intramuscular injections: A major source of variability in analgesic response to meperidine. *Pain, 8*, 47–62.

Austin, K. L., Stapleton, J. V., & Mather, L. E. (1980b). Relationship between blood meperidine concentration and analgesic response: A preliminary report. *Anesthesiology, 53*, 460–466.

Auvil-Novak, S. E. (1992). *Development and testing of a chronobiologic model for pain management in nursing: Efficacy of chronotherapeutic versus traditional administration of patient-controlled analgesia.* Dissertation Abstracts International. 53(04). 1780B (University Microfilms No. 9223310).

Auvil-Novak, S. E. (1997). A middle-range theory of chronotherapeutic intervention for postsurgical pain. *Nursing Research, 46*, 66–71.

Auvil-Novak, S. E., Novak, R. D., & El Sanadi, N. (1996). Twenty-four-hour pattern in emergency department presentation for sickle cell vaso-occlusive pain crisis. *Chronobiology International, 13*, 449–456.

Auvil-Novak, S. E., Novak, R. D., Smolensky, M. H., Kavanagh, J. J., Kwan, J. W., & Wharton, J. T. (1988). Twenty-four hour variation in self-administration of morphine sulfate (MS) and hydromorphone (H) by post-surgical gynecologic cancer patients. *Annual Review of Chronopharmacology, 5*, 343–346.

Auvil-Novak, S. E., Novak, R. D., Smolensky, M. H., Morris, M., & Kwan, J. W. (1990). Temporal variation in self-administration of morphine sulfate via patient-controlled analgesia in postoperative gynecologic cancer patients. *Annual Review of Chronopharmacology, 7*, 253–256.

Beamer, A. D., Lee, T. H., Cook, E. F., Brand, D. A., Rouan, G. W., Weisberg, M. C., & Goldman, L. (1987). Diagnostic implications for myocardial ischemia of the circadian variation of the onset of chest pain. *American Journal of Cardiology, 60*, 998–1002.

Bellamy, N., Sothern, R. B., Campbell, J., & Buchanan, W. W. (1991). Circadian rhythm in pain, stiffness, and manual dexterity in rheumatoid arthritis: Relation between discomfort and disability. *Annals of the Rheumatic Diseases, 50*, 243–248.

Bodnar, R. J., Kelly, D. D., Spiaggia, A., & Glussman, M. (1978). Biophasic alterations of nociceptive threshold induced by food deprivation. *Physiological Psychology, 6*, 391–395.

Bourdalle-Badie, C., Bruguerolle, B., Labreque, G., Robert, S., & Erny, P. (1990). Biological rhythms in pain and anesthesia. *Annual Review of Chronopharmacology, 6*, 155–182.

Bruera, E., Macmillan, K., Kuehn, N., & Miller, M. J. (1992). Circadian distribution of extra doses of narcotic analgesics in patients with cancer pain: A preliminary report. *Pain, 49*, 311–314.

Buchsbaum, M. S., Davis, G. C., & Bunney, W. E. (1977). Naloxone alters pain perception and somatosensory evoked potentials in normal subjects. *Nature, 270*, 620–622.

Buckett, W. R. (1981). Circadian and seasonal rhythm in stimulation produced analgesia. *Experientia, 37*, 878–880.

Cancer Pain Management Guideline Panel. (March, 1994). *Management of cancer pain: Clinical Practice Guidelines* (AHCPR Publication No. 94-0592). Rockville, MD: Agency for Health Care Policy and Research.

Cannon, C. P., McCabe, C. H., Stone, P. H., Schactman, M., Thompson, B., Theroux, P., Gibson, R. S., Feldman, T., Kleinman, N. S., Tofler, G. H., Mueller, J. E., Chaitman, B. R., & Braunwald, E. (1997). Circadian variation in the onset of unstable angina and non-Q-wave acute myocardial infarction (the TIMI III Registry and TIMI IIIB Source). *American Journal of Cardiology, 79,* 253–258.

Clench, J., Reinberg, A., Dziewanowska, Z., Ghata, J., & Smolensky, M. (1981). Circadian changes in the bioavailability and effects of indomethacin in healthy subjects. *European Journal of Clinical Pharmacology, 20,* 359–369.

Closs, S. J. (1990). An exploratory analysis of nurses: Provision of postoperative analgesic drugs. *Journal of Advanced Nursing, 15,* 42–49.

Closs, S. J. (1992). Patient's night-time pain, analgesic provision and sleep after surgery. *International Journal of Nursing Studies, 29,* 381–392.

Crockett, R. S., Bornschein, R. L., & Smith, R. P. (1977). Diurnal variation in response to thermal stimulation mouse hot–plate test. *Physiology & Behavior, 18,* 193–196.

Davis, G. C. (1983). Endorphins and pain. *Psychiatric Clinics of North America, 6,* 473–487.

Davis, G. C., Buchsbaum, M. S., & Bunney, W. E. (1978). Naloxone decreases diurnal variation in pain sensitivity and somatosensory evoked potentials. *Life Sciences, 23,* 1449–1460.

Dent, R. R., Guillemault, C., Albert, L. H., Posner, B. I., Cox, B. M., & Goldstein, A. (1981). Diurnal rhythm of plasma immunoreactive beta-endorphin and its relationship to sleep stages and plasma rhythms of cortisol and prolactin. *Journal of Clinical Endocrinology and Metabolism, 52,* 942–947.

Dunn, M., Blouin, D., & Labreque, G. (1993). Time-dependent variations in morphine-requirements in patients with postoperative pain. In G. Labreque (Ed.), *Proceedings of the 21st Conference of the International Society of Chronobiology, Quebec, Canada* (pp. III–10). Quebec: The International Society for Chronobiology.

Folkard, S., Glynn, C. J., & Lloyd, J. W. (1976). Diurnal variation and individual differences in the perception of intractable pain. *Journal of Psychiatric Research, 20,* 289–301.

Frederickson, R. C. A., Burgis, V., & Edwards, J. D. (1977). Hyperalgesia induced by naloxone follows diurnal rhythm in responsivity to painful stimuli. *Science, 198,* 756–758.

Gobel, H., & Cordes, P. (1990). Circadian variation of pain sensitivity in pericranial musculature. *Headache, 30,* 418–422.

Grabfield, G. P., & Martin, E. G. (1912). Variations in the sensory threshold for faradic stimulation in normal human subjects: I. The diurnal rhythm. *American Journal of Physiology, 31,* 300–308.

Graves, D. A., Batenhorst, R. L., Bennett, R. L., Wettstein, J. G., Griffen, W. O., Wright, B. D., & Foster, T. S. (1983). Morphine requirements using patient-controlled analgesia: Influence of diurnal variation and morbid obesity. *Clinical Pharmacy, 2,* 48–53.

Hamra, J. G., Kamerling, S. G., Wolfsheimer, K. J., & Bagwell, C. A. (1993). Diurnal variations in plasma ir-Beta-endorphin levels and experimental pain thresholds in the horse. *Life Sciences*, *53*, 121–129.

Hausmann, D., Licthlen, P. R., Nikutta, P., Wenzlaff, P., & Daniel, W. G. (1991). Circadian variation of myocardial ischemia in patients with stable coronary artery disease. *Chronobiology International*, *8*, 385–398.

Hindmarsh, K. W., Tan, L., Sankaran, K., & Laxdahl, V. A. (1989). Diurnal rhythms of cortisol, ACTH and beta-endorphin levels in neonates and adults. *Clinical Investigation*, *151*, 153–156.

Jacox, A., Ferrel, B., Heidrich, G., Hester, N., & Miakowski, C. (1992). A guideline for the nation: Managing acute pain. *American Journal of Nursing*, *5*, 49–55.

Jores, A., & Frees, J. (1937). Die tagenchwankungen der schmertzempfindung (The daily variation found in pain). *Deutsche Medizine Wochenshrift*, *63*, 963.

Kavaliers, M., & Hirst, M. (1983). Daily rhythms of analgesia and mice. *Brain Research*, *279*, 387–393.

Kavaliers, M., Hirst, M., & Tesky, G. C. (1983). Aging, opioid analgesic and the pineal gland. *Life Science*, *32*, 2279–2287.

Kavaliers, M., & Ossenkopp, K. P. (1988). Day-night rhythms of opioid and non-opioid stress induced-analgesia: Differential inhibitory effects of exposure to magnetic fields. *Pain*, *32*, 223–229.

Kelly, D. D. (1979). The role of endorphins in stress-induced analgesia. *Annals of the New York Academy of Sciences*, *398*, 260–271.

Labreque, G., Lepage-Savary, D., & Poulin, E. (1988). Time-dependent variations in morphine induced analgesia. *Annual Review of Chronopharmacology*, *5*, 135–138.

Levi, F., Le Louarn, C., & Reinberg, A. (1985). Timing optimizes sustained-release indomethacin treatment of osteoarthritis. *Clinical Pharmacology and Therapeutics*, *37*, 77–84.

Martin, E. G., & Grabfield, G. B. (1914). Variations in the sensory threshold for faradic stimulation in normal human subjects: I. The nocturnal rhythm. *American Journal of Physiology*, *33*, 415–422.

Martinez-Gomez, M., Cruz, Y., Salas, M., Hudson, R., & Pachero, P. (1994). Assessing pain threshold in the rat: Changes with estrus and time of day. *Physiology and Behavior*, *55*, 651–657.

Master, A. M. (1960). The role of effort and occupation (including physicians) in coronary occlusion. *Journal of the American Medical Association*, *174*, 942–948.

Mattioli, G., Cioni, G., & Adreoli, C. (1986). Time sequence of anginal pain. *Clinical Cardiology*, *9*, 165–169.

Moore-Ede, M. C., Czeisler, C. A., & Richardson, G. S. (1983). Circadian timekeeping in health and disease: 1. Basic properties of circadian pacemakers. *New England Journal of Medicine*, *309*, 469–475.

Naber, D., Cohen, R. M., Pickar, D., Kalin, N. H., Davis, G., Pert, B., & Bunney, W. E. (1981). Episodic secretion of opioid activity in human plasma and monkey CSF: Evidence for a diurnal rhythm. *Life Sciences*, *28*, 931–935.

Ostfeld, A. M. (1963). The natural history and epidemiology of migraine and muscle contraction headache. *Neurology*, *13*, 11–15.

Pickard, G. E. (1987). Circadian rhythm of nociception in the golden hamster. *Brain Research, 425,* 395–400.

Pollmann, L., & Harris, P. H. P. (1978). Rhythmic changes in pain sensitivity in teeth. *International Journal of Chronobiology, 5,* 459–464.

Pollmann, L., & Hildebrandt, G. (1987). Circadian profiles and circaseptan periodicity in the frequency of administration of analgetic drugs after oral surgery. *Functional Neurology, 2,* 231–237.

Procacci, P., Della Corte, M., Zoppi, M., & Maresca, M. (1974). Rhythmic changes of the cutaneous pain threshold in man. A general review. *Chronobiologia, 1,* 77–96.

Reinberg, A. (1992). Concepts in chronopharmacology. *Annual Review of Pharmacology and Toxicology, 32,* 51–66.

Reinberg, A., & Smolensky, M. H. (Eds.). (1983). *Biological rhythms and medicine: Cellular, metabolic, physiopathologic and pharmacologic aspects* (1st ed.). New York: Springer Verlag.

Reinberg, A., Smolensky, M. H., & Labreque, G. (1986). The hunting of a wonder pill for resetting all biological clocks. *Annual Review of Chronopharmacology, 4,* 171–200.

Ritschel, W. A., Bykadi, G., Ford, D. J., Bloomfield, S. S., & Levy, R. C. (1983). Pilot study on disposition and pain relief after i.m. administration of meperidine during the day or night. *International Journal of Clinical Pharmacology and Therapeutic Toxicology, 21,* 218–223.

Sittl, R., Kamp, H. D., & Knoll, R. (1990). Zirkadinae rhythmik des Schmerzempfindens bie tumor patienten (Circadian rhythm of pain found in tumor patients). *Nevenheilkunde, 9,* 22–24.

Solomon, G. D. (1992). Circadian rhythms and migraine. *Cleveland Clinic Journal of Medicine, 59,* 326–329.

Spetzler, B., & Anderson, L. (1987). Patient-controlled analgesia in the total joint arthroplasty patient. *Clinical Orthopedics, 215,* 122–125.

Strian, F., Lautenbacher, S., Galfe, G., & Holzl, R. (1989). Diurnal variations in pain perception and thermal sensitivity. *Pain, 36,* 125–131.

Suda, M., Hayaishi, O., & Nakagawa, H. (1979). *Biological rhythms and their central mechanism.* Amsterdam: Elsevier.

Tamsen, A., Hartvig, P., & Dahlstrom, B. (1980). Endorphins and on-demand pain relief. *Lancet, 1,* 769–770.

Tamsen, A., Sakurada, T., & Wahlstrom, A. (1982). Postoperative demand for analgesics in relation to individual levels of endorphins and substance P in cerebrospinal fluid. *Pain, 13,* 171–183.

Thompson, D. R., Sutton, T. W., Jowett, N. I., & Pohl, J. E. (1991). Circadian variation in the frequency of onset of chest pain in acute myocardial infarction. *British Heart Journal, 65,* 177–178.

Vanier, M. C., Labreque, G., & Lepage-Savary, D. (1992). Temporal changes in hydromorphone analgesia in cancer patients. In M. H. Smolensky, G. Labreque, A. Reinberg, B. Lemmer, & E. Haus (Eds.), *Proceedings of the 5th International*

Conference on Biological Rhythms and Medications (pp. xii–8). Houston: Pergamon Press.

Voulteenaho, O., Leppalouoto, J., & Mannisto, P. (1982). Rat plasma and hypothalamic B-endorphin levels fluctuate concomitantly with plasma corticosteroid during the day. *Acta Physiologica Scandanavia, 115,* 515–516.

Wesche, D. L., & Frederickson, R. C. A. (1978). Diurnal differences in opioid peptide levels correlated with nociceptive sensitivity. *Life Science, 24,* 1861–1868.

Wesche, D. L., & Frederickson, R. C. A. (1981). The role of the pituitary in the diurnal variation in tolerance to painful stimuli and brain enkephalin levels. *Life Sciences, 29,* 2199–2205.

Wilder-Smith, C. H., Schimke, J. H., & Bettiga, A. (1992). Circadian pain responses with tramadol (T), a short-acting opioid and alpha-adrenergic agonist, and morphine (M) in cancer pain. In M. H. Smolensky, G. Labreque, A. Reinberg, B. Lemmer, & E. Haus (Eds.), *Proceedings of the 5th International Conference on Biological Rhythms and Medications* (pp. xii–7). Houston: Pergamon Press.

Chapter 7

Chronic Low Back Pain: Early Interventions

Julia Faucett

ABSTRACT

Low back pain is a common and costly social problem. Many of the long term outcomes of chronic low back pain (CLBP), such as those related to occupational and social function or patient and family coping, are sensitive to nursing intervention. To identify potentially productive areas for nursing intervention research, studies from 1990 to 1998 were reviewed that investigated (a) potential early indicators that acute or subchronic low back pain would result in chronic pain and disability, (b) patient perspectives on adaptation to chronic pain, and (c) the value of interventions undertaken during the acute and subchronic phases of back pain to modify long-term outcomes. Sixteen quantitative studies were identified that prospectively investigated the natural history and outcomes of low back pain. Six qualitative studies that investigated the perspectives of patients with back pain were also identified. Ten randomized clinical trials were identified that investigated interventions undertaken during the acute or subchronic stages of back pain.

Clinical interventions that included advice to re-engage in activity, support to develop personalized goals, reinforcement for healthy gains and appropriate functional activities, and physical conditioning exercises tended to be successful in returning patients to work or limiting their self-reported disability and pain. Interventions that promoted communication at the worksite or modified the patient's job were also successful in promoting a faster return to work. Nonetheless, this is a nascent area of research in need of improvements related to the selection of appropriate subjects and controls, the timing and duration of interventions, and the reliability with which interventions are implemented. Furthermore, patients with back pain are most likely to benefit when nursing theories about chronic pain are linked to clinical intervention research.

Keywords: Low Back Pain, Chronic Pain, Disability, Early Intervention, Prevention

Low back pain is a common and costly social problem. Back pain is reported by 31 million Americans and annually accounts for $16 billion in economic costs (Deyo, Cherkin, Conrad, & Volinn, 1991; Snook & Webster, 1986). Chronic low back pain (CLBP) additionally causes considerable suffering to patients and their families, resulting in lost productivity, financial drain, depression, substance abuse, family conflict, social withdrawal, and the risk of dangerous invasive procedures or fruitless alternative treatments. Chronic back pain thus has the potential to result in multiple outcomes, many of which are sensitive to nursing intervention (Larsen et al., 1994). Pain management from the nursing perspective, for example, includes not only pain relief, but also assistance to patients to help them learn to modulate pain in multiple life circumstances and expand their capacity to handle the pain (Davis, 1992). Similar to any patient facing a chronic illness, vulnerable patients are likely to benefit from early identification and assistance with healthy adaptation and accommodation to CLBP. Nursing intervention for patients at risk for CLBP will require research to improve our understanding of how patients learn to cope with chronic pain and to identify patient characteristics or other factors predictive of poor long-term outcomes. The purpose of this chapter is to review recent research literature about patient responses to chronic pain, and the early identification and treatment of vulnerable low back pain patients.

Studies from 1990 to 1998 were reviewed that investigated (a) potential early indicators that acute or subchronic low back pain would result in chronic pain and disability, (b) patient perspectives on adaptation to chronic pain, and (c) the value of interventions undertaken during the acute and subchronic phases of back pain to modify long-term outcomes. The literature for this review was obtained through computer-assisted searches of Medline, the Cumulative Index of Nursing and Allied Health Literature (CINAHL), and PsychInfo. Studies were also referred by experts in the field or identified using an ancestry approach. Back pain studies for the review were identified by using subject headings and keywords pertaining to back pain, back injury, chronic pain, prevention and early intervention, nursing, health and patient education, case management, and outcomes assessment. Keywords also included a variety of specific outcomes of chronic pain such as quality of life, disability, self care, coping, control, depression, pain behavior, substance use, family, nonconventional therapy, and health care utilization.

The search was further limited to prospective studies of the natural history of low back pain, randomized clinical trials of interventions delivered during the first 12 weeks of reporting back pain, and interventions that nurses could potentially implement (e.g., studies of the outcomes of spinal manipulation, surgery, or multidisciplinary pain centers were excluded). Qualitative studies of patient responses to chronic back pain were also included. Sixteen quantitative studies were identified that prospectively investigated the natural history and outcomes of low back pain. Six qualitative studies that investigated the perspectives of patients with back pain were also identified. Ten studies were identified that investigated interventions undertaken during the acute or subchronic stages of back pain.

There are three levels to prevention in low back pain. Simply defined these are: *primary*—the prevention of injury; *secondary*—the prevention of disease progression and modification of severity; and *tertiary*—the prevention of disability and other complications. This review focuses on tertiary, and to some extent on secondary, levels of prevention. Studies investigating the prevention of back injury were not included, although primary prevention strategies to limit the occurrence of back injuries are essential, and roles for nursing are clearly indicated in this area (c.f., Karas & Conrad, 1996). Likewise, there are many ways in which nurses can assist patients to modify pain severity once a back injury has occurred. The major focus of this review, however, is on interventions to modify adverse outcomes of CLBP.

There were several notable exclusion criteria. The review included studies of interventions that could be implemented by nurses, but excluded most multidisciplinary and team-delivered interventions in which nurses might play important roles. There is an important trend towards multidisciplinary intervention for low back pain, but the role of nursing has not been sufficiently distinguished in outcome studies of multidisciplinary intervention to review it purposefully. Numerous quantitative studies about chronic pain patients were excluded because although they included subjects with low back pain, the back pain group was not separated out for comparative analyses. Studies were also excluded if they focused on instrument development or if the interval between the injury and the time of the first consult for pain exceeded 3 months. Additionally, studies about chronic pain that included low back pain patients as a specific comparison group may have been missed if the studies were not indexed under low back pain. Important studies in the scientific journals of non-English speaking countries may also have been missed, as well as studies recently completed but not yet indexed.

The chapter has five sections. First, chronic pain is defined and the societal impact of back pain is discussed. In the second section, longitudinal studies that investigated the natural history of back pain and early prognostic indicators of chronicity and disability are reviewed. The third section reviews qualitative studies that investigated patients' perspectives about adaptation to

chronic pain. The fourth section presents research on early intervention programs to modify the long-term impact of back pain. The final section summarizes the chapter and presents recommendations for future research.

THE PROBLEM OF CHRONIC LOW BACK PAIN

Definitions

Pain has been defined by the International Association for the Study of Pain
as "an unpleasant sensory and emotional experience associated with actual or
potential tissue damage, or described in terms of such damage" (Mersky &
Bogduk, 1994, pp. 209–214). In fact, most back pain is classified as nonspecific, denoting the absence of definite organic pathology or tissue damage.
Low back pain has traditionally been subdivided into acute, subacute or subchronic, and chronic pain syndromes. Chronic pain is generally defined as
pain of greater than 90–180 days duration (Mersky & Bogduk, 1994). Several
of the studies in this review, for example, report changes in the nature of the
back pain experience that occurred after 3 months (e.g., Philips & Grant, 1991).
       Clinical indicators have been studied to refine the diagnoses of acute and
chronic pain for the North American Nursing Diagnosis Association (Simon,
Baumann, & Nolan, 1995). Acute and chronic pain differed on their total
differential diagnostic validity scores as drawn from 125 expert nurses who
reported on 55 clinical indicators. The only statistically significant critical
indicator identified for acute pain, however, was the "communication of pain
descriptors," and no critical indicators were identified for chronic pain. These
findings suggest that the communication of pain between patients and nurses
may be more common in acute than chronic pain conditions, but that overall,
other relevant signs of distress and autonomic response are nonspecific for
pain. These findings reinforce McCaffery's often quoted definition that "Pain
is whatever the experiencing person says it is" (McCaffery, 1979, p. 11).
       Other studies suggest that the division between acute and chronic back
pain is not distinct, since many patients suffer relapse and recurrence (Infante-
Rivard & Lortie, 1997; Robinson, 1998; Von Korff, Deyo, Cherkin, & Barlow,
1993; Wahlgren et al., 1997). There have been recent recommendations to
classify low back pain syndromes based on the relationships between pain
severity and disability outcomes, rather than on the duration of pain (Krause &
Raglund, 1994; Von Korff, 1994). In fact, the proposed subtypes resemble
pain states described by patients (Borkan, Reis, Hermoni, & Biderman, 1995;
Howell, 1994). Nevertheless, definitions for disability and return to work, a

primary indicator of disability, vary throughout the research literature in how they are operationalized, and work status itself may vary considerably over the course of a painful chronic disorder (Robinson, 1998). Thus, since research on alternative subtypes is still in a formative stage, the following definitions will be used for the purposes of organizing the literature review: acute pain lasts under 6 weeks in duration; subchronic pain lasts 6 weeks to 12 weeks; and chronic pain is pain that lasts over 12 weeks.

Prevalence and Incidence of Low Back Pain and Related Disability

It is predicted that low back pain will strike a great majority of us during our lifetimes. Recent studies undertaken in a variety of industrial nations estimated that 16–29% of the adult population will report low back pain on any one day, 39% will have episodes of pain lasting at least one day within the previous month, 48% will report back pain in the previous year, and 59–62% will suffer an episode of low back pain in their lifetime (Bergenudd & Nilsson, 1994; Hillman, Wright, Rajaratnam, Tennant, & Chamberlain, 1996; McKinnon, Vickers, Ruddock, Townsend, & Meade, 1997; Papageorgiou, Croft, Ferry, Jayson, & Silman, 1995). Hurwitz and Morgenstern (1997) estimated a prevalence rate among the general population of 5.7% for any back condition. This somewhat lower estimate is the result of a study of the National Health Interview Survey (n = 84,573) that inquired only about back conditions which restricted activity for at least one day during the 2 weeks preceding the survey. This may represent a more serious experience of back pain. It should be noted, however, that back pain, in combination with arthritis and sciatica, has been found to be more likely than other common illnesses such as asthma, hypertension, diabetes, or cardiovascular conditions to result in role limitations (Lyons, Lo, & Littlepage, 1994).

In terms of chronic pain, investigators have reported that 23–26% of adults may suffer from low back pain of more than 3 months duration, while an additional 21% suffer pain of subchronic duration (Andersson, Ejlertsson, Leden, & Rosenberg, 1993; Hillman et al., 1996). When limited to cases that resulted in functional limitation or more than 25 episodes in the last year, a much smaller annual prevalence of 3.9% was reported in North Carolina for low back pain of greater than 3 months duration (Carey et al., 1995). Of that prevalence group, 34% considered themselves to be permanently disabled.

A large proportion of back pain cases are occupational in etiology and prove costly in terms of lost work time, medical care, and indemnity costs. Occupational low back pain in the U.S. accounts for 149.1 million lost work days and 25% of all worker compensation claims costs (Deyo et al., 1991; Snook & Webster, 1987). Furthermore, back injuries are more likely to occur to relatively predictable populations of workers who are in low-status, physically heavy jobs or who are currently unemployed. Among American workers, national survey results indicated that 17.6% suffered continuous low back pain of 7 days or more during the last year (Guo et al., 1995). Sixty-five percent of those episodes were attributed to occupational causes, with repeated activities considered to be the cause of low back pain in 35.6% of the cases, single events in 21.4%, and a combination of repeated and sudden single events in 20.7%. In contrast, an additional 7.5% of cases were attributed to disease conditions and 2.1% to pregnancy. Construction workers, automobile mechanics, nurses' aides, maids, janitors, farmers, and hairdressers were among the most likely to develop work-related low back pain. Approximately 2.5% of back pain experienced in the previous 12 months was attributed to the worker's recent job, with truck drivers at 7% being the most commonly affected (Behrens, Seligman, Cameron, Mathias, & Fine, 1994). In England, 13.7% of workers reported low back pain related to their jobs and 21.8% took time off from their jobs because of low back pain (Hillman et al., 1996). Thus, the worksite is likely to be an important area for research investigation and intervention.

Studying all types of back pain in the general population in a retrospective manner, Hurwitz and Morgenstern (1997) identified the following risk factors for developing chronic disability: being older than 34 years, male, Black, never married, unemployed, and with less than high school education, weight above the 50th percentile, and traumatic onset of the back condition. These predictors differ from studies of clinical populations, which frequently identify women to be at greater risk (e.g., Carey et al., 1995; Von Korff et al., 1993), although marriage has previously been found to be "protective," as has education (Dionne et al., 1995). The contributions of less education to greater disability rates have been explained, in part, by the likelihood that those with less education will have more physical jobs and a greater tendency to somaticize (Dionne et al., 1995). This chapter reviews prospective studies that investigated early predictors of long-term pain and disability.

Health Care Utilization and Costs

Hart, Deyo, and Cherkin (1995) reported that back pain ranked as the fifth leading reason for seeking medical care, accounting for approximately 2.8% of all office visits. Fifty-six percent of those visits were for nonspecific low back pain. Carey and colleagues reported that, in North Carolina, 73% of adults reporting CLBP sought health care, with 91% of those seeking physician care and 10% receiving surgery (Carey et al., 1995). Carey et al. estimated that costs in North Carolina for CLBP exceeded $300 million. In a one-year prospective study of back pain costs, predictors of high costs were determined to be higher pain severity and disability, greater number of days in pain, depression, receipt of compensation, and disc disease (Engel, Von Korff, & Katon, 1996). Not surprisingly, each of these factors also predicted more visits for back pain, hospital admissions, radiologic procedures, and medication usage, implying that as back pain becomes chronic, it becomes increasingly expensive to treat. Among worker compensation cases, 25% of all cases appear to account for over 90% of the costs (Snook & Jensen, 1984). Furthermore, it is widely presumed that the longer an individual is off work, the less likely he or she is to return to work, and the greater the risk of high claims costs.

Findings from England replicate the higher costs of CLBP there (Hillman et al., 1996). Nonetheless, Hillman et al. also found that chronic and even severe pain did not inevitably result in seeking professional health care. Furthermore, many patients seek alternatives to conventional Western care for back pain. Eight percent of those reporting any type of low back pain sought nonconventional therapies (Hillman et al., 1996). In a survey of randomly selected adults from the community, 20% reported back pain and 36% of those sought nonconventional therapy, primarily for chiropractic or massage therapy (Eisenberg et al., 1993). Although chiropractic treatments are often reimbursed by third-party payers, other nonconventional therapies may be covered out of pocket by patients, and are often overlooked in estimates of patient costs.

The discussion above indicates that CLBP is a common and often diagnostically vague disorder that poses increasing risk through the middle and most productive years and results in profound economic effects on patients and society. Moreover, epidemiological studies such as the ones summarized above suggest that research to identify early indicators of chronic pain and disability might yield future improvements in intervention. The next section discusses research studies that investigated demographic, psychosocial, clinical, and occupational factors for their ability to predict long term outcomes.

EARLY INDICATORS OF LONG-TERM OUTCOMES

Numerous studies were conducted in the 1980s to illuminate the characteristics of patients with chronic pain who were likely to respond well to rehabilitation or tertiary levels of treatment. A prospective study by Gallagher and colleagues, for example, investigated return-to-work outcomes among CLBP patients (Gallagher et al., 1989). The study findings suggested that patients who were more able to perform daily activities, felt more mastery over and responsibility for their own health, had been out of work a shorter time, and had a greater ease of changing occupations were more likely to be working again at 6 months post-treatment. Because of findings such as these, and because chronic pain was known to bring with it changes in attitudes, psychological well-being, coping strategies, physical conditioning, and social interaction, investigators also began to query the potential of intervening before the onset of chronic and disabling pain, at secondary and primary levels of prevention. Thus, Frymoyer and Cats-Baril (1987) began a series of studies to develop a multifactorial model to predict disability outcomes from low back pain. Researchers like Richard Deyo also began to investigate prognostic factors at earlier stages of low back pain. Seventy-eight percent of the subjects in their 1988 study, for example, had acute low back pain at inception (Deyo & Diehl, 1988).

In the 1990s, the number of studies investigating potential early indicators of long-term outcomes of low back pain increased, subject selection criteria tended to be better defined, and prospective designs became more frequent. Sixteen prospective studies published since 1990 that investigated the natural history of back pain were identified for this review. Of these, seven primarily investigated self-reported pain severity, functional status, or wellness outcomes. Among the seven, there were three studies that contacted patients within 3 weeks of their initial visits to the physician for low back pain; two that contacted patients with subchronic pain; and two that contacted a majority of the sample within 7 weeks of their seeking care but included pain of variable duration. Studies that followed patients with mixed types of pain duration were included if the designs were sufficient to draw conclusions about patients whose pain had lasted less than 6 months. In addition, there were nine studies that investigated work loss time or work status. Among these nine, seven studies followed acute low back pain patients or identified patients absent from work for 6 weeks or less, and two followed subchronic or mixed groups of patients.

Predictors of Self-Reported Pain, Disability, and Well-Being

Philips and Grant (1991) successfully followed 92 general practice and emergency department patients reporting a first episode of acute low back pain (79% retention rate) for 6 months to investigate changes in pain and psychological factors. Among the 40% who continued to report pain at 6 months, pain intensity, sickness impact, and disability had declined; work loss, down time, sleep disturbances, anxiety, and frustration had decreased; and exercise had increased, suggesting that patients adjusted to continuing pain. Depression did not distinguish patients with persistent pain from those who had recovered. Patients who developed chronic pain were likely to have widened their search for relief by visiting medical specialists and trying alternative physical therapies, and they were also more likely than those who had recovered to have started litigation in the early stage of their disorder. Philips and Grant concluded that pain, rather than worsening over time, had persisted, with the greatest changes occurring between onset and 3 months, and more gradual changes occurring after 3 months.

In a predictive study of self reported disability, Burton and colleagues followed 186 osteopathy patients (74% retention rate) for one year (Burton, Tillotson, Main, & Hollis, 1995). For acute pain patients (n = 56), coping using catastrophic thinking or praying and hoping, somatic perceptions, impaired straight leg raising, and leg pain together accounted for 69% predicted of the variance in disability scores one year later. For patients with subchronic to chronic pain (n = 59), prediction was less successful, with baseline disability and pain scores accounting for only 18% of the variance in disability scores at follow-up. Pain-related factors, depression, fear and avoidance, and examination factors other than leg pain did not contribute significantly to the follow-up scores for disability. This suggests that early indices of poor coping and nerve involvement may be useful to identify patients at risk for persistent disability from low back pain. For patients in the subchronic or chronic stages of pain, however, predicting changes in disability may become increasingly difficult.

Van den Hoogen and colleagues studied 269 Dutch patients (45% response rate) from 11 general practices in Amsterdam to identify predictors of the length of time to recovery from low back pain (Van den Hoogen, Koes, Deville, van Eijk, & Bouter, 1997). Seventy-eight percent of the sample had pain of less than 7 weeks duration. After 12 weeks, 65% were pain-free and after one year, 90% were pain-free. A longer time to recovery was predicted most strongly by the receipt of physical therapy in the first 5 weeks of treatment, with additional contributions made by baseline pain intensity and previous back surgery—factors which suggest a pain disorder that initially appears more severe or unremitting. Leg pain was predictive in the univariate, but not the multivariate analyses. Otherwise, patient demographics and the investigators' psychosocial and physical assessment measures were noncontributory. It is notable that for patients who attained recovery before the end of the study, 76% had a relapse after being free of pain for at least 1 month. The median time to relapse was 7 weeks and the median duration was of the relapse was 3 weeks.

Wahlgren and colleagues studied Navy men (n = 76) with subchronic daily back pain and followed them for 1 year to assess the outcomes from a first episode of low back pain (Wahlgren et al., 1997). Pain tended to resolve slowly for these men because, at 6 months, 78% reported continued pain with 26% reporting it to be disabling, and at 1 year, 72% reported pain, with 14% reporting it to be disabling. Thus, this study suggests that once pain has lasted 6 to 8 weeks, residual long-term pain and disability are highly probable. In the main, like the patients with unresolved pain studied by Philips and Grant (1991), pain and disability did not worsen; they simply persisted.

Several investigators found that pain grade, or a combination of initial pain and disability scores, was the best predictor of subsequent status (Burton et al., 1995; Von Korff, Deyo, Cherkin, & Barlow, 1993; Wahlgren et al., 1997). Van Korff and colleagues, for example, studied 1128 HMO patients (93% retention rate) who were seeking care for back pain from their primary providers. The authors demonstrated that the distribution of baseline pain grades did not differ between patients with acute or subchronic pain and those with chronic pain at baseline, and that after 1 year of follow-up, pain grade was a better predictor of a poor outcome than the duration of the pain. The authors argued that pain grade is a better predictor of long-term outcomes than the recency of pain onset, and suggested that nomenclature for chronic pain based on duration is not useful in categorizing patients for rehabilitation. They also found that women and patients with low education were more likely to have poor outcomes at 1 year. Nonetheless, compared to chronic pain patients at the 1-year follow-up, patients with acute or subchronic pain were less likely to report pain in the previous month, more likely to have been pain-free in the prior 6 months, reported lower frequency of pain, and differed significantly in terms of pain grades. Even among patients who were dysfunctional at baseline, half improved and one third experienced good outcomes, demonstrating that pain states are variable even after a long duration.

Two studies investigated work-related variables as predictors of persistent pain and disability and psychological status. Hadler followed 1306 workers (96% response rate) within a week of first seeking care for their back pain to investigate the effect of worker compensation (Hadler, Carey, Garrett, & the North Carolina Back Project, 1995). Patients receiving disability compensation and those who had a duration of pain longer than 2 weeks at baseline, evidence of sciatica, higher baseline disability, or lower education or income were slower to regain their sense of wellness, but not slower to return to work or regain function. Williams investigated the effect of job satisfaction among 82 Navy men who reported subchronic back pain (Williams et al., 1998). After controlling for baseline pain and disability scores and ethnicity, orthopedic impairment scores and job satisfaction were entered into multiple regression analyses to identify their value in predicting 6-month scores for pain, disability, and distress. In these analyses, orthopedic impairment provided a significant contribution to explain the variation in scores for pain, disability, and distress. Job satisfaction provided an additional significant contribution for pain and disability, but not distress. Military rank and type of work, however, were not associated with outcomes.

In summary, this cluster of studies suggests that it may take longer to recover from acute back pain than previously reported, and that as pain becomes subchronic or chronic, it may be less likely to resolve, but it is unlikely to worsen. Furthermore, although patients with a long duration of pain may still improve, patients who recover continue to have substantial risk of relapse or recurrence. It also appears to be more difficult to predict future disability among patients whose pain has passed the acute phase. Nonetheless, in the early stages of pain, these studies indicate that a problematic course may be more likely for patients with evidence of greater baseline pain and disability; low levels of education; poor coping; leg pain, sciatica, or other nerve impingement; lower job satisfaction; and legal involvement through worker compensation or case litigation. Job or worksite characteristics, however, have not been well investigated in this group of studies. The findings from these studies support further research to define subgroups of patients who might benefit from early intervention.

Predictors of Work Loss Time and Return to Work

Gatchel reported on a study that followed specialty clinic patients with acute back pain (n = 394) for 1 year to study predictors of their return to work (Gatchel, Polatin, & Kinney, 1995; Gatchel, Polatin, & Mayer, 1995). At 6 months, 12% of those enrolled continued to be off work because of their back pain. At one year, 7% continued to be disabled from work. Employment status at 1 year was predicted by baseline pain severity and disability, receipt of compensation, female gender, and Scale 3 of the Minnesota Multiphasic Personality Inventory. Scale 3 measures the presence of somatic complaints in combination with a denial of emotional or interpersonal difficulties, and was interpreted by the authors to indicate a passive attitude towards disability following injury. Studying primary care patients, Coste et al. also found baseline pain and disability and compensation status predictive of poor recovery (Coste, Delecoeuillerie, Cohen de Lara, Le Parc, & Paolaggi, 1994). The addition of a previous history of low back pain and employment status further improved the prediction of poor recovery, and the subsequent addition of male gender and low job satisfaction also improved the prediction of greater work loss time. The Coste et al. investigation followed 92 French patients with acute back pain (89% retention rate) for 3 months. These patients had a better recovery rate than those in the Gatchel study, with 90% recovering within 2 weeks, and only two continuing to have persistent pain at 3 months. Compensation and job status, but not psychological factors, were again found to be predictive of time off work in a study of 55 primarily blue-collar workers (92% retention rate) referred by occupational medicine physicians to a spine consultant (Lehmann, Spratt, & Lehmann, 1993). Litigation status and single married status in addition predicted the length of time off work in this study for patients who did not undergo surgery ($n = 47$). At referral, the average subject had been out of work for 4 weeks; over the 6-month course of the study, over 76% returned to work. The findings from these three studies suggest that by 6 months, most acute back pain patients recover enough to return to work. Those with more severe injuries, or a history of back injury, and those with work-related injuries are likely to have a more problematic course.

Abenheim and colleagues completed a prospective review of Canadian patients' charts (n = 1848) to identify the association between the physician's initial diagnosis and the chronicity of the patient's back disorder (Abenhaim et al., 1995). Files were randomly selected from the provincial worker compensation board and physician diagnoses made within 7 days of the onset of absence from work were noted. Chronicity was defined as 6 months of work absence within the 2-year study period, thus including relapse and recurrence. Approximately 9% of patients received a specific diagnosis for their back problem, although most patients presented without definitive pathology. These 9% accounted for 31% of workers who became chronic over the course of the study. A specific diagnosis and older age each rendered patients five times more likely to become chronic. The amount of compensation again was a significant predictor of chronicity. Abenhaim et al. (1995) suggested that the diagnostic label itself may affect the course of care and compensation status.

Five studies investigated work-related factors as predictors of future work status in greater depth. Goertz (1990) completed a chart review of 207 patients who presented to an occupational medicine clinic with work-related low back pain. After 2 months, six patients (3%) remained on modified duty, but all were back at work. Analyses of variance demonstrated that several factors noted at the presentation of the patient were significantly associated with the number of days that patients eventually spent away from their jobs: older age; the presence of spasm, reflex changes, facet or disc involvement, radicular pain or pain below the knee; past history of pain; the patient's employer not being an airline; physical aspects of the job; and the availability of modified duty positions. Gender in this study and the nature of symptom onset were not found to be contributory. It is of note that in this study, approximately 65% of all patients spent some time on limited duty before returning to their jobs.

Infante-Rivard and Lortie (1996) studied 291 Canadian patients (72% response rate) attending rehabilitation clinics for first compensated episodes of back pain. Fifty percent had returned to work within 112 days of initiating treatment. Separate analyses were undertaken for demographic, job-related, and clinical factors. In those analyses, less work loss time was associated with working for a public employer or a larger employer, at a job with a longer duration of employment, regular employment, less repetitive work tasks, and more flexible work breaks. A variety of clinical factors were also found to be significantly associated with the time to return to work, such as absence of radiating pain, good flexion, absence of disc disease and neurological signs, and earlier care-seeking. Gender, age, and marital status were noncontributory, as were physical efforts on the job, job satisfaction, other medical problems, being overweight, and a history of back problems. A final multivariate model demonstrated significant associations between less work loss time and younger age, absence of disc disease, earlier care-seeking, better flexion, absence of neurological signs, and having a public employer, longer employment duration, and flexible break time.

Oleinick and colleagues investigated acute and subchronic disability separately within a cohort of 8628 workers with occupational back injuries incurred in 1986 (Oleinick, Gluck, & Guire, 1996). During the first 8 weeks after injury, 74.7% of the workers had returned to work. In the second analysis, which considered only the 2184 workers who had not returned to work within 8 weeks, 10.7% had not returned to work after approximately 4 years of follow-up. Factors that predicted earlier return to work within the 8-week window included male gender, younger age, fewer dependents, injury not from a fall, white-collar work, not being in construction, and lower compensation rates. Marital status and employer size were noncontributory. Factors that predicted earlier return to work after the acute 8-week window included younger age, employer size, and having the lowest or highest compensation rates.

Finally, continuing the work of Frymoyer and Cats-Baril (1987) to identify predictors of long-term disability, Reid investigated workers with acute occupational back pain (n = 207, 30% response rate) for the time it took them to return to work (Reid, Haugh, Hazard, & Tripathi, 1997). By the first week, 69.4% had returned to work, by 3 months, 93.7% had returned. In terms of early predictors of chronicity, in this study, workers over 50 returned to work significantly earlier than younger workers, but gender, wage levels, length of employment, and weekly hours of work were not found to be significant. As in the Goertz study (1990), many of those who went back to work returned to modified jobs or changed their work hours, job, or employer. Using the same sample of injured workers (n = 163, 23% response rate), Hazard and his associates investigated the predictive efficacy of a brief screening inventory (Hazard, Haugh, Reid, Preble, & MacDonald, 1996). The 11-item inventory included items about job demand and coworker relationships, patient attitudes about future work status, previous back injuries, marital status, and pain. A variety of cutoff scores for the inventory were tested for sensitivity and specificity in predicting which patients would be off work at follow-up. The results demonstrated a range of sensitivity of 1.00 to 0.62 and specificity from 0.70 to 0.91. Cats-Baril and Frymoyer (1991) also tested a similar version of their model with a 6-month follow-up period, but that study was not reviewed because it recruited patients in the chronic stage of back pain.

Similar to the studies in the previous section, these studies found that significant baseline predictors of return to work included self-reports of less pain and disability, not having positive examination findings or specific back diagnoses, and no involvement with worker compensation or case litigation. The studies in this section were more likely to include job factors as predictors. Job factors found to be predictive of return to work included longer job duration, no job termination, the availability of modified duty or flexible break time, white-collar work or less physical duties, and employer size or type. Results for age and gender remain unclear, with the studies differing on the findings for men vs. women or older vs. younger aged workers. Likewise, the few studies that investigated psychological factors found differing results.

The prospective study is a better design than the cross-sectional study for investigating temporal and causal relationships. The biggest threat to the validity of the prospective studies above instead affects generalizability and is related to the representativeness of the samples. For example, the studies differed in whether patient participants were drawn from a community-wide selection of clinical sites or a single provider or clinic. In general, the community-based study is more widely representative; furthermore, it limits bias related to practice variations that may influence the course of patients' pain disorders during the follow-up period. Diminishing subject retention over time also poses a potential threat to generalizability. One risk of sample attrition, for example, is that the surviving sample of patients may have worse pain or disability than those who drop out, thus artificially inflating outcome scores. Investigators may be able to defend the lack of differences between surviving sample members and dropouts on the basis of demographics, but they rarely have access to information that allows them to compare these groups on meaningful clinical factors. Thus, results should be interpreted conservatively for studies in which the attrition is high, or in which the initial sample may not adequately represent the population of affected patients. It is additionally difficult to compare these studies because of variations in the sample inclusion criteria based on the duration of pain or work loss time. Taken together, these studies indicated that different predictors may be important for acute as compared with subchronic pain patients, and that subsamples should be separately investigated.

These studies represent exploratory efforts to investigate prognostic indicators of chronic pain and disability. There is still little agreement on which personal, psychosocial, clinical, or job-related factors are important to include as potential predictors, or how to define relevant outcome variables and measure them in a standard manner. Return to work, for example, may be evaluated as how long it took the patient to return to work or simply whether the patient has ever returned to any job, without regard for job modification or part time work. For example, few investigators recorded whether a patient returned to the same job and same employer, a different job or employer, or a job that had been modified in terms of work tasks or hours worked per week. Likewise, it is uncommon to investigate how long injured workers stay on the job once they return; thus, the issue remains that workers may return too soon and face a greater risk for relapse. Additionally, if return to work is evaluated by the closure of an insurance claim, efforts must be made to determine whether a financial settlement was made in order to close the case or whether in fact the worker rejoined the workforce (Oleinick et al., 1996).

ADAPTATION TO CHRONIC LOW BACK PAIN: PATIENT PERSPECTIVES

Qualitative research allows the investigator to use open-ended interviews, group discussions, and participant observation to obtain a broad set of data to describe the experience of chronic pain. Qualitative techniques used in the studies reviewed for this chapter included grounded theory, phenomenology, content analysis, and feminist approaches. Six studies reporting on the perspectives of CLBP patients were reviewed. One study of chronic musculoskeletal pain and one study of mixed chronic pain were included to enrich the discussion. The need for qualitative research to describe the patient's perspective of the pain experience has not been well appreciated, as can be seen by the low number of studies in this area. Nonetheless, a really satisfactory quantitative method to predict outcomes from low back pain, as described above, has largely defied identification. There is a clear need to utilize other techniques to understand the problem of low back pain, and especially the disability and distress that it evokes.

The major themes of the chronic pain experience identified by qualitative researchers focused on transition from an acute disorder to a chronic one; vulnerability, losses and distress related to the past, more active self; and the development of new conceptualizations of self and one's life potential while living with chronic pain. The relative emphasis on the adverse vs. healthier outcomes of chronic pain varied depending upon the sample. Howell (1994) and Schlesinger (1996) elected to study women (n = 19 and n = 28, respectively) from the community with chronic pain. Strong, Large, and Franz (1995) and Large and Strong (1997) also studied community members (n = 15; n = 19, respectively) and selected those who had sought treatment but not from a pain management center. Other researchers drew patient samples from clinical settings. Tarasuk and Eakin (1994), for example, studied injured workers (n = 15) from Canadian rehabilitation centers, while Bowman (1991) selected patients (n = 15) from a pain management center. Borkan et al. (n = 66 in focus groups, n = 10 in interviews) and Skelton (n = 52) studied primary care patients (Borkan et al., 1995; Skelton, Murphy, Murphy, & O'Dowd, 1996).

Patients who are distressed about their pain experience may be more likely to seek care from secondary-level sources, such as pain management or rehabilitation clinics. Thus, themes identified by Bowman (1991) focused more on the despair, struggle, and helplessness that accompanied the loss of productive and important activities, and the dominating grip that pain held on subjects' lives. Likewise, themes identified by Tarasuk and Eakin (1994) focused on the development of a sense of permanent vulnerability and fear of reinjury. Vulnerability and the need for caution were reinforced by health-care providers who cast doubt on the potential for recovery and conveyed the impression that major changes in lifestyle were essential to reduce the risk of future injury. Others identified the impact that pain had on daily activities and the need for occasionally major adaptations in work, family, and self-care activities (Skelton et al., 1996). In addition to identifying the losses and changes related to chronic pain, Howell (1994), by contrast, was also able to identify healthy coping styles that resulted from having the physical pain experience validated by oneself and others. Such validation was likely to lead to accepting one's limitations and initiating self-care activities to maximize pain relief and well-being. Borkan and colleagues discussed the demoralization and self-criticism that can complicate the pain problem if this validation is lacking or if the reality of the pain is challenged (Borkan et al., 1995). Similarly, Strong et al. (1995) identified healthy accommodation to chronic pain as finally accepting it as irremediable and actively managing it, through decision making and planning.

For subjects in Howell's (1994) and Strong et al.'s (1995) studies, acknowledgement of the physical or somatic nature of the pain and listening to the body appeared to be fundamental to successfully coping with it. Howell also suggested that, among the women in her sample, healthy progression was accompanied by gains in wisdom, compassion, and empathy. Similarly, Borkan and his group suggested that coping, for some, included allowing the pain to govern at least some aspects of living, and this was interpreted as participating in the sick role at least occasionally. Their study also suggested, however, that coping for others involved masking the pain and enduring it to pursue one's routine (Borkan et al., 1995). This contrasting view of coping is also evident in the study by Large and Strong (1997) in which coping was associated with mastery, stoicism, and maintaining appropriate social interaction and appearances. It is possible that there are gender- or situation-related (e.g., public vs. private settings) aspects of coping that need further investigation. Coping was poorly differentiated from self-care in this group of studies. Thus, self-care and coping both included individual techniques such as meditation, relaxation, or exercise, and also changes in attitudes about one's role in managing the pain and maintaining general well-being (Borkan et al., 1995; Howell, 1994; Strong et al., 1995). Further research will be needed to more clearly define these aspects of adaptation.

Qualitative and quantitative studies report complementary findings about coping with chronic pain. Several of the qualitative studies identified uncertainty related to the prognosis of chronic pain and its impact; changes or deficits in social relationships; and the need to manage multiple symptoms, including distress, depression and thoughts of suicide, as fundamental issues in coping with chronic pain (Borkan et al., 1995; Bowman, 1991; Schlesinger, 1996). These same factors have been affirmed by surveys of patients with pain by nurse researchers (Hitchcock, Ferrell, & McCaffrey, 1994; Pellino & Oberst, 1992). Qualitative and quantitative researchers have also both noted the associations of less mood disturbance and better pain management with having multiple coping strategies to respond to a variety of situations, actively managing the pain, and feeling in control (Hitchcock et al., 1994; Large & Strong, 1997; Lin & Ward, 1996; Pellino & Oberst, 1992; Strong et al., 1995). Studies of the community have illustrated that not all persons with chronic pain experience the need to consult a physician. Furthermore, a substantial minority prefer alternative therapy or providers, often because of better communication skills and empathic listening (Borkan et al., 1995; Eisenberg et al., 1993; Hitchcock et al., 1994; Howell, 1994; Skelton et al., 1996). Men and women may differ, however, in how they personally cope with pain and what stimulates them to seek professional care. Weir and colleagues, for example, have found that adaptation to chronic pain varies by gender such that confident support, the perceived burden of the pain, and work status are more important for men, while cognitive factors, such as self-evaluations of resilience or the pain's impact on quality of life are more important for women (Weir, Browne, Tunks, Gafni, & Roberts, 1996). Furthermore, Weir and colleagues found these social and cognitive factors differentially influenced not only psychosocial adaptation to chronic pain, but also health care utilization and costs.

Criteria which allow the reader to determine the quality of a study are equally important in qualitative and quantitative research. Minimally, reports of qualitative research should provide enough information about the methodology that analytical processes and decisions can be retraced and subsequent reinterpretations generated if one desired to review the data. The reports in this section varied widely in terms of how clearly the authors defended the credibility of their data and analyses. Howell (1994) and Borkan, for example, carefully detailed their data collection and analysis methods (Borkan et al., 1995). Other reports lacked information about how themes were identified or confirmed by the researchers, and only rarely did authors report rechecking their findings with subjects. Additionally, theoretical sampling and the concomitant use of different data collection methods, such as using both focus groups and interviews, often enriches the efforts of qualitative researchers to derive concepts and build theories from their work. Several of the studies reported above, however, used convenience samples from clinics or the community rather than more conceptually driven subject recruitment strategies. Such sampling strategies may reflect the early nature of research in this area, but more methical techniques will be needed to improve theories about back pain. Qualitative research which investigates the patient's perspective on living with CLBP could benefit, for example, from samples that allowed comparisons between men and women, community and clinical settings, and patients with back pain and those with other types of chronic illnesses.

Qualitative studies are likely to substantially enrich theoretically driven research about patient coping and the transition from acute to chronic pain. Qualitative research offers information on the contextual nature of adaptation to chronic pain and the multiple situations in which the patient must cope with pain, including work, family, and health care settings.

EARLY INTERVENTION TO MODIFY THE IMPACT OF CHRONIC LOW BACK PAIN

The randomized clinical intervention trials reviewed in this section varied in terms of the outcome variables that were investigated. Most early interventions were targeted at reducing work absence and long-term disability. Additional outcomes studied included health care utilization and costs, pain severity, pain behaviors, self-reported disability and its impact, coping, and patient satisfaction with care. Studies also varied in terms of the selection criteria that were used to identify patients eligible for early intervention. Although some included patients with acute pain or subchronic pain only, many selected patients on the basis of the duration of their sick leave or accumulated absenteeism from work. In most cases, the time spent away from work would parallel the duration of the pain; in a case of repeated recurrences, however, it may not be possible to determine the length of time a patient has had a painful disorder from the information provided in the study. The studies investigated patients with nonspecific back pain for the most part; patients with nerve involvement or specific diagnoses tended to be excluded. All but one of these studies followed patients for 1 year or more after the intervention.

Interventions reviewed in this section fell primarily into two types. The first, education and counseling, involved educating patients about various aspects of pain, back care, and activity management; counseling them to resume normal activities without fear and providing positive reinforcement; and establishing an exercise regimen. This set of interventions varied in terms of the number of encounters between provider and patient, the formalization of reinforcement methods, the nature of the exercise plan, and the training required to prepare the provider to assess the patient and deliver the intervention. The second type of intervention tended to include similar components, but added worksite assessment and intervention, and was more likely to include multiple providers.

Education and Counseling

Five studies provided brief education and counseling interventions that averaged three sessions or less (Indahl, Velund, & Reikeraas, 1995; LeClaire et al., 1996; Malmivaara et al., 1995; Philips, Grant, & Berkowitz, 1991; Underwood & Morgan, 1998). They ranged from a 1-hour educational session with a patient pamphlet (Underwood & Morgan, 1998) to three 90-minute sessions of "back school" (LeClaire et al., 1996). Of the five, three reported no significant improvement for the treatment group as compared to the control group in terms of return to work (LeClaire et al., 1996; Philips et al., 1991; Underwood & Morgan, 1998). These three interventions were targeted primarily at patients with acute pain and provided structured approaches including back school or a specific exercise regimen. Others, in fact, have found mixed results or little effect for back school interventions alone (Cohen et al., 1994; Koes, van Tulder, van der Windt, & Bouter, 1994). Likewise, Cherkin found little effect for a similar brief approach with patients whose back pain was of varying duration (Cherkin, Deyo, Street, Hunt, & Barlow, 1996). Malmivaara et al. (1995) on the other hand, reported that a control group, who were counseled to return to normal activities, had significantly fewer sick leave days and were more able to return to work as compared to a group given a modest back exercise program or one given 2 days on bed rest. Similarly, for a group of subchronic patients, Indahl et al. (1995) reported that counseling patients to return to their normal activities without fear and assisting them to set practical and individualized goals was more successful than usual care.

Three studies that provided more intensive intervention to patients who reported acute back pain reported significant improvements for the intervention groups. Stankovic and Johnell (1990) provided patients with daily sessions for a week to teach a specific exercise program based on the McKenzie system. They demonstrated the efficacy of this program in comparison with a two-session back school program in terms of return to work, work loss time during the initial episode, pain, and movement, but not patient self-help or work loss during recurrences. Additionally, in a 5-year follow-up, they demonstrated consistent advantages of the exercise program in terms of fewer recurrences and fewer patients on sick leave (Stankovic & Johnell, 1995). Linton, Hellsing, and Andersson (1993) provided an individually determined range of sessions with the provider, potentially up to 12 weeks of sessions with an actual median of 3 sessions, to assist the patient to maintain daily activities, reinforce healthy behaviors, and allow practice of specific training activities. Finally, Faas and colleagues provided two exercise-centered sessions per week over 5 weeks and contrasted the intervention group with an attention-control placebo group who received ultrasound treatments and a no-intervention control group (Faas, Chavannes, van Eijk, & Gubbels, 1993). The intervention group and the placebo group each demonstrated significantly less time to recover as compared to the control group, suggesting that attention from the provider was the active element of these interventions. None of the other studies in this section provided attention controls, and thus, attention effects cannot be ruled out, despite the apparent better success of more intensive intervention programs.

Worksite Assessment and Intervention

Two additional studies were reviewed that offered more complex and highly structured interventions of even greater duration and included worksite assessment and intervention (Lindström et al., 1992; Lindström, Öhlund, & Nachemson, 1995; Loisel et al., 1997). Lindström and colleagues provided worksite assessment, back school, functional capacity testing, and individualized graded activity resumption with operant reinforcement until the patient had returned to work. Loisel and colleagues also provided worksite assessment and intervention and back school, and for particularly difficult cases, added work hardening and therapeutic return to work. Both of these intervention programs are considerably more costly to implement than those reported above, but both demonstrated convincing long-term improvement for patients in terms of early return to work and reduced rates of recurrence. Loisel et al., for example, demonstrated that patients returned to work 2.4 times faster if they received the intervention. Furthermore, in the Loisel study, the worksite assessment and intervention proved to be the most effective component. In addition to informing the provider about the patient's work situation, it included team meetings with the patient, supervisor, management and labor representatives, physician and ergonomist to discuss recommendations for job modification and ergonomic redesign.

It would be difficult to replicate many of these studies based on the information about the interventions provided in the research reports. The studies also uniformly lacked sufficient information to judge the reliability with which interventions were implemented across the study sample, and little information is provided about the training or testing of providers who implemented the interventions. Subject inclusion criteria varied from one study to another, and in many cases, selection based on the accumulation of sick leave was insufficient to entirely determine whether the interventions were in fact offered to patients in the acute or subchronic stages of back pain or whether patients were suffering an exacerbation of a chronic condition. Such distinctions may be important. The study by Linton et al. (1993) demonstrated, for example, that an intervention may be successful for patients with first-time back pain, but not those with a history of back pain. Most of the studies drew subjects from a wide variety of clinics or practices, or from worker compensation rolls, and this diversity contributed to the generalizability of their findings. As with other prospective studies, however, subject attrition over the course of the follow-up period was an important consideration; the studies varied in terms of how well they retained subjects in the various comparison groups. Control groups varied from treatment-as-usual to alternative treatments and placebo controls. Most studies used standard and well-known measures of outcomes. Many also provided data on a variety of outcomes of interest to nurses, such as patient satisfaction, self-care knowledge, and disability impact, in addition to pain and return to work variables.

SUMMARY AND RECOMMENDATIONS FOR RESEARCH

In sum, recent quantitative and qualitative studies have been reviewed to identify critical features of the transition from acute to chronic back pain conditions. Such studies are promising in terms of their potential to characterize patients at risk for suboptimal psychological, social, occupational, and clinical outcomes. Classifications that are based more on the patient's experience of pain and disability, rather than simply the duration of the injury, are likely to facilitate the identification of patients who will benefit most from selected interventions (Krause & Ragland, 1994; Von Korff, 1994). Most patients with an episode of low back pain will never have to face the challenge of chronic pain, because many recover and major functional limitations are rare. For others, the process of adapting to chronic pain is like adaptation to any chronic illness; it requires new and multiple skills, coping with loss, redefinitions of the self as vulnerable, and the ability to share concerns with and learn from others, whether they are professionals, family members, or coworkers.

Patients often have no control over constraints related to physical impairment and disease severity, the availability or modifiability of a job, and the nature of the disability compensation and legal systems—factors shown to be related to back pain outcomes. On the other hand, patients with a greater sense of control and self-efficacy, a variety of coping skills and resources, and who feel validated about the physical nature of their disorder are likely to be more successful throughout the course of adapting to chronic back pain. Furthermore, for the most part, clinical interventions in which providers advised patients to re-engage in activity without fear, supported them in developing personalized goals, reinforced healthy gains and appropriate functional activities including returning to modified work, and promoted physical conditioning tended to be successful in returning patients to work or limiting their self-reported disability and pain. Intermittent provider interactions with the patient during critical transition phases may facilitate better coping (Frank et al., 1998). It is additionally probable that patients who are able to return more quickly to work and family activities will be less likely to have poor psychosocial and economic outcomes. In fact, interventions that promoted communication among the patient, employer, and provider, or modified the patient's job were successful in promoting a faster return to work (Frank et al., 1998). Recent reviews of job redesign and modification provide additional support for the importance of pursuing worksite programs (Krause, Dasinger, & Neuhauser, 1998; Snook, 1988).

The types of interventions reviewed in this chapter fall within the scope of nursing practice. Nurses already offer patients counseling, guidance, support, training, case management, and worksite consultation and intervention. Special training may be required for nurses to implement some interventions in primary care or occupational health environments. Special training may be needed, for example, to acquire specific skills in physical and functional assessment, worksite and job analyses, and operant behavioral reinforcement. Nonetheless, nurses perform or direct similar activities in a variety of settings currently.

Prospective research to identify early predictors of long-term outcomes might benefit from including variables that characterize the work setting and job, and health care setting and provider, in addition to the physical disorder and patient. Organizational system issues that pose constraints for the patient may potentially contribute to poor outcomes as much as personal, psychosocial, or clinical factors inherent to the patient or disorder. The supervisor who is reluctant to allow an injured worker to return (cf. Linton, 1991) or the provider who is frustrated by the patient's lack of response to treatment may have considerable impact upon the vulnerable patient. In addition to identifying subtypes of patients at risk for poor outcomes, qualitative research might facilitate the identification of important setting and contextual variables. Theoretical sampling in qualitative studies might also be used to investigate critical aspects of the patient's self-perception, coping, and needs for support and information within each of the stages of acute, subchronic, and chronic pain.

Thus, nurses need to know what characterizes vulnerable patients with back pain, what transition phases during the development of subchronic and chronic pain might provide opportunities for intervention, and how to develop interventions that are contextually meaningful. Prescriptive nursing theory about chronic painful conditions and patient adaptation should be the goal of future intervention research. In fact, nurses are currently publishing theories about patient responses to chronic illness, pain management, and quality of life for patients with pain that may guide research (e.g., Davis, 1992; Dluhy, 1995; Ferrell, Grant, Padilla, Vemuri, & Rhiner, 1991; Larsen et al., 1994). CLBP patients are likely to benefit most when there are iterative linkages between research and theory.

ACKNOWLEDGMENT

My thanks to Judith Spiers, RN, MN who completed the computer assisted literature search and located the articles reviewed for this chapter.

REFERENCES

Abenhaim, L., Rossignol, M., Gobeille, D., Bonvalot, Y., Fines, P., & Scott, S. (1995). The prognostic consequences in the making of the initial medical diagnosis of work-related back injuries. *Spine, 20*, 791–795.

Andersson, H. I., Ejlertsson, G., Leden, I., & Rosenberg, C. (1993). Chronic pain in a geographically defined general population: Studies of differences in age. *The Clinical Journal of Pain, 9*, 174–182.

Behrens, V., Seligman, P., Cameron, L., Mathias, C. G. T., & Fine, L. (1994). The prevalence of back pain, hand discomfort, and dermatitis in the US working population. *American Journal of Public Health, 84,* 1780–1785.

Bergenudd, H., & Nilsson, B. (1994). The prevalence of locomotor complaints in middle age and their relationship to health and socioeconomic factors. *Clinical Orthopaedics and Related Research, 308,* 264–270.

Borkan, J., Reis, S., Hermoni, D., & Biderman, A. (1995). Talking about the pain: A patient-centered study of low back pain in primary care. *Social Science and Medicine, 40,* 977–988.

Bowman, J. (1991). The meaning of chronic low back pain. *AAOHN Journal, 39,* 381–384.

Burton, A. K., Tillotson, K. M., Main, C. J., & Hollis, S. (1995). Psychosocial predictors of outcome in acute and subchronic low back trouble. *Spine, 20,* 722–728.

Carey, T. S., Evans, A., Hadler, N., Kalsbeek, W., McLaughlin, C., & Fryer, J. (1995). Care-seeking among individuals with chronic low back pain. *Spine, 20,* 312–317.

Cats-Baril, W. L., & Frymoyer, J. W. (1991). Identifying patients at risk of becoming disabled because of low-back pain: The Vermont Rehabilitation Engineering Center Predictive Model. *Spine, 16,* 605–607.

Cherkin, D. C., Deyo, R. A., Street, J. H., Hunt, M., & Barlow, W. (1996). Pitfalls of patient education: Limited success of a program for back pain in primary care. *Spine, 21,* 345–355.

Cohen, J. E., Goel, V., Frank, J. W., Bombardier, C., Peloso, P., & Guillemin, F. (1994). Group education interventions for people with low back pain: An overview of the literature. *Spine, 19,* 1214–1222.

Coste, J., Delecoeuillerie, G., Cohen de Lara, A., Le Parc, J. M., & Paolaggi, J. B. (1994). Clinical course and prognostic factors in acute low back pain: An inception cohort study in primary care practice. *BMJ, 308,* 577–580.

Davis, G. (1992). The meaning of pain management: A concept analysis. *Advances in Nursing Science, 15,* 77–86.

Deyo, R. A., Bass, J. E., Walsh, N. E., Schoenfeld, L. S., & Ramamurthy, S. (1988). Prognostic variability among chronic pain patients: Implications for study design, interpretation, and reporting. *Archives of Physical Medicine and Rehabilitation, 69,* 174–178.

Deyo, R. A., Cherkin, D., Conrad, D., & Volinn, E. (1991). Cost, controversy, crisis: Low back pain and the health of the public. *Annual Review of Public Health, 12,* 141–156.

Deyo, R. A., & Diehl, A. K. (1988). Psychosocial predictors of disability in patients with low back pain. *The Journal of Rheumatology, 15,* 1557–1564.

Dionne, C., Koepsell, T. D., Von Korff, M., Deyo, R. A., Barlow, W. E., & Checkoway, H. (1995). Formal education and back-related disability. In search of an explanation. *Spine, 20,* 2721–2730.

Dluhy, N. (1995). Mapping knowledge in chronic illness. *Journal of Advanced Nursing, 21,* 1051–1058.

Eisenberg, D. M., Kessler, R. C., Foster, C., Norlock, F. E., Calkins, D. R., & Delbanco, T. L. (1993). Unconventional medicine in the United States: Prevalence, costs, and patterns of use. *The New England Journal of Medicine, 328,* 246–252.

Engel, C. C., Von Korff, M., & Katon, W. J. (1996). Back pain in primary care: Predictors of high health-care costs. *Pain, 65*, 197–204.

Faas, A., Chavannes, A. W., van Ejik, J. T. M., & Gubbels, J. W. (1993). A randomized, placebo-controlled trial of exercise therapy in patients with acute low back pain. *Spine, 18*, 1388–1395.

Ferrell, B., Grant, M., Padilla, G., Vemuri, S., & Rhiner, M. (1991). The experience of pain and perceptions of quality of life: Validation of a conceptual model. *The Hospice Journal, 7*, 9–24.

Frank, J., Sinclair, S., Hogg-Johnson, S., Shannon, H., Bombadier, C., Beaton, D., & Cole, D. (1998). Preventing disability from work-related low back pain. *Canadian Medical Association Journal, 158*, 1625–1631.

Frymoyer, J. W., & Cats-Baril, W. (1987). Predictors of low back pain disability. *Clinical Orthopaedics and Related Research, 221*, 89–97.

Gallagher, R. M., Rauh, V., Haugh, L. D., Milhous, R., Callas, P. W., Langelier, R., McClallen, J. M., & Frymoyer, J. (1989). Determinants of return-to-work among low back pain patients. *Pain, 39*, 55–67.

Gatchel, R. J., Polatin, P. B., & Kinney, R. K. (1995). Predicting outcome of chronic back pain using clinical predictors of psychopathology: A prospective analysis. *Health Psychology, 14*, 415–420.

Gatchel, R. J., Polatin, P. B., & Mayer, T. G. (1995). The dominant role of psychosocial risk factors in the development of chronic low back pain disability. *Spine, 20*, 2702–2709.

Goertz, M. (1990). Prognostic indicators for acute low-back pain. *Spine, 15*, 1307–1310.

Guo, H. R., Tanaka, S., Cameron, L. L., Seligman, P. J., Behrens, V. J., Ger, J., Wild, D. K., & Putz-Anderson, V. (1995). Back pain among workers in the United States: National estimates and workers at high risk. *American Journal of Industrial Medicine, 28*, 591–602.

Hadler, N. M., Carey, T. S., Garrett, J., & The North Carolina Back Project. (1995). The influence of indemnification by workers' compensation insurance on recovery from acute backache. *Spine, 20*, 2710–2715.

Hart, L. G., Deyo, R. A., & Cherkin, D. C. (1995). Physician office visits for low back pain: Frequency, clinical evaluation, and treatment patterns from a U.S. National survey. *Spine, 20*, 11–19.

Hazard, R. G., Haugh, L. D., Reid, S., Preble, J. B., & MacDonald, L. (1996). Early prediction of chronic disability after occupational low back injury. *Spine, 21*, 945–951.

Hillman, M., Wright, A., Rajaratnam, G., Tennant, A., & Chamberlain, M. A. (1996). Prevalence of low back pain in the community: Implications for service provision in Bradford, UK. *Journal of Epidemiology and Community Health, 50*, 347–352.

Hitchcock, L. S., Ferrell, B. R., & McCaffery, M. (1994). The experience of chronic nonmalignant pain. *Journal of Pain and Symptom Management, 9*, 312–318.

Howell, S. L. (1994). A theoretical model for caring for women with chronic nonmalignant pain. *Qualitative Health Research, 4*, 94–122.

Hurwitz, E. L., & Morgenstern, H. (1997). Correlates of back problems and back-related disability in the United States. *Journal of Clinical Epidemiology, 50*, 669–681.

Indahl, A., Velund, L., & Reikeraas, O. (1995). Good prognosis for low back pain when left untampered: A randomized clinical trial. *Spine, 20,* 473–477.

Infante-Rivard, C., & Lortie, M. (1996). Prognostic factors for return to work after a first compensated episode of back pain. *Occupational and Environmental Medicine, 53,* 488–494.

Infante-Rivard, C., & Lortie, M. (1997). Relapse and short sickness absence for back pain in the six months after return to work. *Occupational and Environmental Medicine, 54,* 328–334.

Karas, B. E., & Conrad, K. M. (1996). Back injury prevention interventions in the workplace: an integrative review. *AAOHN Journal, 44,* 189–196.

Koes, B. W., van Tulder, M. W., van der Windt, D. A. W. M., & Bouter, L. M. (1994). The efficacy of back schools: A review of randomized clinical trials. *Journal of Clinical Epidemiology, 47,* 851–862.

Krause, N., Dasinger, L. K., & Neuhauser, F. (1998). Modified work and return to work: A review of the literature. *Journal of Occupational Rehabilitation, 8,* 113–139.

Krause, N., & Ragland, D. R. (1994). Occupational disability due to low back pain: A new interdisciplinary classification based on a phase model of disability. *Spine, 19,* 1011–1020.

Large, R., & Strong, J. (1997). The personal constructs of coping with chronic low back pain: Is coping a necessary evil? *Pain, 73,* 245–252.

Larsen, P., Carrieri, V., Dodd, M., Faucett, J., Froelicher, E., Gortner, S., Halliburton, P., Janson-Bjerklie, S., Lee, K., Miaskowski, C., Savedra, M., Stotts, N., Taylor, D., & Underwood, P. (1994). A model for symptom management. *Image: The Journal of Nursing Scholarship, 26,* 272–276.

Leclaire, R., Esdaile, J. M., Suissa, S., Rossignol, M., Proulx, R., & Dupuis, M. (1996). Back school in a first episode of compensated acute low back pain: A clinical trial to assess efficacy and prevent relapse. *Archives of Physical Medicine and Rehabilitation, 77,* 673–679.

LeFort, S. M., Gray-Donald, K., Rowat, K. M., & Jeans, M. E. (1998). Randomized controlled trial of a community-based psychoeducation program for the self-management of chronic pain. *Pain, 74,* 297–306.

Lehmann, T. R., Spratt, K. F., & Lehmann, K. K. (1993). Predicting long-term disability in low back injured workers presenting to a spine consultant. *Spine, 18,* 1103–1112.

Lin, C. C., & Ward, S. E. (1996). Perceived self-efficacy and outcome expectancies in coping with chronic low back pain. *Research in Nursing & Health, 19,* 299–310.

Lindström, I., Öhlund, C., Eek, C., Wallin, L.-E., Peterson, L., Fordyce, W. E., & Nachemson, A. L. (1992). The effect of graded activity on patients with subacute low back pain: A randomized prospective clinical study with an operant-conditioning behavioral approach. *Physical Therapy, 72,* 281–290.

Lindström, I., Öhlund, C., & Nachemson, A. (1995). Physical performance pain, pain behavior and subjective disability in patients with subacute low back pain. *Scandinavian Journal of Rehabilitation Medicine, 27,* 153–160.

Linton, S. J. (1991). The manager's role in employees' successful return to work following back injury. *Work & Stress, 5*, 189–195.

Linton, S. J., Hellsing, A. L., & Anderson, D. (1993). A controlled study of the effects of an early intervention on acute musculoskeletal pain problems. *Pain, 54*, 353–359.

Loisel, P., Abenhaim, L., Durand, P., Esdaile, J. M., Suissa, S., Gosselin, L., Simard, R., Turcotte, J., & Lemaire, J. (1997). A population-based, randomized clinical trial on back pain management. *Spine, 22*, 2911–2918.

Lyons, R. A., Lo, S. V., & Littlepage, B. N. C. (1994). Comparative health status of patients with 11 common illnesses in Wales. *Journal of Epidemiology and Community Health, 48*, 388–390.

Malmivaara, A., Häkkinen, U., Aro, T., Heinrichs, M. L., Koskenniemi, L., Kuosma, E., Lappi, S., Paloheimo, R., Servo, C., Vaaranen, V., & Hernberg, S. (1995). The treatment of acute low back pain: Bed rest, exercises, or ordinary activity? *The New England Journal of Medicine, 332*, 351–355.

McCaffery, M. (1979). *Nursing management of the patient with pain* (2nd ed.). Philadelphia: Lippincott.

McKinnon, M. E., Vickers, M. R., Ruddock, V. M., Townsend, J., & Meade, T. W. (1997). Community studies of the health service implications of low back pain. *Spine, 22*, 2161–2166.

Mersky, H., & Bogduk, N. (Eds.). (1994). *Classification of chronic pain: Descriptions of chronic pain syndromes and definitions of pain terms* (2nd ed.). Seattle, WA: IASP Press.

Oleinick, A., Gluck, J. V., & Guire, K. E. (1996). Factors affecting first return to work following a compensable occupational back injury. *American Journal of Industrial Medicine, 30*, 540–555.

Papageorgiou, A. C., Croft, P. R., Ferry, S., Jayson, M. I. V., & Silman, A. J. (1995). Estimating the prevalence of low back pain in the general population: Evidence from the South Manchester Back Pain Survey. *Spine, 20*, 1889–1894.

Pellino, T. A., & Oberst, M. T. (1992). Perception of control and appraisal of illness in chronic low back pain. *Orthopaedic Nursing, 11*, 22–27.

Philips, H. C., & Grant, L. (1991). The evolution of chronic back pain problems: A longitudinal study. *Behavior Research and Therapy, 29*, 435–441.

Philips, H. C., Grant, L., & Berkowitz, J. (1991). The prevention of chronic pain and disability: A preliminary investigation. *Behavior Research and Therapy, 29*, 443–450.

Reid, S., Haugh, L. D., Hazard, R. G., & Tripathi, M. (1997). Occupational low back pain: Recovery curves and factors associated with disability. *Journal of Occupational Rehabilitation, 7*, 1–14.

Robinson, J. P. (1998). Disability in low back pain: What do the numbers mean? *American Pain Society Bulletin, 8*, 9–13.

Scheer, S. J., Radack, K. L., & O'Brien, D. R. (1995). Randomized controlled trials in industrial low back pain relating to return to work: Part 1. Acute interventions. *Archives of Physical Medicine and Rehabilitation, 76*, 966–973.

Schlesinger, L. (1996). Chronic pain, intimacy, and sexuality: A qualitative study of women who live with pain. *The Journal of Sex Research, 33,* 249–256.

Simon, J. M., Baumann, M. A., & Nolan, L. (1995). Differential diagnostic validation: Acute and chronic pain. *Nursing Diagnosis, 6,* 73–79.

Skelton, A. M., Murphy, E. S., Murphy, R. J. L., & O'Dowd, T. C. (1996). Patients' views of low back pain and its management in general practice. *British Journal of General Practice, 46,* 153–156.

Snook, S. H. (1988). Approaches to the control of back pain in industry: Job design, job placement and education/training. *Occupational Medicine, 3,* 45–59.

Snook, S. H., & Jensen, R. C. (1984). Cost of occupational low back pain. In M. H. Pope, J. W. Frymoyer, & G. Andersson (Eds.), *Occupational low back pain* (pp. 115–121). New York: Prager.

Snook, S. H., & Webster, B. S. (1986). The cost of disability. *Clinical Orthopaedics and Related Research, 221,* 77–84.

Stankovic, R., & Johnell, O. (1990). Conservative treatment of acute low back pain: A prospective randomized trial: McKenzie method of treatment versus patient education in "mini back school." *Spine, 15,* 120–123.

Stankovic, R., & Johnell, O. (1995). Conservative treatment of acute low back pain. *Spine, 20,* 469–472.

Strong, J., Large, R. G., & Franz, C. P. (1995). Coping with chronic low back pain: An idiographic exploration through focus groups. *International Journal of Psychiatry in Medicine, 25,* 371–387.

Tarasuk, V., & Eakin, J. (1994). Back problems are for life: Perceived vulnerability and its implications for chronic disability. *Journal of Occupational Rehabilitation, 4,* 55–64.

Underwood, M. R., & Morgan, J. (1998). The use of a back class teaching extension exercises in the treatment of acute low back pain in primary care. *Family Practice, 15,* 9–15.

van den Hoogen, H. J. M., Koes, B. W., Deville, W., van Eijk, J. T. M., & Bouter, L. M. (1997). The prognosis of low-back pain in general practice. *Spine, 22,* 1525–1521.

Von Korff, M. (1994). Studying the natural history of back pain. *Spine, 19,* 2041s–2046s.

Von Korff, M., Deyo, R. A., Cherkin, D., & Barlow, W. (1993). Back pain in primary care: Outcomes at 1 year. *Spine, 18,* 855–862.

Wahlgren, D. R., Atkinson, J. H., Epping-Jordan, J. E., Williams, R. A., Pruitt, S. D., Klapow, J. C., Patterson, T. L., Grant, I., Webster, J. S., & Slater, M. A. (1997). One-year follow-up of first onset low back pain. *Pain, 73,* 213–221.

Weir, R., Browne, G., Tunks, E., Gafni, A., & Roberts, J. (1996). Gender differences in psychosocial adjustment to chronic pain and expenditures for health care services used. *The Clinical Journal of Pain, 12,* 277–290.

Williams, R. A., Pruitt, S. D., Doctor, J. N., Epping-Jordan, J. E., Wahlgren, D. R., Grant, I., Patterson, T. L., Webster, J. S., Slater, M. A., & Atkinson, J. H. (1998). The contribution of job satisfaction to the transition from acute to chronic low back pain. *Archives of Physical Medicine and Rehabilitation, 79,* 366–374.

PART III

Other Research

Chapter 8

Wandering in Dementia

DONNA L. ALGASE

ABSTRACT

In this paper, published research studies addressing the phenomenon of wandering in dementia are reviewed. Empirical findings of 108 studies are categorized and summarized to reveal dimensions of wandering behavior, significance of wandering as a clinical phenomenon, correlates of wandering, and tested intervention strategies. Implications for improving methodological rigor of future studies are offered and gaps in the current knowledge base are identified.

Keywords: Wandering, Ambulation Behavior, Dementia

Wandering is among the most intriguing, potentially hazardous, and least understood of dementia-related behaviors. Recently, interest in wandering has increased, and pressure for identifying appropriate management strategies has intensified due both to a government mandate reducing restraint use in nursing homes and to family preference for less restrictive alternatives. Efficient development of effective interventions requires well-substantiated, empirically based theory. Thus, the goals of this literature review are to summarize and synthesize findings of published research studies addressing the phenomenon of wandering and to clarify direction for future empirical work.

Wandering studies are plagued by missing or ambiguous definitions. In structuring a literature search for this review, "wandering" was applied broadly to refer to problematic ambulatory behavior of persons with dementia, regardless of by whom or for whom ambulation was considered problematic. The only ambulatory problem specifically excluded was gait disturbance. The intent was to encompass a sufficiently wide range of definitions so that all facets of wandering could be captured. Improved conceptual clarity for the term "wandering" was an intended outcome. Care was exercised to cast a net broadly enough to encompass the full range of applicable studies, yet to bind the limits of the search sufficiently for excluding studies which might further dilute usefulness of the term. Key terms used were: abscond, ambulation, ambulatory behavior, AWOL, egress, elopement, exit behavior, hyperactivity, locomotion or locomotor activity, pacing, psychomotor agitation, spatial disorientation, walking, wandering or wandering behavior, and wayfinding. Limiting terms (dementia, most recent 5 years) were applied when the number of citations for a key term was extraordinarily large or a term was known to have alternative meanings in non-dementia contexts. A notable exclusion is "sundowning." Studies of sundowning often capture ambulation data of demented persons, but these data are usually mixed with other behaviors, and their inclusion was thought to confound the review.

This review covers only research studies published as professional journal articles. Although the author is aware of relevant dissertations, book chapters, monographs, and conference proceedings, they are not included for two reasons. First, equivalent standards of scientific rigor could not be assumed for such publications as can be expected for professional journals. Second, resources needed to search and retrieve such material were beyond those available to this effort.

Three databases (Cumulative Index to Nursing and Allied Health Literature [CINAHL], 1982 through 1997; Medline, 1966 through 1997; and PSYCHInfo, 1967 through 1997) were searched using software by Ovid Technologies. A benefit of this software is that it scans not only titles and key terms, but also abstracts and text of the article itself, when available online. However, this program cannot isolate research articles. Thus, the search was limited to citations having abstracts.

This search strategy yielded a total of 896 citations which were reviewed against three inclusion criteria:

(a) a research study, including case studies, involving human adults with any dementia;
(b) contains data specific to wandering, as defined above, however labeled or defined by the author; and
(c) is written in English.

In cases where a decision to include an article could not be made from the abstract, the article itself was reviewed. Most exclusions were made because the article was not a research study or did not apply to dementia; a smaller proportion was eliminated because these used animal models, studied adolescents or children, were dissertations, did not report data specific to wandering, or were written in a foreign language. Resulting citations were then entered into a database to eliminate duplicates. These procedures yielded 93 studies for review. Attesting to the lack of standard terminology and clarity on the concept of wandering in dementia, these procedures failed to elicit 15 additional, salient, published, research studies known to the author as meeting inclusion criteria. By including these, the review encompasses a total of 108 studies and contains two sections: (a) a summary of empirical findings and (b) a critique of methods and recommendations for further work.

EMPIRICAL FINDINGS

While a sizable number of studies reveal information about wandering behavior, only 40 have wandering as a major focus. Rather, the bulk of included works report wandering data gathered in the course of investigating a related issue. Some studies also captured wandering data in measures for psychiatric symptoms, hyperactivity, agitation, or disruptive behavior. However, these studies were excluded whenever wandering data were compiled along with other items in a measure and no analyses were particular to wandering. Findings from all studies with discrete measures of wandering were culled and grouped broadly into four areas: empirical characterizations, clinical significance, correlates, and interventions. Each area was further elaborated according to available information. Thus, the structure of the following section reflects the current range of empirical knowledge about wandering behavior. However, given the small number of studies directly addressing wandering, this structure should not be taken to encompass all aspects of the phenomenon that can or should be studied empirically.

Empirical Characterizations

Research characterizes wandering in three ways: in terms and definitions used; through measures employed to capture wandering behavior; and by descriptions afforded through the previous two means. A summary of what each way contributes to an understanding of wandering follows.

Terms and definitions.   Researchers, even in studies focused directly on wandering, use a variety of terms and definitions for it. In many studies, whether it is a major focus or not, wandering is undefined, but terms and definitions were explicitly stated in 24 studies. When compiled and analyzed, they reflected four dimensions, which characterize wandering as ambulating behavior of demented persons that:

(a) occurs in large volume, that is at a high frequency, rate, or amount (Algase, 1992b; Dawson & Reid, 1987; Hewawasam, 1996b; Hussian & Brown, 1987; Namazi, Rosner, & Calkins, 1989; Satlin et al., 1991; Snyder, Rupprecht, Pyrek, Brekhus, & Moss, 1978);

(b) has a seemingly aimless, lapping, or random quality or pattern (Algase, Kupferschmid, Beel-Bates, & Beattie, 1997; Dawson & Reid, 1987; Gilley, Wilson, Bennett, Bernard, & Fox, 1991; Hewawasam, 1996; Martino-Saltzman, Blasch, Morris, & McNeal, 1991; Monsour & Robb, 1982; Mungas, Weiler, Franzi, & Henry, 1989; Namazi et al., 1989; Snyder et al., 1978);

(c) exceeds or transgresses environmental limits, i.e., into hazardous or unauthorized territory or with oblivion to some physical barriers, such as furniture (Chafetz, 1990; Cumming, Cumming, Titus, Schmelzle, & MacDonald, 1982; Gurwirz, Sanchez-Cross, Eckler, & Matulis, 1994; Hewawasam, 1996a; Hussain & Brown, 1987; Hwang, Yang, Tsai & Liu, 1997; Jozsavi, Richards, & Leach, 1996; Mungas et al., 1989); and

(d) reflects spatial disorientation or navigational deficits, such as getting lost, being impaired in learning new or following old routes, and shadowing others (Ballard, Mohan, Bannister, Handy, & Patel, 1991; Henderson, Mack, & Williams, 1989; Hussain, 1982; Hwang et al., 1997; Liu, Gauthier, & Gauthier, 1991; Monsour & Robb, 1982; Mungas et al., 1989).

Less clear is the distinction or overlap between wandering and pacing. In some instances, they mean the same thing (e.g., Cohen-Mansfield, Werner, Marx, & Freedman, 1991; Lachs, Backer, Siegal, Miller, & Tinetti, 1992; Satlin et al., 1991). Yet, wandering and pacing have also been viewed as distinct (Mungas et al., 1989) or only partially overlapping phenomena (Algase et al., 1997; Martino-Saltzman et al., 1991).

Measures.   Although operational definitions of wandering are often unspecified, multiple means to quantify wandering are available, including rating scales and checklists, observational strategies, activity monitors, and functional assessment techniques. In many studies, wanderers and nonwanderers are compared (e.g., Cornbleth, 1977; Monsour & Robb, 1982; Snyder et al., 1978) or wandering is reported to occur in some subset of the sample (e.g., Conn, Lee, Steingart, & Silberfeld, 1992; Mungas et al., 1989; Riter & Fries, 1992). Such classifications are rarely made using a guiding definition or criteria for distinguishing groups; with rare exceptions (see Algase, 1992b; Thomas, 1997), examination of the validity or reliability of groupings is lacking. Most often decisions about wandering status are based on a priori judgments of staff or caregivers or on retrospective medical record reviews reflecting the clinical judgments of a variety of health professionals. Thus, caution is warranted when interpreting results of such works.

Rating scales and checklists are the most frequently employed means to quantify wandering; formal or informal caregivers are the usual data source. Except for one brief checklist (Algase, 1992a), no scale exclusive to wandering behavior exists. However, a number of scales designed to evaluate a wider range of behaviors associated with dementia include items on wandering. Some are scored by indicating presence or absence of a behavior (e.g., Dementia Behavior Disturbance Scale) (Baumgarten, Becker, & Gauthier, 1990); others provide rankings of frequency and/or severity (e.g., Cohen-Mansfield Agitation Inventory) (Cohen-Mansfield, 1986; Cohen-Mansfield, Marx, & Rosenthal, 1989), Berlin Rating Scale for Assessing Psychomotor Restlessness) (Gutzmann, Kuhl, Kanowski, & Khan-Boluki, 1997). Although evidence supporting validity and reliability of many of these scales exists for the overall concept they tap (see Davis, Buckwalter, & Burgio, 1997 for a recent review), psychometric properties with regard to wandering are unknown.

The Present Behavioral Examination (PBE) (Hope & Fairburn, 1992) is an interview guide covering eight behavioral domains of dementia-related behavior. Of all scales containing items on wandering, the walking (or activity disturbance) domain of the PBE includes the widest range of behaviors (11 items). Designed for use in an interview format with caregivers of community-dwelling persons with dementia, items are rated on an ordinal scale in either seven- or three-point versions (Hope & Fairburn, 1992; Hope, Tilling, Gedling, & Keene, 1994). Inter-rater reliability for the walking domain was reported as mean kappa scores of .77 (median = .87) and .48 (median = .57) when used with two independent samples, $N = 40$ and $N = 39$ respectively (Hope & Fairburn, 1992).

Staff and nurse ratings, such as those used by Dawson and Reid (1987) or Fisher, Fink, and Loomis (1993), reflect a more a limited range of wandering behaviors, but they also afford a means to judge how problematic wandering is perceived to be. Ratings are usually based on recall, and no published evaluation addressing the extent to which ratings match objective accounts of wandering was found.

With the exception of the PBE, scales and checklists reflect a narrow and imprecise view of wandering. Each captures only one or two dimensions of the behavior (most often volume or spatial disorientation) and many are subject to interpretation by raters. However, some of these measures add a temporal dimension: daytime versus nighttime occurrence. Although not explicit in definitions of wandering, this is an important fifth dimension. Knowledge of wandering's temporal aspects could help to elucidate the role of neurological mechanisms mediating the behavior.

Proposed for clinical assessment, the Queen Elizabeth Behavioral Assessment Graphical System (QBAGS), is a rating scale that could be adapted to provide a temporal picture (Prodger, Hurley, Clark, & Bauer, 1992). Accordingly, an ordinal ranking for wandering is plotted each hour; a daily distribution is produced by examining hourly fluctuations. Unfortunately, rankings proposed for wandering reflect a mixture of wandering dimensions that may not be ordinal in nature. However, using dimensions explicated in this review, a more refined rating system could be developed.

Wandering is observable and, thus, accessible through observational techniques. Both direct and indirect approaches have been used. Several researchers used direct observation with a variety of behavior mapping techniques (Cohen-Mansfield, Werner, & Marx, 1991; Goldsmith, Hoeffer, & Rader, 1995; Hussain, 1982; Lucero, Hutchinson, Leger-Krall, & Wilson, 1993; Matteson & Linton, 1996; Snyder et al., 1978). Mapping techniques vary in the number of wandering dimensions tapped and in the set of associated contextual and/ or behavioral variables noted, but none has a clear theoretical basis. Mapping captures presence or type of behavior occurring within brief time periods, usually lasting several minutes. Reports using these techniques often lack reliability estimates for raters. When reported, inter-rater reliability ranges from .87 to 1.00 (Cohen-Mansfield et al., 1991; Matteson & Linton, 1996).

Using a time-study approach, Algase et al. (1997) employed direct, real-time, continuous observation within a rhythm framework to count the frequency of cycles (or episodes), to time duration in phases (locomoting and non-locomoting), and to classify pattern using Martino-Saltzman's typology (1991). Other features of a cycle, such as impetus (self-initiated or other-directed), location, presence of others at the start or stop of cycles and their phases, and hour of the day have been incorporated into this methodology (Algase, 1992a; Algase et al., 1997). Strong inter- and intra-rater reliability is reported for these methods.

Researchers have also used a variety of indirect strategies. Martino-Saltzman et al. (1991) applied an automatic detection system to videotape episodes of ambulation. Subjects wore electronic ankle tags to trigger the system, activating recordings (one frame per second) in one of several detection zones where surveillance cameras were mounted. Tapes were later coded for travel patterns; raters obtained a kappa of .79 ($z = 13.2$, $p < .0001$). Chafetz (1990) provides another example. Using an existing door alarm to alert staff, he was able to count door openings (i.e., exit attempts); staff on the study unit also recorded whenever they intervened to prevent an exit. Observational approaches provide a better picture of wandering than rating scales or checklists. However, their validity is affected by the mapping or coding scheme used, because no scheme reviewed captures all five dimensions of wandering: volume, quality, environmental limits, navigational deficit, and temporal distribution.

Only recently have activity measuring devices been used to quantify wandering. Satlin, Volicer, Stopa, and Harper (1995) and Satlin et al. (1991) measured locomotor activity with a piesoelectric monitor worn at the waist over 48 to 72 hours. Algase et al. (1997) used mechanical sensing devices worn at the waist and ankle to estimate movement over periods up to 24 hours. Since neither device sorts ambulation from other movement of the trunk or limb, both instruments provide only an estimate of the amount of ambulation and its approximate distribution over time. Further, neither instrument taps other dimensions of wandering, such as quality or navigational deficit. Thus, their validity for measuring wandering is partial, and both require further evaluation of the extent to which they reflect actual wandering activity. However, these devices offer promise in advancing the study of wandering, as they are highly reliable and may be suitable to index amount and temporal distribution of wandering in some instances.

Although many researchers have equated wandering and navigational deficits, efforts to directly measure this functional aspect of ambulation are rare. In one effort, Liu et al. (1991) adapted and developed several tasks requiring subjects to find their way through large-scale space. Although it reflects only a partial view of wandering, this approach places it within a navigational paradigm. In two other studies, researchers also developed navigational paradigms that could be applied to the study of wandering in nursing home settings (Herman & Bruce, 1981; Weber, Brown, & Weldon, 1978). Results of these works are not reported here, as findings were not particular to demented subjects.

Descriptions.   Descriptive studies of wandering range from single-case observational studies (Rossby, Beck, & Heacock, 1992) to large-scale surveys based on rating scales completed by caregivers (Nasman, Bucht, Erikkson, & Sandman, 1993). In all but two of samples (Hope & Fairburn, 1990; Hope et al., 1994), subjects were institutionalized. Across studies dementia status of subjects was generally established against some standard (e.g., Mini-Mental Status Exam or DSM-III criteria for dementia); only one sample was limited to persons with Alzheimer's disease (AD) (Satlin et al., 1991).

In several studies, descriptive data elaborates aspects of wandering's dimensional structure. In a single case study of disruptive behavior, several dimensions (volume, quality, environmental transgressions, temporal distribution) were documented in a White male (age 71 years) with a primary degenerative dementia (Rossby et al., 1992). Seventeen instances of aimless walking and 21 instances of ambulating into inappropriate places occurred during 24 hours of observation capturing all hours of the day. Even while seated in a geri-chair, the subject used his feet to propel himself into inappropriate places twice and "walked" aimlessly seven times. Comparing documented episodes to observed ones, staff over-reported aimless walking and under-reported entries into inappropriate locations.

Data reported by Rantz and McShane (1994) reflected four dimensions of wandering. Using a focus group design, 58 staff members from three nursing home settings described care situations for residents with dementia. Content analysis resulted in four groupings, one of which was "wandering behavior disturbances." Items in that grouping were: paces for hours, unable to sit down (volume); unable to focus on eating, walks off during meals (quality/pattern); wandering in and out of residents' rooms, wanting to leave, attempting to get outside, eloping (transgresses environmental limits), and cannot find own room/bathroom, looking/searching for others, and unable to find what they are seeking (spatial disorientation). Two general behaviors were also reported: restlessness and wandering in halls.

In a large-scale survey, Nasman et al. (1993) gathered data on the prevalence of behavioral symptoms in an institutionalized sample ($N = 1350$). Staff reported the relative frequency of 22 behaviors for each resident on the Multi-Dimensional Dementia Assessment Scale for the Elderly (MDDAS) (Sandman, Adolfsson, Norberg, Nystrom, & Winblad, 1988). Factor analysis (principal components) yielded six factors, two of which are congruent with dimensions of wandering. Three items comprising the factor "escape behavior" (packs up things/is often on the way home, hides things, often stands at the outer door wanting to go out) is similar to the dimension of transgressing environmental limits. The four items of the "wandering behavior" factor (lies in other patients beds, piles up chairs/pushes tables/upends furniture, wanders back and forth alone or with others, eats others' food) reflect spatial disorientation.

One group of related studies explicitly examined the structure of wandering. In the initial investigation, researchers interviewed caregivers for each of 29 community-dwelling wanderers using the PBE (Hope & Fairburn, 1990). Caregivers reported that 59% of subjects showed increased walking activity (most of the day); 55% walked away from home and had to be brought back; 52% walked aimlessly; 48% walked with an inappropriate purpose (e.g., to find a dead relative); 38% displayed checking and/or trailing behavior; 34% made attempts to leave (thwarted by caregivers); 31% were inappropriately active at night; 21% pottered; and 14% walked with appropriate purpose but inappropriate frequency (e.g., "goes to the post office many times daily"). Overlap in the occurrence of behaviors was also found. Most of those with aimless walking also showed increased activity (87%) as did a majority (78%) of those who were active at night. Although they offered no analysis in support of this hypothesis, authors suggested that wandering may encompass up to five constructs with different etiologies, any combination of which may operate simultaneously. Components were: overall amount of wandering, avoidance of being alone, diurnal rhythm disturbance, navigational ability, and faulty goal-directed behavior.

Albert (1992) subjected Hope and Fairburn's data to a Guttman scaling analysis to evaluate whether a hierarchically structured latent variable (purposeless behavior) could account for the distribution of the data. Albert obtained a coefficient of reproducibility of .78, while Guttman (1974) established the cut-point of .90 for a hierarchical scale. However, by examining the hierarchy obtained, certain behaviors (not necessarily those with greatest frequency) are shown as more or less indicative of wandering than others. Accordingly, Albert reported that "needing to be brought back home" is most indicative because subjects with this behavior were most likely to have performed all others. Purpose-appropriate behavior done excessively was the poorest indicator.

In response, Hope et al. (1994) obtained PBE data from a second set of caregivers ($N = 83$). Item analysis revealed that "trying to leave home" and "being brought back home" did not correlate well with other items. When remaining items were subjected to a principal axis factor analysis, a four factor solution accounted for 54.5% of the variance. Factors were: checking and trailing, increased and aimless walking, pottering, and inappropriate and overappropriate walking. In scaling analyses, criteria for reproducibility and scalability were *not* met. Although these factors are not an exact match to dimensions revealed in sections on definitions and measures, findings support a multidimensional view of wandering.

Several descriptive studies offer findings that can be organized by the five-dimensional structure of wandering. Five investigators described volume. Increased ambulation among wanderers was found by Snyder and associates (1978) who reported that wanderers moved about during 32.5% of 18 10-minute observations (versus 4.2% for non-wanderers). Mid-stage dementia residents in one nursing unit spent 2/3 of their unstructured time walking around and socializing and the other 1/3 either walking alone or sitting (Lucero et al., 1993). During 679 3-minute observation periods for each of six wanderers, pacing was seen 55% of the time and continued throughout the entire period in 77% of observations where it occurred at all (Cohen-Mansfield et al., 1991). Satlin et al. (1991) compared overall diurnal activity output of 19 institutionalized, ambulatory AD subjects with that of eight non-demented controls. Raw values were not noticeably different, 463 units for AD versus 489 for controls, but the standard deviation was much higher for AD subjects, 321 versus 116. A subgroup of eight AD subjects, identified as pacers (on the criteria of spending greater time in non-goal-directed walking and inability to be distracted from this activity), had 720 units of activity (± 292), or 66% higher than controls and about 2.5 times that of non-pacing AD subjects.

Yet, high levels of ambulation may not be a universal characteristic of wanderers. In a group of ambulatory, demented, nursing home residents (N = 49), standing (5%) and pacing (3%) were seen less often, than sitting (15%) or lying down (13%) (Matteson & Linton, 1996). Among 158 residents who paced, 38 did so less than daily, 72 paced several times daily, and only 48 paced at least hourly (Cohen-Mansfield et al., 1991). Algase et al. (1997) reported estimates of wandering during 24 hours of observation for a sample of 25 ambulatory, demented nursing home residents. Number of cycles ranged widely (120; x = 19.7, $S.D.$ = 27.5) as did total time wandering (199.1 minutes; x = 42.9, $S.D.$ = 53.2). However, amount of wandering (frequency and total duration) is moderately stable (tau = .34 to .41, p < .05) over a 3-day period at both standard and individualized 2-hour epochs.

The quality or pattern of wandering is also described in several studies. In a narrative description of the unstructured time of mid- and late-stage dementia residents, a meandering quality emerges, whereby subjects move between activities in a happenstance fashion (Lucero et al., 1993). More objectively, routes of wanderers traced on floor plans were more complex and circuitous than those of nonwanderers (Snyder et al., 1978). However, not all walking of demented persons is convoluted. Martino-Saltzman et al. (1991) reported that 81.3% of walking episodes of wanderers were direct (vs. 94% for nonwanderers); random, pacing, and lapping patterns constituted 1%, 0.1%, and 17.3% respectively. Using the same typology, Algase et al. (1997) found a much higher proportion (47%) of the nondirect patterns: wandering episodes were 77.2% random, 12.1% lapping, and 7.2% pacing; differences from Martino-Saltzman's data were attributed to the range of locations for observation.

Several studies describe environmental transgressions. Most wandering occurs in corridors (Cohen-Mansfield et al., 1991; Lucero et al., 1993), where wanderers tend to enter rooms or test doors located at the ends; it is also seen in large communal areas, where subjects circle the perimeter (Lucero et al., 1993). Wanderers may also exit through unlocked doors (Lucero et al., 1993). Exit or near-exit behavior is well-documented (Chafetz, 1990; Hewawasam, 1996a, 1996b; Hussain, 1982; Hussain & Brown, 1987; Namazi et al., 1989), but natural conditions fostering exits have not been elucidated.

Spatial disorientation is a cardinal feature in many definitions and scales for wandering, but descriptions of this dimension are few. Liu et al. (1991)

compared 15 AD patients with mild impairment (mean MMSE = 22.9) to controls (mean MMSE = 29.5) on a range of spatial tasks. AD subjects did significantly worse on 8 of 12 perceptual spatial orientation tasks and all nine higher cognitive spatial orientation tasks, three of which involved ambulating in large-scale space. Compared to nonwandering nursing home residents with a provisional diagnosis of AD ($n = 16$), wanderers ($n = 5$) performed significantly worse on tests reflecting parietal lobe function (deLeon, Potegal, & Gurland, 1984), a brain region including the hippocampus, where spatial memories are formed (O'Keefe & Nadel, 1978). However, none of the parietal tasks used by deLeon et al. involved wayfinding or ambulating. Travel efficiency (direct episodes as a percent of all independent ambulation episodes) declines significantly with cognitive impairment ($F = 5.76$, $p < .01$), from 96.8% among mildly impaired subjects to 73.9% among severely impaired ones (Martino-Saltzman et al., 1991).

Temporal aspects of wandering have been described in four studies. From among a total of 1764 observations of 49 ambulatory demented nursing home residents, Matteson and Linton (1996) report a total of 24 pacing observations during the day shift, 16 during the evening shift, and 12 during the night shift. Martino-Saltzman et al. (1991) calculated rates of travel inefficiency for ambulatory demented subjects by time periods of varying duration over the course of a day. Subjects with mild cognitive impairments ($n = 12$) had an average inefficiency rating of 5% (range 2 to 15% per time period), while only two periods have efficiencies over the mean: 2 to 5 p.m. (7%) and 7 to 10 p.m. (15%). Those with moderate impairments ($n = 11$) averaged 7% inefficient travel (range 1–13%) with two periods exceeding the mean: 4 to 7 a.m. (13%) and 7 to 10 p.m. (12%). Severely-impaired subjects ($n = 9$) averaged 28% inefficient travel (range 15 to 32%); four periods exceeded the mean: 10 p.m. to 4 a.m. (31%), 9 a.m. to noon (31%), 2 to 5 p.m. (32%), and 7 to 10 p.m. (31%). Travel inefficiency was below the mean only in the early morning (4 to 7 a.m.) and during mealtimes for the severely impaired.

Algase et al. (1997) graphed the frequency and total time in motion by hour for each travel pattern for a group of 25 ambulatory demented nursing home residents. The proportion of wandering increased as the day progressed, 23% during the night shift, 39% during the day, and approximately 57% during the evening. Whether considered by episodes or time in motion, lapping and pacing had similar distributions at low rates and with relatively small hourly fluctuations across the entire 24-hour period. Random wandering and direct (nonwandering) episodes also had similar distributions. While rates and fluctuations were also low and small during nighttime hours, random and direct ambulation rose rapidly beginning at 0600 hours and remained at high levels throughout the day and evening. Peak times for frequency of wandering episodes were 1700 and 1800 hours and for minutes wandering were 0900 and 1800 hours. Peak times for frequency of direct ambulation were 1400 and 1800 hours and for minutes in direct ambulation were 0900 and 1400 hours.

Finally, in analyses evaluating circadian rhythm of locomotion, Satlin and associates (1991) compared AD pacers with AD non-pacers and non-demented controls. Pacers had a 22% lower relative circadian amplitude for activity (an index of circadian rhythm stability) than controls and non-pacers. Although AD subjects differed from controls on several indices of circadian rhythm, pacers and non-pacers were not substantially different from each other, except for overall amount of activity.

Significance

The significance of wandering as a clinical problem has been described in terms of prevalence and incidence, contribution to caregiver stress, association with negative outcomes, and resource consumption. Research findings elaborating each area are summarized in the following section.

Prevalence and incidence. Prevalence estimates of wandering vary widely. Its incidence has not been determined either in dementia overall or in any one type of dementia. Comparison of prevalence estimates across studies is complicated by inconsistent definitions and diverse samples, some composed of only persons with dementia and others with more mixed cognitive problems. Further, most samples are nonrandom, and the target population to which they apply is not always clear. Findings are summarized below for community-residing and institutionalized samples.

The overall proportion of community-residing persons with dementia identified as wanderers ranges from 2 to 50% (unweighted mean across studies = 19%), based largely on family caregiver reports across eight studies encompassing 1576 subjects (Ballard et al., 1991; Baumgarten et al., 1990; Cohen-Mansfield, Werner, Watson, & Pasis, 1995; Cooper, Mungas, & Weiler, 1990; Koss et al., 1997; Patterson et al., 1990; Teri, Hughes, & Larson, 1990; Teri, Larson, & Reifler, 1988). The majority of subjects in these samples met established criteria for AD. In purely AD samples, prevalence rates ranged from 2 to 49% (unweighted mean = 25%) (Baumgarten et al., 1990; Cooper et al., 1990; Koss et al., 1997; Teri et al., 1990). Most often, a positive response to a single question resulted in classification as a wanderer. In a few studies, prevalence of specific wandering behaviors were reported (Ballard et al., 1991; Baumgarten et al., 1990; Cohen-Mansfield, Werner, Watson, et al., 1995), revealing that nighttime wandering was somewhat less frequent (5 to 16%;

unweighted mean 12%) than daytime wandering (2 to 30%; unweighted mean 17%). Wandering prevalence rates have also been estimated by level of cognitive impairment; rates were 12 to 18% for mild, 22–24% for moderate, and 38 to 50% for severe impairment (Cooper et al., 1990; Teri et al., 1988).

In institutionalized samples encompassing over 7,000 residents, wanderers constituted between 5 and 100% (unweighted mean = 31%) of the population (Algase, 1992b; Algase et al., 1997; Burns, Jacoby, & Levy, 1990; Cumming et al., 1982; Everitt, Fields, Soumerai, & Avorn, 1991; Hwang et al., 1997; Kirk, Donnelly, & Compton, 1991; Mann, Graham, & Ashby, 1984; Marin et al., 1997; Nasman et al., 1993; Patterson et al., 1990; Riter & Fries, 1992; Rosin, 1977). In most studies, estimates were based on subjects with dementia, but the proportion of subjects able to walk independently is unknown. However, in three studies (total N = 5842), samples represented a general long-term care population; wanderers constituted between 13 and 22% of these subjects (unweighted mean = 17%). Thus, the proportion of ambulatory, demented nursing home residents who wander is likely higher than the unweighted mean of 31% derived across studies. Classification as a wanderer was often based on some assessment using an identified scale or measure. Interestingly, when based on observations of ambulatory demented residents in two settings, Algase et al. (1997) found that 100% of subjects did wander. Using a far narrower definition which equated wandering only with elopement from the facility, Gurwitz et al. (1994) calculated an annual rate of three incidents per 100 beds.

Source of stress.   Wandering is distressing to family and staff, and this distress is not culture-bound. Forty percent of U.S. families reported it as a problem (Rabins, Mace, & Lucas, 1982), often leading to institutionalization (Sanford, 1975), at least among British subjects. In a Taiwanese sample of 29 family caregivers, 17.5% reported concern with wandering (Shyu, Yip, & Chen, 1996). Further, wandering is consistently included in staff surveys of difficult behaviors and is usually in the top half of behaviors rated (Bright, 1986; Fisher et al., 1993; Haley, 1983). Canadian physicians and nurses reported wandering as the second most frequent behavior problem in nursing homes and ranked it second only to physical aggression as the behavior of greatest concern to them (Conn et al., 1992). Of 15 behaviors evaluated, wandering was the fifth most difficult to manage (Fisher et al., 1993). It was also among seven behaviors causing significant stress for staff (Bright, 1986) and 50% of staff identified wandering as producing mild to severe stress for them (Everitt et al., 1991). Of 126 patients new to a Canadian geropsychiatric service, 35% reported wandering as a problem; however, caregivers of those subjects did not tolerate wandering in approximately 90% of cases, a rate much higher than for five of the other six behaviors reported as causes for admission (Rockwood, Stolee, & Brahim, 1991).

Negative outcomes. Commonly, falls, restraints use, and early mortality are thought to accompany wandering. Number of falls was correlated, $r = .15$, $p < .01$, with frequency of pacing in a nursing home population (Cohen-Mansfield et al., 1991). Wanderers also are likely to sustain fractures (odds ratio = 3.6), but not more so than subjects with poor balance, cataracts, or musculoskeletal problems (Buchner & Larson, 1987). Further, 53% of wanderers sustained a fracture during 3 years of follow-up. In particular, a very strong association between wandering and hip fractures was demonstrated (odds ratio = 6.9, 95% confidence interval = 1.66 to 28.6, $p = .005$). However, fall and fracture rates in relation to amount or pattern of wandering remain unknown.

Restraints and wandering have received more study. Nursing home staff cited prevention of wandering as the reason for restraints in 20% of new applications (Tinetti et al., 1991). Examined in the first month after admission and throughout the following year, wandering was a significant predictor of restraint use (standardized regression coefficients = .14 to .33, $p \geq .05$) in nursing homes with both high use and low use rates (Burton et al., 1992). However, high use may be a U.S. phenomenon. In a recent Swedish study, wandering was not likely to lead to restraint; 9% of subjects in geriatric facilities who were restrained were wanderers, while 14% of the unrestrained also wandered (Karlsson et al., 1996). Further, in a study of restraints in an acute care setting in Britain, only bedrails were used and, of 56 reported instances of use, only one was to prevent wandering (O'Keeffe, Jack, & Lye, 1996).

Restraints are an important issue for wanderers. Negative outcomes associated with restraint use in general are well known. Over 20 years ago, Cornbleth (1977) offered clear evidence for the value of a restraint-free environment for wanderers by demonstrating better range of motion among them when on a ward permitting free ambulation. Interestingly, nonwanderers with cognitive impairments had better range of motion on traditional units where wanderers may be restrained. This finding argues for the benefits of a special care unit (SCU) for wanderers especially. Sand, Yeaworth, and McCabe (1992) offer more recent support. In a state survey of 203 long-term care facilities, only 3% with SCUs saw daytime wandering in AD patients as a significant problem, while 12% of facilities without SCUs viewed it as problematic. Further, no SCU used restraints to manage wandering, but 12% of facilities without SCUs did.

The connection between wandering and mortality has been evaluated in two studies. In a sample of 126 AD outpatients who were followed for at least 6 years, the combination of wandering and falling reduced survival rates by more than 3 years, likely related to morbidity from hip fractures (Walsh, Welch, & Larson, 1990). As a separate category, behavioral problems alone (of which wandering was one) reduced survival rates by over 1 year. In more recent work, wandering was associated with shortened survival in a univariate analysis (Bowen et al., 1996). In multivariate analyses of the same data, controlling for the effects of age, gender, and dementia severity, wandering had no independent effect on survival.

Resource consumption.   Not only does wandering lead to institutional care (Sanford, 1975), it often results in costlier care. In a study examining magnitude of unacceptable behavior in facilities for the aged in British Columbia, Cumming et al. (1982) determined that one in six persons nominated for transfer to special behavioral units were named due to intrusive, wandering behavior. Wandering is a frequently cited reason for admission to geropsychiatric services (Lam, Sewell, Bell, & Katona, 1989; Moak, 1990; Rockwood et al., 1991). Lam and associates determined that wandering (along with aggression and incontinence) more often resulted in hospitalization than in placement in less costly homes for old people in Britain (Lam et al., 1989). Surprisingly, however, wandering did not explain assignment to a SCU according to a study by Riter and Fries (1992) in which wanderers were over two times more prevalent in SCUs than in general nursing units. Although significant in a univariate analysis, it was not a predictor of SCU placement in multivariate analyses that controlled for other independent variables, particularly ability to transfer independently. This conclusion can be challenged on a logical basis. Demented persons are not placed on SCUs because they are better able to transfer independently; rather, this ability more likely reflects their capacity to wander! Not only is wandering associated with costlier forms of care, it is also a reason precluding discharge to the community from hospital-based geropsychiatric services in over 9% of patients (Vieweg, Blair, Tucker, & Lewis, 1995).

Correlates

An array of factors has been examined in efforts to explain wandering. Results of these studies are organized and presented in this section according to cognitive and neurological factors, personal characteristics of wanderers, and environmental conditions under which wandering occurs.

Cognitive and neurological factors.   Early studies did not reveal associations between level of cognitive impairment and wandering (Monsour & Robb,

1982; Snyder et al., 1978). Now 16 studies using better measures of cognitive impairment and more robust sampling strategies offer compelling evidence for this association (Algase, 1992b; Baker, Kokmen, Chandra, & Schoenberg, 1991; Ballard et al., 1991; Buchner & Larson, 1987; Burns et al., 1990; Cohen-Mansfield, Marx, & Rosenthal, 1989; Cooper et al., 1990; Cooper & Mungas, 1993; Devanand et al., 1997; Gilley et al., 1991; Hwang et al., 1997; Jost & Grossberg, 1995; Marin et al., 1997; Martino-Saltzman et al., 1991; Miller, Tinklenberg, Brooks, Fenn, & Yesavage, 1993; Teri et al., 1988, 1990).

Wanderers' scores on global measures of cognitive performance are significantly lower than non-wanderers (Algase, 1992b; Buchner & Larson, 1987; Burns et al., 1990). Wanderers also show poorer discrete cognitive skills, including memory, language, concentration/attention, visual-spatial/construction tasks, orientation, judgment, conceptualization, and initiation/perseveration (Algase, 1992b; Burns et al., 1990; Martino-Saltzman et al., 1991; Miller et al., 1993), although evidence for orientation, recall, and language repetition is conflicting (Miller et al., 1993).

Studies reveal increasing proportions of wanderers among subjects at each level of dementia ranging from 0–18% (unweighted mean = 8.0%) among mildly demented, 3–26% (unweighted mean = 13.6%) among moderately demented, and 0–67% (unweighted mean = 29.5%) among severely demented subjects (Ballard et al., 1991; Cooper et al., 1990; Cooper & Mungas, 1993; Hwang et al., 1997; Teri et al., 1988, 1990); when tested, differences in proportions between levels of impairment were significant (Cooper et al., 1990; Teri et al, 1988). Disease severity and duration correlates with wandering, $r = .18–.56$, $p = .01$ to $.05$ (Devanand et al., 1997; Gilley et al., 1991; Marin et al., 1997; Martino-Saltzman, 1991) and explains 29% of its variance (Gilley et al., 1991). Yet, in at least one study, no association was found between disease severity and status as a wanderer (Ryan et al., 1995). Wandering usually manifests *late* in a dementing process (Baker et al., 1991; Jost & Grossberg, 1995; Miller et al., 1993) and, if present, is associated with a faster rate of cognitive decline (Miller et al., 1993; Teri et al., 1990). Yet early spatial disorientation is one of twelve features signifying Alzheimer's disease, as compared to vascular dementia or Pick's disease (Gustafson & Nilsson, 1982).

Above analyses of cognitive impairment and wandering rely on classification of subjects as wanderers or nonwanderers based largely on caregiver reports. In only one work was actual wandering behavior observed at each level of dementia severity; random and lapping patterns of wandering increased as a percent of overall ambulation as cognitive function declined, while the pacing pattern remained stable through all levels of impairment (Martino-Saltzman et al., 1991).

Most studies of wandering and cognitive impairment (or disease severity) were done in AD samples. Among AD patients, a younger age at onset is also significantly associated with wandering, characterized as pacing and motor activity (Gilley et al., 1991). However, among subjects with other dementias, similar prevalence rate also were found. Data from a sample of 1312 subjects revealed that wanderers constituted 9.0% of AD subjects and 10.8% of those with vascular dementia (Cooper & Mungas, 1993). For both diagnoses, rates were low (9–12% in the early stages) and higher as each disease progressed (17–37% in the later stages). In a comparison of demented subjects with AD and Parkinson's disease (PD), the proportion of wanderers were not significantly different, 15% AD versus 13% PD (Bliwise et al., 1995). Of 318 HIV-related dementia subjects, 15% wandered (Boccellari & Dilley, 1992). Wandering was significantly associated (49%) with the severe impairment, $X^2 = 42, p \geq .0001$, and was correlated with substantial residential placement difficulty, $r = .37, p \geq .001$). Among subjects with Down's syndrome, daytime wandering occurred with significantly greater frequency ($p = .013$) among those who were demented; prevalence of wandering among the demented Down's subjects was five of 15 cases, with three of these occurring at the moderate level of impairment (Prasher & Filer, 1995). Although wandering has been associated with mixed impairment, that is, having both reversible and irreversible causes (Algase, 1992b), a significant association with AD, compared to vascular and other dementias, was also reported (Thomas, 1997).

However, some investigators argue that wandering is not due to global cognitive decline, but is a function of one (or several) more discrete neurological mechanisms. Among these, mechanisms underlying spatial orientation have been a prime focus. In addition to work by deLeon et al. (1984) and Liu et al. (1991) cited earlier, others have shown deficits in spatial capacities (or neuroanatomical substrates for same) among wanderers. Henderson et al. (1989) determined that neuropsychological tests of memory and visouconstructive ability, but not of disease severity, attention, or language impairment, were significant predictors of spatial disorientation for 28 ambulatory AD subjects. They suggested that these results may implicate dysfunction of neocortical areas in the right hemisphere concerned with visuospatial processes. Shown through positron emission tomography (PET), wanderers ($n = 9$) had a relative deficit in regional metabolic rate for glucose in the right parietal lobe as compared to the left parietal lobe, temporo-parieto-occipital region, and occipital lobe, bilateral frontal lobes, and cerebellum (Meguro et al., 1996); wanderers were inpatients with vascular dementia who wandered out of their rooms, got lost inside the hospital, or would not return to their rooms on 7 of 14 consecutive days. Still, in a comparison of wanderers and nonwanderers with probable AD on spatial orientation, attention/concentration, and perseveration, Ryan et al. (1995) found differences only for perseveration, which was greater both overall and as more recurrent and continuous. Failure to find an expected difference in spatial orientation was thought due to milder severity of illness in their sample compared to that of Henderson et al. (1989) and/or to the possibility that wandering may result from impaired visuospatial attention, rather than orientation, in early stages of AD. Further, they suggested that difficulty in shifting visuospatial attention (i.e., inability to disengage), may be a form of continuous perseveration (Sandson & Albert, 1987).

Reduced higher-order cognitive and planning abilities may also play a role in wandering (Passini, Rainville, Marchand, & Joanette, 1995). Fourteen early to mid-stage AD subjects and 28 controls (matched for age, gender and education) did a complex wayfinding task in an unfamiliar environment. Accompanied by an observer, subjects found their way to a standard location within a hospital from a nearby bus stop (and back). In addition to observing general performance, observers gathered data on the planning abilities and decision processes used by subjects. All AD subjects made significantly more errors both in reaching the destination and in returning from it; and their error rate did not improve significantly on the return trip. Analysis of their decision-making processes revealed reduced ability to form (or to actively retain) an overall plan for reaching the goal; inability to detect relevant from irrelevant information, which quickly overloaded their active problem-solving capacity; impulsive responses to stimuli, which drew them off course or task; and inability to stop the search when the desired destination was identified, a form of perseveration. So, in addition to tapping spatial representations (a function of the hippocampus), it is necessary to perform spatio-cognitive operations (a problem-solving task or frontal lobe function) for effective wayfinding. Since these higher-order operations are affected early in AD, they may account for early spatial disorientation.

Circadian rhythm disturbances, particularly sleep disturbances, have also been investigated as a basis for wandering. In a study comparing 28 male AD subjects with 10 healthy controls, AD subjects displayed circadian cycles with a lower amplitude for locomotor activity, indicating a greater proportion of nighttime activity; no difference in amplitude of core-body temperature occurred (Satlin et al., 1995). However, the acrophase of AD subjects' temperature cycles was delayed by 4.5 hours. A subgroup of AD patients having a large mean difference in acrophases of activity and temperature cycles were also found; these subjects had even lower temperature amplitudes ($p = .001$) and a greater proportion of nighttime locomotion ($p = .008$), indicating impairment in the endogenous pacemaker synchronizing these rhythms. As the suprachiasmatic nucleus, which mediates activity and temperature rhythms, shrinks in AD (Swaab, Fliers, & Partiman, 1985), circadian rhythm disturbances may account for nighttime wandering. Primary sleep disorders, such as sleep apnea, do not appear to affect wandering. Pacing was negatively correlated with indices of sleep apnea, $r = -.15$, $p < .01$, but positively related to myocolonic movements, $r = .16$, $p < .01$ (Cohen-Mansfield, Werner, & Freedman, 1995). Although lower rates of pacing were seen after sleep periods than immediately before them, differences were insignificant, suggesting that fatigue is not a factor in wandering.

Lastly, wandering is associated with psychiatric phenomena that may overlay dementia. It is more prevalent in the face of depression (Mann et al., 1984), but its association with delusions is conflicting (Berrios & Brook, 1985; Lachs et al., 1992). Although psychiatric conditions are likely not a primary etiology for wandering, their association with the behavior is not surprising, given that psychiatric disorders may further cloud cognitive capacities.

Personal characteristics.   Wanderers and nonwanderers do not differ by gender, education, or race (Burns et al., 1990; Cohen-Mansfield et al., 1991; Cooper et al., 1990; Henderson et al., 1989; Hwang et al., 1997; Ryan et al., 1995; Thomas, 1997). However, gender differences may apply to specific dimensions of wandering. Wandering behaviors were more common in men and escape behaviors more common in women in one sample (Nasman et al., 1993). In all but two samples, evidence for lack of an age difference between wanderers and nonwanderers is fairly robust (Cohen-Mansfield et al., 1991; Henderson et al., 1989; Hwang et al., 1997; Martino-Saltzman et al., 1991; Ryan et al., 1995). Thomas (1997) found wanderers to be significantly younger while Cooper et al. (1990) reported them as significantly older. As samples were non-random, demographic findings should be viewed with caution.

Wanderers are in better general health than nonwanderers. Wandering is negatively related to pain and eating impairment and positively related to appetite and to fewer medications and medical diagnoses; relationships to cardiovascular disease, incontinence, diabetes, and depressed affect were not shown (Cohen-Mansfield et al., 1991). Martino-Saltzman et al. (1991) found no association between low travel efficiency and use of drugs (diuretics, laxatives, major or minor tranquilizers, or any combination of these). In another study, escape behavior was positively correlated with ADL ability, and both wandering and escape behaviors were related to lower physical workload for staff (Nasman et al., 1993). Yet, small positive correlations ($r = .11$ to $.14$) were found between wandering and impaired grooming, dressing, and bathing ability (Cohen-Mansfield et al., 1991).

Wandering may coexist with other behavior problems. A significant relationship to other agitated behaviors, specifically verbal agitation, $r = .16$;

physical aggression, $r = .19$; and other nonaggressive physical behaviors (such as hoarding), $r = .23$, has been reported (Cohen-Mansfield et al., 1991). Yet, Dawson and Reid (1987) found no differences between wanderers and nonwanderers on a measure of agitation/aggression, but they did find associations between hyperactivity and the frequency and degree of wandering. Wandering was also reported in eight of 14 coprophagics; but no test of significance was applied (Ghaziuddin & MacDonald, 1985).

The role of life experience and personality in wandering has also been examined. Evidence suggests that wandering may follow from a high level of pre-morbid life stress to which wanderers reacted with more motor behaviors (Cohen-Mansfield et al., 1991; Monsour & Robb, 1982). The pre-morbid personality of wanderers was also more active and sociable than that of nonwanderers (Monsour & Robb, 1982; Thomas, 1997). Wanderers had higher scores on warmth, gregariousness, positive emotion, altruism, and activity on the NEO Five-Factors Personality Inventory (Thomas, 1997).

Environmental conditions.   In only two studies were environmental conditions conducive to wandering examined; both were observational and conducted under naturally occurring conditions. Wandering may increase when an environment is unfamiliar. Evidence supporting this conclusion rests in the positive correlation of increased wandering to presence of residents from other units and to relocating to another unit and in its negative correlation to length of stay (Cohen-Mansfield et al., 1991; Cohen-Mansfield & Werner, 1995). Wandering declines during structured activities and ADLs and when a subject is alone (Cohen-Mansfield & Werner, 1995). If noise is low, wandering increases, but it is not associated to exposure to television or music; conversely, when lighting and temperature are normal, wandering increases. Few features of the social environment have been examined. Wandering increases when subjects are more than three feet away from others or when there are two to five other persons present. However, neither type of person in the immediate environment nor presence of visitors appears to play a role.

Interventions

Researchers have investigated a range of interventions for wandering. Unfortunately, few are based on a guiding theory or explanation for the behavior itself. Most strive to contain wandering within an acceptable area or to reduce its frequency while disregarding benefits that may ensue from it.

Pharmacological means.   A variety of drugs have been used to "treat" wandering. Even after implementing regulations intended to eliminate inappropriate use of psychoactive drugs in nursing homes, a fair number of wanderers continue to receive these medications. One large nursing home survey revealed that neuroleptics were given to 15% of wanderers, benzodiazepines to 10%, and antidepressants to 7% (Everitt et al., 1991). Yet, the efficacy of these drugs for managing wandering has not been evaluated in well-controlled studies.

The range of drugs evaluated for wandering reflects a palliative approach and measures of treatment efficacy presume a goal of eradicating the behavior. Subjective improvements were seen in case studies using anti-androgens (Amadeo, 1996) and (for nighttime wandering) a sedative, zolpidem (Shelton & Hocking, 1997). In more formal works aimed at anxiety control, alprazolam (Szwabo, Woodward, Grossberg, & Shen, 1991) and propranolol (Shankle, Neilson, & Cotman, 1995) reduced wandering, but raters were not blinded and no control groups were used. Comparing two neuroleptics (tiapride and melperone) revealed similar efficacy in reducing wandering (over 1 point on a 6-point scale), but their efficacy in relation to placebo is unknown (Gutzman et al., 1997). Tacrine improved baseline pacing scores in 70% and stabilized them in 81% of AD subjects in a double-blind study; differences in rates compared to the placebo group were significant (Raskind, Sadowski, Sigmund, Beitler, & Auster, 1997). In two well-designed case studies of vascular dementia, mild wandering was eliminated with fasudil hydrochloride (Kamei, Oishi, & Takasu, 1996).

Egress control methods.   Various camouflage techniques and grid patterns affixed to the floor have been evaluated for their effectiveness in deterring exits, based on visual agnosia and other visual deficits in AD which convey a three-dimensional appearance to a two dimensional surface (Hinton, Sadun, Blanks, & Miller, 1986; Hutton, 1985; Nissen et al., 1985; Steffes & Thralow, 1987). Hussian and Brown (1987) demonstrated that eight horizontal stripes beginning 3 feet from a closed door significantly reduced doorway contact among demented males to 30% from 98% at baseline; for one subject, no pattern of stripes had any effect. A repetition of this technique in front of glass doors was ineffective (Chafetz, 1990). In another replication testing the eight-stripe design in both horizontal and vertical configurations, reductions in doorway contacts and exits were noted for each subject ($n = 10$; females $= 7$) under each condition, but were significant only for AD subjects and for one person with Parkinson's dementia (Hewewasam, 1996a, 1996b). Again, the horizontal design was the more effective one. Several additional grid designs and doorknob concealment strategies were evaluated by Namazi et al. (1989). A cloth panel across the width of the door, regardless of color, reduced exits to zero, a finding validated by Dickinson, McLain-Kark, and Marshall-Baker (1995). A full-length mirror positioned a foot in front of a door also lowered the number of door contacts and exits significantly, but not entirely (Mayer & Darby, 1991). Researchers cautioned that approaches toward the doorway may increase by attraction to the mirror.

Despite frequent use of alarms and other security systems in clinical settings, only one study evaluating them was found. Five patients were observed as a closed locked door was converted to an open door fitted with an electronic sensor and audio alarm (Negley, Molla, & Obenchain, 1990). Two subjects had few passbys or exits regardless of condition. For the remaining three, the open door alone attracted increased passbys and exits. Once the alarm was activated, passbys remained elevated from baseline for one subject, but exits decreased for those who had any previous attempts. Reduced exits continued even when the alarm was deactivated, but counts reflect only a one-week follow-up period.

Behavioral techniques.   Behavioral strategies have been applied to manage banned entries and exits of wanderers. Although effective in the short run, behavioral techniques meet with difficulty in sustaining behavior change. The intrusive wandering behavior of one demented woman was handled by simply trading rooms with another resident to accommodate the subject's travel patterns (Donat, 1984). By conditioning three subjects to supernormal visual stimuli, Hussain (1982) reduced their entries into unauthorized areas; but, as cues were faded, the behavior returned, necessitating both booster training sessions and persistent display of cues to sustain the behavior change. Using a strategy termed differential reinforcement of other behaviors (DRO), Jozsvai et al. (1996) reduced exit attempts (and two other behaviors) for one male with Creutzfeld-Jacob disease. Yet, without monitoring, staff subverted gains by lapsing into a variable reinforcement schedule for undesired behaviors or by failing to reinforce desired behaviors, thereby programming extinction.

Group strategies.   Groups for wanderers have been tried to affect wandering and to improve the milieu on nursing units where wanderers reside (Holmberg, 1997; Rosswurm, Zimmerman, Schwartz-Fulton, & Norman, 1986; Smith-Jones & Francis, 1992). Generally, groups were designed to provide structured activities; one focused on periods of planned walking. Two were groups limited to wanderers (Holmberg, 1997; Rosswurm et al., 1986), while a larger program included residents with a range of disruptive behaviors. In addition, the program described by Rosswurm et al. included changes to the dining area to permit freer access to residents and the addition of residents' pictures to their doors. Length of sessions varied from 1 to 2 hours each; frequency of sessions varied between twice daily to three times per week over periods ranging from 5 weeks to one year. All programs reported subjective improvements to the milieu. Holmberg (1997) reported significantly fewer ($p = .03$) incidents of aggressive behavior on weekdays when the group met as compared to weekdays and to all days (including weekends and holidays) when it did not meet. Differences were not accounted for by a mere reduction in number of residents left on the unit during group meetings. Reports of reduced wandering were also subjective (Smith-Jones & Francis, 1992). In a more objective estimate of the impact on wandering, time spent walking increased but entries into other residents' rooms remained stable (Rosswurm et al., 1986). Daytime sleeping decreased and interactions with staff increased, although most of these were staff-initiated. Wanderers also spent more time in the halls and activity-dining area and less in their own rooms and those of other residents. Unfortunately, these changes were not evaluated statistically.

Milieu therapies.   Design of whole environments or programs of care have been considered for their impact on wandering. In fact, the first study of wandering was such an evaluation. In a quasi-experiment comparing a locked ward with a traditional unit, range of motion was significantly ($p < .04$) improved for wanderers on the locked ward and for nonwanderers on the traditional one at twelve weeks post-intervention (Cornbleth, 1977). A major benefit of today's SCU, as perceived by both families and staff, is freedom to wander (Dupuis, Dobbelsteyn, & Ericson, 1996). Perceptions are supported by the finding that SCUs are more likely ($p < .01$) to allow nighttime wandering and to use distraction and alternative activities as means to manage wandering, than are general nursing home units (Sand et al., 1992). In the same survey, these researchers revealed that no SCU used restraints to control wandering. Further evidence of increased tolerance for wandering on units with more flexible programming was shown by Matthews, Farrell, and Blackmore (1996). When staff changed from a task-oriented to a client-oriented approach to care, the number of residents who paced frequently increased by an average of 4.5% and those who frequently tried to get to another place grew by an average of 7%. However, in one study, the goal of a "comprehensive approach" to managing wandering was to reduce it (Goldsmith et al., 1995). Evaluation of a single subject for changes in wandering associated with this approach showed the opposite to be the case. This result is not entirely surprising, as the "comprehensive approach" actually includes increased opportunity for safe wandering and decreased emphasis on physical and chemical restraint. While ambulating alone increased during and after the intervention period, exit attempts remained stable and, as could be expected with increased ambulating, instances of entering into unsafe locations also rose.

White noise.   Young, Muir-Nash, and Ninos (1988) examined the impact of white noise for its effects on nighttime wandering on a group of eight subjects with a history of the behavior admitted to an inpatient hospital unit. With subjects serving as their own controls, the treatment effect was not significant for the group. However, two subjects demonstrated substantially less wandering during the treatment phase. Characteristics differentiating these two subjects from the others were not delineated.

Caregivers' approaches. Management approaches used by family caregivers duplicate many of those seen in institutional settings. Restraint (both physical and chemical, including alcohol), diversion through activity, reality orientation, ignoring the behavior (when it does not pose a hazard), and getting assistance in finding a missing member, are examples offered by Dodds (1994). However, restraint was generally passive (e.g., locking exterior doors) and limited to times when activity was perceived as excessive. On occasion, a family locked their relative in the house alone when they needed to go out, resulting in substantial guilt. Families also sought respite from constantly being followed, colluded with inaccurate beliefs of their family member to avoid confrontation, and used verbal and physical aggression when their frustration mounted. Three strategies emerged from focus groups of Taiwanese caregivers: environmental management, monitoring, and guidance as means to manage wandering (Shyu et al., 1996). In a similar study, U.S. caregivers also reported using environmental adjustments and reassurance to manage wandering (Richter, Roberto, & Bottenberg, 1995). These caregivers also reported that reality orientation was ineffective and often increased agitation.

SUMMARY AND DIRECTIONS FOR FUTURE RESEARCH

Research on the phenomenon of wandering is ripe with opportunity for improvement. Of prime importance is the need to move beyond current conceptual ambiguity in meanings of the term. Simply classifying subjects as wanderers or nonwanderers is no longer acceptable; fuller portrayal of subjects, at least as to amount, quality, and temporal nature of their ambulatory behavior, is the emerging norm. Effort to capture navigational abilities or deficits of subjects and to typify their environmental transgressions should also be considered in designing future studies.

Studies of wandering would also benefit from clarification of the intended target population. The value of knowledge gleaned from existing studies is weakened by inconsistencies in comparing wanderers to nonwanderers who may represent a general nursing home population, institutionalized and/or community-residing demented elderly, or those with mixed ambulatory status and/or medical basis for cognitive impairment. Current evidence suggests that, although wandering occurs in many dementias, its features, and likely its neurological basis, may vary with underlying pathology. Future studies should take this into account, if possible. Additionally, researchers should avoid using small, non-probability samples, except in preliminary studies, and control for degree of cognitive decline.

Intervention studies for wandering are generally weak, suffering conceptually from imprecise thinking about goals of intervention and appropriateness of the theory (if any) behind it. Designs are often single case studies, few comparisons or controls are used, and outcome measures are often ill-defined and poorly operationalized. While these studies are premature by some scientific standards, the author appreciates the clinical need to press forward with intervention work, and urges the use of well-constructed, multiple case studies for initially evaluating promising ideas.

Many gaps in our knowledge of wandering persist. Researchers are only beginning to describe wandering in ways that mesh with advances in cognitive and neurosciences. Continued work in this direction is essential for linking aspects of wandering to neural mechanisms that may mediate it. Such knowledge can enlighten our understanding about aspects of the behavior that may or may not be appropriate for or amenable to alteration and can point toward possible intervention strategies.

Knowledge of noncognitive characteristics of persons who display various amounts and kinds of wandering is also warranted. If needs, such as hunger or fatigue; physical conditions, such as pain; and/or psychological states, such as boredom or tension, also contribute to the behavior, clearer goals of and avenues for intervention may emerge. For the same reason, expansion of our knowledge of environmental factors, both physical and social, that impede or induce wandering is required. Studies evaluating multifactorial etiologies (i.e., cognitive, noncognitive, and environmental factors), are most desirable.

Outcomes of wandering are virtually unknown. Although clinical impressions and a few studies suggest that both positive results (e.g., increased range of motion) and negative results (e.g., falls) occur, documentation of these outcomes and the circumstances producing them is very limited, and the degree to which various aspects of wandering (i.e., amount vs. quality), contribute to these outcomes is totally unknown. For instance, the impact of wandering on weight and nutritional status has not been studied, although a potential connection is logical.

Examination of the impact of wandering on caregivers and other residents of care environments should also be extended. An assumption that wandering is stress-producing or negatively affects some others in a setting permeates several studies reviewed; yet precisely that which is troublesome about wandering has not been delineated. Thus, an appropriate target for intervention, wanderer versus caregiver, staff, or other residents, remains unclear.

Finally, as suggested above, the need to develop a sound theoretical explanation for wandering is imperative as a basis for designing and testing rational interventions. Given that resources will always be limited and the number of active investigators is small, priority should be given to explanation over intervention at this stage of the science on wandering.

ACKNOWLEDGMENT

Acknowledgment is given to Barbara Harrison, doctoral student, for conducting the literature search and assisting in screening articles for inclusion in this work.

REFERENCES

Albert, S. M. (1992). The nature of wandering in dementia: A Guttman scaling analysis of an empirical classification scheme. *International Journal of Geriatric Psychiatry, 7*, 783–787.

Algase, D. L. (1992a). A century of progress: Today's strategies for managing wandering behavior. *Journal of Gerontological Nursing, 18*, 23–34.

Algase, D. L. (1992b). Cognitive discriminants of wandering among nursing home residents. *Nursing Research, 41*, 78–81.

Algase, D. L., Kupferschmid, B., Beel-Bates, C. A., & Beattie, E. R. (1997). Estimates of stability of daily wandering behavior among cognitively impaired long-term care residents. *Nursing Research, 46*, 172–178.

Amadeo, M. (1996). Antiandrogen treatment of aggressivity in men suffering from dementia. *Journal of Geriatric Psychiatry & Neurology, 9*, 142–145.

Baker, F. M., Kokmen, E., Chandra, V., & Schoenberg, B. S. (1991). Psychiatric symptoms in cases of clinically diagnosed Alzheimer's disease. *Journal of Geriatric, 4*, 71–78.

Ballard, C. G., Mohan, R. N. C., Bannister, C., Handy, S., & Patel, A. (1991). Wandering in dementia sufferers. *International Journal of Geriatric Psychiatry, 6*, 611–614.

Baumgarten, M., Becker, R., & Gauthier, S. (1990). Validity and reliability of the dementia behavior disturbance scale. *Journal of the American Geriatrics Society, 8*, 221–226.

Berrios, G. E., & Brook, P. (1985). Delusions and the psychopathology of the elderly with dementia. *Acta Psychiatrici Scandinavica, 72*, 296–301.

Bliwise, D. L., Watts, R. L., Watts, N., Rye, D. B., Irbe, D., & Hughes, M. (1995). Disruptive nocturnal behavior in Parkinson's disease and Alzheimer's disease. *Journal of Geriatric Psychiatry & Neurology, 8*, 107–110.

Boccellari, A. A., & Dilley, J. W. (1992). Management and residential placement problems of patients with HIV-related cognitive impairment. *Hospital & Community Psychiatry, 43,* 32–37.

Bowen, J. D., Malter, A. D., Sheppard, L., Kukull, W. A., McCormick, W. C., Teri, L., & Larson, E. B. (1996). Predictors of mortality in patients diagnosed with probable Alzheimer's disease. *Neurology, 47,* 433–439.

Bright, R. (1986). The use of music therapy and activities with demented patients who are deemed "difficult to manage." *Clinical Gerontologist, 6,* 131–144.

Buchner, D. M., & Larson, E. B. (1987). Falls and fractures in patients with Alzheimer-type dementia. *Journal of the American Medical Association, 257,* 1492–1495.

Burns, A., Jacoby, R., & Levy, R. (1990). Psychiatric phenomena in Alzheimer's disease. IV: Disorders of behavior. *British Journal of Psychiatry, 157,* 86–94.

Burton, L. C., German, P. S., Rovner, B. W., Brant, L. J., & Clark, R. D. (1992). Mental illness and the use of restraints in nursing homes. *Gerontologist, 32,* 164–170.

Chafetz, P. K. (1990). Two-dimensional grid is ineffective against demented patients' exiting through glass doors. *Psychology and Aging, 5,* 146–147.

Cohen-Mansfield, J. (1986). Agitated behaviors in the elderly: II. Preliminary results in the cognitively deteriorated. *Journal of American Geriatrics Society, 34,* 722–727.

Cohen-Mansfield, J., Marx, M. S., & Rosenthal, A. S. (1989). A description of agitation in a nursing home. *Journal of Gerontology, 44,* M77–84.

Cohen-Mansfield, J., & Werner, P. (1995). Environmental influences on agitation: An integration summary of an observation study. *The American Journal of Alzheimer's Care and Related Disorders and Research, 10,* 32–39.

Cohen-Mansfield, J., Werner, P., Marx, M., & Freedman, L. (1995). Sleep and agitation in agitated nursing home residents: An observational study. *Sleep, 18,* 674–680.

Cohen-Mansfield, J., Werner, P., & Marx, M. S. (1991). Two studies of pacing in the nursing home. *Journal of Gerontology: Medical Sciences, 46,* M77–83.

Cohen-Mansfield, J., Werner, P., Watson, V., & Pasis, S. (1995). Agitation among elderly persons at adult day-care centers: The experiences of relatives and staff members. *International Psychogeriatrics, 7,* 447–458.

Conn, D. K., Lee, V., Steingart, A., & Silberfeld, M. (1992). Psychiatric services: A survey of nursing homes and homes for the aged in Ontario. *Canadian Journal of Psychiatry, 37,* 525–530.

Cooper, J. K., & Mungas, D. (1993). Risk factor and behavioral differences between vascular and Alzheimer's dementias: The pathway to end-stage disease. *Journal of Geriatric Psychiatry & Neurology, 6,* 29–33.

Cooper, J. K., Mungas, D., & Weiler, P. G. (1990). Relation of cognitive status and abnormal behaviors in Alzheimer's disease. *Journal of the American Geriatrics Society, 38,* 867–870.

Cornbleth, T. (1977). Effects of a protected hospital ward area on wandering and nonwandering geriatric patients. *Journal of Gerontology, 32,* 573–537.

Cumming, J., Cumming, E., Titus, J., Schmelzle, E., & MacDonald, J. (1982). The episodic nature of behavioral disturbances among residents of facilities for the aged. *Canadian Journal of Public Health, 73,* 319–322.

Davis, L. L., Buckwalter, K., & Burgio, L. D. (1997). Measuring problem behaviors in dementia: Developing a methodological agenda. *Advances in Nursing Science, 20,* 40–55.

Dawson, P., & Reid, D. (1987). Behavioral dimensions of patients at risk of wandering. *The Gerontologist, 27,* 104–107.

de Leon, M., Potegal, M., & Gurland, B. (1984). Wandering and parietal signs in senile dementia of Alzheimer's type. *Neuropsychobiology, 11,* 155–157.

Devanand, D. P., Jacobs, D. M., Tang, M. X., Del Castillo-Castaneda, C., Sano, M., Marder, K., Bell, K., Bylsma, F. W., Brandt, J., Albert, M., & Stern, Y. (1997). The course of psychopathologic features in mild to moderate Alzheimer disease. *Archives of General Psychiatry, 54,* 257–263.

Dickinson, J. I., McLain-Kark, J., & Marshall-Baker, A. (1995). The effects of visual barriers on exiting behavior in a dementia care unit. *Gerontologist, 35,* 127–130.

Dodds, P. (1994). Wandering: A short report on coping strategies adopted by informal carers. *International Journal of Geriatric Psychiatry, 9,* 751–756.

Donat, D. C. (1984). Modifying wandering behavior: Dementia assessment. *Clinical Gerontologist, 3,* 41–43.

Dupuis, M., Dobbelsteyn, J., & Ericson, P. (1996). Special care units for residents with Alzheimer's (investigating the perceptions of families and staff). *Canadian Nursing Home, 7,* 4–7, 9.

Everitt, D. E., Fields, D. R., Soumerai, S. S., & Avorn, J. (1991). Resident behavior and staff distress in the nursing home. *Journal of the American Geriatrics Society, 39,* 792–798.

Fisher, J. E., Fink, C. M., & Loomis, C. C. (1993). Frequency and management difficulty of behavioral problems among dementia patients in long-term care facilities. *Clinical Gerontologist, 13,* 3–12.

Ghaziuddin, N., & McDonald, C. (1985). A clinical study of adult coprophagics. *British Journal of Psychiatry, 147,* 312–313.

Gilley, D. W., Wilson, R. S., Bennett, D. A., Bernard, B. A., & Fox, J. H. (1991). Predictors of behavioral disturbance in Alzheimer's disease. *Journal of Gerontology, 46,* 362–371.

Goldsmith, S. M., Hoeffer, B., & Rader, J. (1995). Problematic wandering behavior in the cognitively impaired elderly: A single-subject case study. *Journal of Psychosocial Nursing & Mental Health Services, 33,* 6–12.

Gurwitz, J. H., Sanchez-Cross, M. T., Eckler, M. A., & Matulis, J. (1994). The epidemiology of adverse and unexpected events in the long-term care setting. *Journal of the American Geriatrics Society, 42,* 33–38.

Gustafson, L., & Nilsson, L. (1982). Differential diagnosis of presenile dementia on clinical grounds. *Acta Psychiatrica Scandinavica, 21,* 194–209.

Guttman, L. L. (1974). The basis for scalgram analysis. In G. M. Maraneel (Ed.), *Scaling: A sourcebook for behavioral scientists* (pp. __). Chicago: Aldine.

Gutzmann, H., Kuhl, K. P., Kanowski, S., & Khan-Boluki, J. (1997). Measuring the efficacy of psychopharmacological treatment of psychomotoric restlessness in dementia: Clinical evaluation of tiapride. *Pharmacopsychiatry, 30,* 6–11.

Haley, W. E. (1983). Priorities for behavioral intervention with nursing home resident. *International Journal of Behavioral Geriatrics, 1,* 47–51.

Henderson, V., Mack, B., & Williams, B. W. (1989). Spatial disorientation in Alzheimer's disease. *Archives of Neurology, 46,* 391–394.

Herman, J. F., & Bruce, P. R. (1981). Spatial knowledge of ambulatory and wheelchair-confined nursing home residents. *Experimental Aging Research, 7,* 491–496.

Hewawasam, L. (1996a). Floor patterns limit wandering of people with Alzheimer's. *Nursing Times, 92,* 41–44.

Hewawasam, L. (1996b). The use of two-dimensional grid patterns to limit hazardous ambulation in elderly patients with Alzheimer's disease. *NtResearch, 1,* 217–228.

Hinton, D. R., Sadun, A. A., Blanks, J. C., & Miller, C. A. (1986). Optical nerve degeneration in Alzheimer's disease. *The New England Journal of Medicine, 315,* 485–487.

Holmberg, S. K. (1997). Evaluation of a clinical intervention for wanderers on a geriatric nursing unit. *Archives of Psychiatric Nursing, 11,* 21–28.

Hope, R. A., & Fairburn, C. G. (1990). The nature of wandering in dementia: A community-based study. *International Journal of Geriatric Psychiatry, 5,* 239–245.

Hope, R. A., & Fairburn, C. G. (1992). The present behavioral examination (PBE): The development of an interview to measure current behavioral abnormalities. *Psychological Medicine, 22,* 223–230.

Hope, T., Tilling, K., Gedling, K., & Keene, J. (1994). The structure of wandering in dementia. *International Journal of Geriatric Psychiatry, 9,* 149–155.

Hussian, R. A. (1982). Stimulus control in the modification of problematic behavior in elderly institutionalized patients. *International Journal of Behavioral Geriatrics, 1,* 47–51.

Hussian, R. A., & Brown, D. C. (1987). Use of two-dimensional grid patterns to limit hazardous ambulation in demented patients. *Journal of Gerontology, 42,* 558–560.

Hutton, J. T. (1985). Eye movements in Alzheimer's disease: Significance and relationship to visuospacial confusion. In J. T. Hutton & A. D. Kenny (Eds.), *Senile dementia of the Alzheimer's type* (pp. 3–33). New York: Alan R. Liss.

Hwang, J. P., Yang, C. H., Tsai, S. J., & Liu, K. M. (1997). Behavioural disturbances in psychiatric inpatients with dementia of the Alzheimer's type in Taiwan. *International Journal of Geriatric Psychiatry, 12,* 902–906.

Jost, B. C., & Grossberg, G. T. (1995). The evolution of psychiatric symptoms in Alzheimer's disease: A natural history study. *Journal of the American Geriatrics Society, 44,* 1078–1081.

Jozsvai, E., Richards, B., & Leach, L. (1996). Behaviour management of a patient with Creutzfeld-Jacob disease. *Clinical Gerontologist, 16,* 11–17.

Kamei, S., Oishi, M., & Takasu, T. (1996). Evaluation of fasudil hydrochloride treatment for wandering symptoms in cerebrovascular dementia with 31P-magnetic resonance spectroscopy and Xe-computed tomography. *Clinical Neuropharmacology, 19,* 428–438.

Karlsson, S., Bucht, G., Eriksson, S., & Sandman, P. O. (1996). Physical restraints in geriatric care in Sweden: Prevalence and patient characteristics. *Journal of the American Geriatrics Society, 44,* 1348–1354.

Kirk, S., Donnelly, M. E., & Compton, S. A. (1991). A profile of residents of old people's homes. *Ulster Medical Journal, 60,* 154–158.

Koss, E., Weiner, M., Ernesto, C., Cohen-Mansfield, J., Ferris, S. H., Grundman, M., Schafer, Sano, M., Thal, L. J., Thomas, R., & Whitehouse, P. J. (1997). Assessing patterns of agitation in Alzheimer's disease patients with the Cohen-Mansfield Agitation Inventory: The Alzheimer's Disease Cooperative Study. *Alzheimer Disease & Associated Disorders, 11 Suppl 2,* S45–50.

Lachs, M. S., Becker, M., Siegal, A. P., Miller, R. L., & Tinetti, M. E. (1992). Delusions and behavioral disturbances in cognitively impaired elderly persons. *Journal of the American Geriatrics Society, 40,* 768–773.

Lam, D., Sewell, M., Bell, G., & Katona, C. (1989). Who needs psychogeriatric continuing care? *International Journal of Geriatric Psychiatry, 4,* 109–114.

Liu, L., Gauthier, L., & Gauthier, S. (1991). Spatial disorientation in persons with early senile dementia of the Alzheimer type. *American Journal of Occupational Therapy, 45,* 67–74.

Lucero, M., Hutchinson, S., Leger-Krall, S., & Wilson, H. S. (1993). Wandering in Alzheimer's dementia patients. *Clinical Nursing Research, 2,* 160–175.

Mann, A. H., Graham, N., & Ashby, D. (1984). Psychiatric illness in residential homes for the elderly: A survey in one London borough. *Age and Ageing, 13,* 257–265.

Marin, D. B., Green, C. R., Schmeidler, J., Harvey, P. D., Lawlor, B. A., Ryan, T. M., Aryan, M., Davis, K. L., & Mohs, R. C. (1997). Noncognitive disturbances in Alzheimer's disease: Frequency, longitudinal course, and relationship to cognitive symptoms. *Journal of the American Geriatrics Society, 45,* 1331–1338.

Martino-Saltzman, D., Blasch, B. B., Morris, R. D., & McNeal, L. W. (1991). Travel behavior of nursing home residents perceived as wanderers and nonwanderers. *Gerontologist, 31,* 666–672.

Matthews, E. A., Farrell, G. A., & Blackmore, A. M. (1996). Effects of an environmental manipulation emphasizing client-centred care on agitation and sleep in dementia sufferers in a nursing home. *Journal of Advanced Nursing, 24,* 439–447.

Matteson, M. A., & Linton, A. (1996). Wandering behaviors in institutionalized persons with dementia. *Journal of Gerontological Nursing, 22,* 39–46.

Mayer, R., & Darby, S. (1991). Does a mirror deter wandering in demented older people? *International Journal of Geriatric Psychiatry, 6,* 607–609.

Meguro, K., Yamaguchi, S., Yamazaki, H., Itoh, M., Yamaguchi, T., Matsui, H., & Sasaki, H. (1996). Cortical glucose metabolism in psychiatric wandering patients with vascular dementia. *Psychiatry Research, 67,* 71–80.

Miller, T. P., Tinklenberg, J. R., Brooks, J. O., III., Fenn, H. H., & Yesavage, J. A. (1993). Selected psychiatric symptoms associated with rate of cognitive decline in patients with Alzheimer's disease. *Journal of Geriatric Psychiatry & Neurology, 6,* 235–238.

Moak, G. S. (1990). Characteristics of demented and nondemented geriatric admissions to a state hospital. *Hospital and Community Psychiatry, 41,* 799–801.

Monsour, N., & Robb, S. S. (1982). Wandering behavior in old age: A psychosocial study. *Social Work, 27,* 411–416.

Mungas, D., Weiler, P., Franzi, C., & Henry, R. (1989). Assessment of disruptive behavior associated with dementia: The Disruptive Behavior Rating Scales. *Journal of Geriatric Psychiatry & Neurology, 2,* 196–202.

Namazi, K. H., Rosner, T. T., & Calkins, M. P. (1989). Visual barriers to prevent ambulatory Alzheimer's patients from exiting through an emergency door. *Gerontologist, 29,* 699–702.

Nasman, B., Bucht, G., Eriksson, S., & Sandman, P. (1993). Behavioural symptoms in the institutionalized elderly: Relationship to dementia. *International Journal of Geriatric Psychiatry, 8,* 843–849.

Negley, E. N., Molla, P. M., & Obenchain, J. (1990). No exit: The effects of an electronic security system on confused patients. *Journal of Gerontological Nursing, 16,* 21–25, 36–37.

Nissen, M. J., Corkion, S., Buonanno, F. S., Growdon, J. H., Wray, S. H., & Bauer, J. (1985). Spatial vision in Alzheimer's disease. *Archives of Neurology, 42,* 667–671.

O'Keeffe, S., Jack, C. I., & Lye, M. (1996). Use of restraints and bedrails in a British hospital. *Journal of the American Geriatrics Society, 44,* 1086–1088.

O'Keefe, J., & Nadel, L. (1978). *The hippocampus as a cognitive map.* Oxford, England: Clarendon Press.

Passini, R., Rainville, C., Marchand, N., & Joanette, Y. (1995). Wayfinding in dementia of the Alzheimer's type: Planning abilities. *Journal of Clinical and Experimental Neuropsychology, 17,* 820–832.

Patterson, M. B., Schnell, A., Martin, R. J., Mendez, M., Smith, K. A., & Whitehouse, P. (1990). Assessment of behavioral and affective symptoms in Alzheimer's disease. *Journal of Geriatric Psychiatry and Neurology, 3,* 21–30.

Prasher, V. P., & Filer, A. (1995). Behavioural disturbance in people with Down's syndrome and dementia. *Journal of Intellectual Disability Research, 39,* 432–436.

Prodger, N., Hurley, J., Clarke, C., & Bauer, D. (1992). Queen Elizabeth Behavioural Assessment Graphical System. *Australian Journal of Advanced Nursing, 9,* 4–11.

Rantz, M. J., & McShane, R. E. (1994). Nursing-home staff perception of behavior disturbance and management of confused residents. *Applied Nursing Research, 7,* 132–140.

Raskind, M. A., Sadowsky, C. H., Sigmund, W. R., Beitler, P. J., & Auster, S. B. (1997). Effect of tacrine on language, praxis, and noncognitive behavioral problems in Alzheimer disease. *Archives of Neurology, 54,* 836–840.

Richter, J. M., Roberto, K. A., & Bottenberg, D. J. (1995). Communicating with persons with Alzheimer's disease: Experiences of family and formal caregivers. *Archives of Psychiatric Nursing, 9,* 279–285.

Riter, R. N., & Fries, B. E. (1992). Predictors of the placement of cognitively impaired residents on special care units. *Gerontologist, 32,* 184–190.

Rockwood, K., Stolee, P., & Brahim, A. (1991). Outcomes of admission to a psychogeriatric service. *Canadian Journal of Psychiatry, 36,* 275–279.

Rosin, A. J. (1977). The physical and behavioural complex of dementia. *Gerontology, 23,* 37–46.

Rossby, L., Beck, C., & Heacock, P. (1992). Disruptive behaviors of a cognitively impaired nursing home resident. *Archives of Psychiatric Nursing, 6,* 98–107.

Rosswurm, M. A., Zimmerman, S. L., Schwartz-Fulton, J., & Norman, G. A. (1986). Can we manage wandering behavior? *Journal of Long Term Care Administration, 14,* 5–8.

Ryan, J. P., McGowan, J., McCaffrey, N., Ryan, G. T., Zandi, T., & Brannigan, G. G. (1995). Graphomotor perseveration and wandering in Alzheimer's disease. *Journal of Geriatric Psychiatry & Neurology, 8,* 209–212.

Sand, B. J., Yeaworth, R. C., & McCabe, B. W. (1992). Alzheimer's disease: Special care units in long-term care facilities. *Journal of Gerontological Nursing, 18,* 28–34.

Sandman, P. O., Adofsson, R., Norberg, A., Nystrom, L., & Winblad, B. (1988). Long-term care of the elderly. *Comprehensive Gerontology, Section A, 2,* 120–132.

Sandson, J., & Albert, M. L. (1987). Perseveration in behavior neurology. *Neurology, 37,* 1736–1741.

Sanford, J. (1975). Tolerance of disability in elderly dependents by supporters at home: Its significance for hospital practice. *British Medical Journal, 3,* 471–473.

Satlin, A., Teicher, M. H., Lieberman, H. R., Baldessarini, R. J., Volicer, L., & Rheaume, Y. (1991). Circadian locomotor activity rhythms in Alzheimer's disease. *Neuropsychopharmacology, 5,* 115–126.

Satlin, A., Volicer, L., Stopa, E. G., & Harper, D. (1995). Circadian locomotor activity and core-body temperature rhythms in Alzheimer's disease. *Neurobiology of Aging, 16,* 765–771.

Shankle, W. R., Nielson, K. A., & Cotman, C. W. (1995). Low-dose propranolol reduces aggression and agitation resembling that associated with orbitofrontal dysfunction in elderly demented patients. *Alzheimer Disease & Associated Disorders, 9,* 233–237.

Shelton, P. S., & Hocking, L. B. (1997). Zolpidem for dementia-related insomnia and nighttime wandering. *Annals of Pharmacotherapy, 31,* 319–322.

Shyu, Y., Yip, P. K., & Chen, R. C. (1996). Caregiving experiences of family caregivers of elderly persons with dementia in northern Taiwan. *Kaohsiung Journal of Medical Sciences, 12,* 50–61.

Smith-Jones, S. M., & Francis, G. M. (1992). Disruptive, institutionalized elderly: A cost-effective intervention. *Journal of Psychosocial Nursing & Mental Health Services, 30,* 17–20, 38–39.

Snyder, L. H., Rupprecht, P., Pyrek, J., Breckhus, S., & Moss, T. (1978). Wandering. *The Gerontologist, 18,* 272–280.

Steffes, R., & Thralow, J. (1987). Visual field limitation in the patient with dementia of the Alzheimer's type. *Journal of the American Geriatrics Society, 35,* 198–204.

Swaab, D. F., Fliers, F., & Partiman, T. S. (1985). The suprachiasmatic nucleus of the human brain in relation to sex, age and senile dementia. *Brain Research, 342,* 37–44.

Szwabo, P., Woodward, V., Grossberg, G. T., & Shen, W. W. (1991). The use of Alprazolam for decreasing problem wandering in geriatric patients. *The American Journal of Alzheimer's Care and Related Disorders and Research, 6,* 33–36.

Teri, L., Hughes, J. P., & Larson, E. B. (1990). Cognitive deterioration in Alzheimer's disease: Behavioral and health factors. *Journal of Gerontology, 45,* 58–63.

Teri, L., Larson, E. B., & Reifler, B. V. (1988). Behavioral disturbance in dementia of the Alzheimer's type. *Journal of the American Geriatrics Society, 36,* 1–6.

Thomas, D. W. (1997). Understanding the wandering patient: A continuity of personality perspective. *Journal of Gerontological Nursing, 23,* 16–24.

Tinetti, M. E., Liu, W. L., Marottoli, R. A., & Ginter, S. F. (1991). Mechanical restraint use among residents of skilled nursing facilities: Prevalence, patterns, and predictors. *Journal of the American Medical Association, 265,* 468–471.

Vieweg, V., Blair, C. E., Tucker, R., & Lewis, R. (1995). Factors precluding patients' discharge to the community: A geropsychiatric hospital survey. *Virginia Medical Quarterly, 122,* 275–278.

Walsh, J. S., Welch, H. G., & Larson, E. B. (1990). Survival of outpatients with Alzheimer-type dementia. *Annals of Internal Medicine, 113,* 429–434.

Weber, R., Brown, L., & Weldon, J. K. (1978). Cognitive maps of environmental knowledge and preference in nursing home patients. *Experimental Aging Research, 4,* 157–174.

Young, S. H., Muir-Nash, J., & Ninos, M. (1988). Managing nocturnal wandering behavior. *Journal of Gerontological Nursing, 14,* 6–12.

Chapter 9

Cognitive Interventions Among Older Adults

GRAHAM J. MCDOUGALL, JR.

ABSTRACT

This chapter reviews psychoeducational and/or psychosocial interventions designed to improve cognitive function in adults without cognitive impairment. Included are sections on (a) meta-analyses and other reviews; (b) cognitive aging and cognitive improvement; (c) memory training; (d) depression and memory improvement; (e) self-efficacy and aging memory; (f) maintenance of gains and subject retention; (g) comprehensive memory improvement program; and (h) future research. Several aspects of memory training now known to influence outcomes, i.e., memory performance, need to be considered in future studies. First, follow-up instruction (booster sessions) facilitates the use of these newly learned memory strategies in elders' everyday lives. Second, elders' memory self-efficacy (beliefs and confidence) impacts performance. Third, the inclusion of subjective measures in memory training is recommended. Fourth, greater emphasis needs to be placed on the modification of participants' attitudes toward aging-related memory loss. Fifth, designs must emphasize the long-term outcomes of the memory training. Sixth, establishing a relationship between a memory intervention and functional ability (IADLs) is the next step in assisting older adults to remain independent. If early failure in cognitive ability can be improved through intervention, perhaps early decline in functional independence and the need for formal services, e.g., nursing home placement, can be delayed.

Keywords: Cognitive Interventions, Memory Improvement, Memory Self-Efficacy, Depression

The burgeoning elderly population over 65 years of age in the U.S.—some 33 million people as estimated by the 1990 Census—represents one of the biggest challenges facing the nation today in health care. Memory loss is a reality of aging and individuals are known to experience cognitive changes during the age span of 65 to 85 (Rinn, 1988; Schaie, 1989). In laboratory tests, when adults over 60 years of age are compared to 20-year-olds, the seniors' performance is lower in free recall, cued recall, and recognition memory for lists of words or sentences. The elders score lower on everyday memory tests with ecological validity as well (Light, 1991). Adults in general have major concerns about losing their memory, the negative consequences of memory loss, and the reality that memory functioning declines with age (Poon, 1985; Rinn, 1988; Schaie, 1989). Women have a higher risk of becoming mentally frail and/or developing dementia than men, especially at very old ages (Ford, Haug, Roy, Jones, & Folmar, 1992; Fratiglioni et al., 1997; McDougall & Balyer, 1998).

The emphasis of this chapter is to review psychoeducational and/or psychosocial interventions designed to improve cognitive function in adults without cognitive impairment. An intervention may be defined as a programmatic attempt at altering the course of life span developmental phenomena. Interventions may be classified as concrete technologies involving such parameters as the goal (enrichment, prevention, or alleviation); the target behavior (attention, cognition, memory, perception); the setting (family, classroom, community, or hospital); and the mechanism (training, practice, or health delivery) (Baltes & Danish, 1980). Cognitive interventions are designed to change some aspect of cognitive function such as attention, concentration, or memory. These interventions may be applied to many patient or client populations, such as the elderly in long-term care and young head-injured individuals in rehabilitation settings. The literature reviewed for this chapter was identified using computerized abstracting services (e.g., CINAHL, Psychlit, etc.). The review was limited to published referred journal articles in nursing and multidisciplinary sources, and no limit was placed on the age of the publication, so as to not exclude a seminal reference.

Interventions to improve cognitive function have a long history; however, it was not until the 1950s that interventions specifically designed to improve the cognitive performance in adults were documented in the research literature. Major conceptual issues include (a) meta-analyses and other reviews; (b) cognitive aging and cognitive improvement; (c) memory training; (d) depression and memory improvement; (e) self-efficacy and aging memory; (f) maintenance of gains and subject retention; (g) comprehensive memory improvement programs; and (h) future research.

Numerous investigators have published reviews on interventions designed to improve cognitive performance. The reviews may be broadly classified by the cognitive status of the participant: impaired or intact. The emphases of the reviews are: delirium (Cronnin-Stubbs, 1996); depression and memory impairment (Burt, Zembar, & Niederehe, 1995); memory performance (Verhaeghen et al., 1992); and subjective memory functioning (Floyd & Scogin, 1997).

The two meta-analytic reviews of healthy community-dwelling elderly participants indicated that memory training improved memory performance with large effect sizes of $d = .66$ and $.73$, and improved subjective memory functioning with a small effect size of $d = .19$ (Floyd & Scogin, 1997; Verhaeghen, Marcoen, & Goossens, 1992). The overall findings were positive, since the elderly benefited more from mnemonic training than from either control or placebo treatments. Treatment gains were negatively impacted as the participants increased in age and as the sessions decreased in length from an optimum 90 minutes. The inclusion of pretraining had a positive impact on memory performance in both analyses. Seventy percent of the sample in the meta-analysis did not include comparisons with a no-treatment control group. Many studies did not include target (sensitive) measures related to the mnemonic strategy taught to participants in the intervention.

COGNITIVE AGING AND COGNITIVE IMPROVEMENT

Rowe and Kahn in their review "Human Aging: Usual and Successful" (1987) documented that the effects of the aging process itself have been exaggerated, and the modifying effects of diet, exercise, personal habits, and psychosocial factors underestimated. Woodruff-Pak in her review "Aging and Intelligence: Changing Perspective in the 20th Century" (1989) documented that research on aging and intelligence can be organized into four distinct phases. In Phase I, emerging in the 1920s and predominating until the 1950s, the view of intelligence and aging proceeded to a steep and inevitable decline. The Phase II perspective, from the 1950s to the 1960s, developed as a result of the contradictions in the research literature between the cross-sectional and longitudinal studies—demonstrating stability in intelligence. The Phase III era, dominating until the 1970s, illustrated the influence of context in which intelligence is expressed, and led investigators to explore new means of measuring different abilities such as fluid and crystallized measures of intelligence in adulthood. In this post-Great Society period of the 1970s, interventions to ameliorate intelligence in the aged were undertaken. In Phase IV, a rejection emerged of traditional psychometric measures of academic success in favor of competence in the everyday world. This phase also included the search for abilities that develop in adulthood and old age. Contemporary research on aging and intelligence continues to be undertaken from at least three of the four perspectives. The current Phase IV is viewed as the culmination of almost 70 years of research in which positive stereotypes are beginning to become a reality.

National efforts, such as "Decade of the Brain, 1990–2000" to study human brain function have relevance for cognitive aging research, since there is great variability in memory performance in aging (Subcommittee on Brain and Behavioral Sciences, 1989). Therefore, learning more about the processes of aging memory and the methods to improve memory performance in older adults is crucial. Mortimer's review "Brain Reserve and the Clinical Expression of Alzheimer's Disease" (1997) hypothesized how findings from studies of older nondemented individuals, who have plaques and tangles, to meet diagnostic criteria for Alzheimer's Disease during life may have greater brain reserve which buffered the clinical expression of the disease. Three types of brain reserve were examined: first, the number of neurons and/or the density of their interconnections in youth; second, the collection of cognitive strategies for solving problems and taking neuropsychological tests; and third, the amount of functional brain tissue remaining at any age. Mortimer's conclusion that approximately one-third of individuals meeting neuropathologic criteria for AD are not demented prior to death encourages the view that while the disease may not be preventable, its clinical expression is likely susceptible to intervention, such as early-life nutrition, prevention of cerebrovascular disease, and intellectual stimulation.

MEMORY TRAINING

Treatment for memory complaints in normal healthy elderly persons takes two forms. The most frequent intervention is to simply tell the individual, "Don't worry, there is nothing wrong with you." This advice is rarely heeded, and the person either continues to seek help or silently remains concerned. The second approach is for the older adult to attend a memory-training program designed to improve memory performance. Participants are taught to use mnemonic devices, which are learning strategies that may enhance their learning and future recall of information.

Early research on intellectual training in aging individuals has provided support for ongoing research into modifying older adults' cognitive abilities (Plemons, Willis, & Baltes, 1978; Willis, Blieszner, & Baltes, 1981). Studies show that older adults have a substantial reserve capacity in their fluid intelligence and that training may activate cognitive skills already available in their repertoire (Baltes, Kliegel, & Dittmann-Kohli, 1988; Kliegel, Smith, & Baltes, 1989).

Cognitive aging research indicates that the elderly are interested in memory improvement techniques, but often are at a loss as to how to acquire and implement these skills in their daily lives (McDougall, 1994). Older adults tend to become more dependent on external memory strategies and rely less on their own thinking and remembering ability (Herrmann & Petro, 1990). The use of cognitive strategies has been shown to improve memory performance. These strategies are broadly classified as internal (effort, elaboration, and rehearsal) and external (calendars, lists, and place) (McDougall, 1995a, 1995b). When given appropriate instructions, older adults are capable of using both internal and external strategies to noticeably improve their memory performance.

Memory training programs for older adults usually rely on the teaching of mnemonics, defined as any mental strategy or technique that aids the learning of the desired material by using other, initially extraneous, material to aid learning and future recall (Bellezza, 1981; Brown & Deffenbacher, 1975; Roberts, 1983; Yesavage, 1985). Investigators have recommended that the memory improvement training be multifactorial and go beyond simply teaching one or two mnemonic strategies (Stigsdotter Neely & Backman, 1993a, 1993b; Stigsdotter Neely & Backman, 1995; West, 1989). Because mnemonic strategies are often seen as useful only for classical episodic memory tasks, older adults may have problems and difficulty in transferring the use of these strategies to their everyday lives. Simply teaching mnemonics to elders has no relationship to their everyday memory performance. Older adults often encounter great difficulty transferring mnemonic strategies into their daily lives when mnemonics are the major emphasis of a unifactorial memory training program, e.g., teaching only one or two mnemonic strategies (Brooks, Friedman, & Yesavage, 1993; Kliegel et al., 1990). In previous studies of memory training with older adults, subjects reported on follow-up that they used the memory strategies inconsistently in their everyday lives. For example, Anschutz, Camp, Markley, and Kramer (1987) reported only 10% ongoing use; Hayslip, Maloy, and Kohl (1995) reported 44 and 51%; Stigsdotter Neely and Backman (1993b) reported 39%; and finally Scogin and Bienias (1988) reported 28% ongoing use.

Interestingly, these studies indicated that group instruction provided positive effects in the form of mutual support, reinforcement, and enhanced motivation. Also, visual imagery and relaxation components persisted, rather than mnemonic skills. Memory programs often include training in visual imagery skills to facilitate learning mnemonic devices because it is unusual for older adults to use this technique in their daily lives (Camp, Markley, & Kramer, 1983; Turnure & Lane, 1987). For example, individuals may be taught to increase the elaboration of details during the processing of visual-image associations used in a mnemonic device. In one study, older adults in the stress inoculation group remembered letter sets learned in the program, but did not remember how to use the mnemonic strategy (Hayslip et al., 1995).

Prototype of a Memory Improvement Study

The effects of a 4-session group intervention designed to improve metamemory (both knowledge and beliefs), and memory performance in community-dwelling elders was tested (Dellefield & McDougall, 1996). The association of depression with memory performance and metamemory was also evaluated. A total of 145 community-dwelling older adults (M = 71 years) participated in the study. The memory program was a 2-week, four-session (1 1/2 hours per class) intervention designed to increase memory awareness and knowledge. Each session included lectures, group exercises, and homework assignments. Topics included:

(a)   how memory serves us;
(b)   factors that affect how people remember;
(c)   techniques for remembering names;
(d)   thoughts and feelings when one forgets;
(e)   normal changes in memory with age;
(f)   how memory works (registering, retaining, and retrieving);
(g)   emphasizing memory skills (self-instruction, active observation, making associations, visualization, method of loci, linking, first letter cues, categorization); and
(h)   coping and self-evaluation following memory failures.

An important component of the intervention was providing feedback on their overall memory performance. In addition, memory testing during the first session gave the participants feedback about their initial level of memory performance. The memory performance test was readministered during the last session of the intervention to indicate the degree of change. The course content was based on a combination of sources, primarily from published guides for leading a memory course for the elderly.

Metamemory was operationalized with the Metamemory in Adulthood Questionnaire (MIA), a measure of affect, beliefs, and knowledge. For both experimental and control groups, pre-tests (T1) were administered during the first group intervention session, the first post-test (T2) was scheduled on the date of the last session (10 days following the pretest), and the follow-up test (T3) was scheduled for 2 weeks after the last session (approximately 24 days after the pretest). Both the intervention and the control groups took the pretest, the posttest, and the follow-up test at the same time. The intervention significantly improved both metamemory and memory performance in the treatment group (n = 74). The control group (n = 71) did not improve; in fact, the control group experienced a significant decline in metamemory scores over time. Memory performance was not significantly related to metamemory. The intervention had no effect on this relationship. Although those individuals with depression who scored a mean of 7.5 as measured by the short Geriatric Depression Scale had significantly lower metamemory scores than those without depression, there was no difference in memory performance between the depressed and nondepressed subjects. From the post-test (T2) to the follow-up period (T3), depressed subjects receiving the intervention showed a significant decrease in metamemory scores, while nondepressed subjects showed no change. The dose of the intervention was not strong enough, since subjects had little opportunity to practice in class (enactive mastery experiences). Thus, subjects had enough exposure to memory techniques to see that the techniques could work, but not enough practice to observe actual changes in their memory in everyday situations.

DEPRESSION AND MEMORY IMPROVEMENT

Depression is a significant mental health problem in 15% of the elderly population. Major depressive disorders along with dementia are by far the most serious psychiatric disorders in later life (Blazer, 1990; Fitz & Teri, 1994; Hoch et al., 1993; Poon, 1992). One review of cognitively impaired adults indicated that depression and memory impairment are associated in studies of recall (N = 99) and recognition (N = 48) (Burt et al., 1995). These findings should be interpreted with caution, since memory impairment is not always linked to depression, and the analyses includes only laboratory and diagnostic tests of memory, not tests of everyday memory. Cronnin-Stubbs (1996) reviewed nine studies of delirium in patients in acute care settings and determined that the phenomenon is underdiagnosed.

Greater memory complaints have been found with increasing age in depressed individuals than in nondepressed individuals (Lichtenberg, Ross, Millis, & Manning, 1995; McDougall, 1993; Nussbaum & Sauer, 1993). Depression in the elderly has also been shown to be associated with poor memory efficiency and response (West, Boatwright, & Schleser, 1984; Williams, Little, Seates, & Blockman, 1987). Depression has been found to be a factor in the memory performance of older adults participating in memory training classes (Dellefield & McDougall, 1996; Hayslip, Kennelly, & Maloy,

1990; Scogin, Storandt, & Lott, 1985). However, the relationship between memory complaints and memory performance and between complaints and affective states are perplexing because complaints are positively related to depression, but inversely related to actual performance (Helkala et al., 1997). Interestingly, one team (Gilewski, Zelinski, & Schaie, 1990) reported that depressed elders were less inclined than the nondepressed to use systematic approaches to recall information, while another team predicted the use of mnemonic strategies more often in the cognitively impaired elderly than in the elderly with depression (Niederehe & Yoder, 1989).

In one community sample of 1,491 older adults, self-reported memory performance was negatively related to depression and cognitive rigidity (Herzog & Rodgers, 1989). On the other hand, in a recent study of 2,495 adult volunteers, age, not depression, was consistently a significant predictor of everyday memory performance, followed by vocabulary and gender (West, Crook, & Barron, 1992). However, depression in these studies was assessed with screening instruments [Center for Epidemiological Studies Depression (CESD), Geriatric Depression (GDS), and Zung Self-Rating Depression (SDS) scales] where high scores do not indicate clinical depression. Additionally, the level of depression in these samples was below the cutoff scores for diagnosis of depression.

SELF-EFFICACY AND AGING MEMORY

Bandura's (1977, 1982) general self-efficacy construct provides a useful explanation for ways in which people influence their own motivation and behavior. Perceived self-efficacy refers to the strength of a person's belief that they possess the capabilities to organize and execute whatever courses of action may be required to reach a goal. The influence of self-efficacy may entail regulating one's own motivation, thought processes, affective states, and actions, or it may involve changing environmental conditions, depending on what one seeks to manage (Bandura, 1997). Self-efficacy judgments determine the behavior that is chosen and affect the amount of effort devoted to a task. Bandura (1997) postulated four principal sources of self-efficacy information:

1) enactive mastery experiences that serve as validators of capability;
2) vicarious experiences that alter efficacy beliefs through transmission of competencies and comparison with the attainments of others;
3) verbal persuasion and allied types of social influences that reinforce the possession of a certain capability; and

4) personal recognition of physiological and affective states that are used in part to judge capableness, strength, and vulnerability to dysfunction.

According to Bandura, efficacy beliefs vary across activity domains, levels of demands within the domains, and different environmental circumstances affecting performance. Thus, self-efficacy is task-specific, and influences one's persistence when difficulties are encountered, e.g., cognitive tasks such as remembering (Bandura, 1993).

Memory self-efficacy is defined as beliefs in one's own capacity to use memory effectively in various situations. Knowledge about memory is distinct from memory self-efficacy. Therefore, it is possible that an older individual may have extensive and accurate knowledge about how memory functions, but may also believe that his or her ability to remember in a given context is poor (Hertzog, Dixon, Schulenberg, & Hultsch, 1987). Many older adults have poorer memory confidence than younger adults, and this lower memory confidence may have a number of adverse consequences (Bandura, 1989). It is clear that memory self-efficacy beliefs and memory performance are related constructs.

Decreased confidence and weak motivational processes activated by counterproductive beliefs may impair memory performance (Cornelius & Caspi, 1986; Lachman & Jelalian, 1984; Luszcz, 1993; McDougall, 1994; Ryan & See, 1993; Seeman, Rodin, & Albert, 1993; Willis & Schaie, 1993). If an individual perceives that memory decreases with age, then he or she is quick to interpret faulty performance as a further indicator of declining memory capacity. Individuals with low confidence may stop trying to remember because of doubts about achieving a desired level of performance. Older adults' beliefs were not emphasized in other training programs, but their confidence in their ability to remember had been augmented, resulting in an unplanned outcome (Dittmann-Kohli, Lachman, Kliegel, & Baltes, 1991; Hill, Sheikh, & Yesavage, 1988; Rebok & Offerman, 1983). Beliefs were addressed in several memory improvement studies, but have been used primarily as a control for memory training, or as a training component without pre- and post-measurements.

In one often-quoted study designed specifically to change memory self-efficacy beliefs, the training did not reduce initial age-related performance differences or differences in memory self-efficacy (Rebok & Balcerak, 1989). Correlations between memory self-efficacy and memory performance were not significant, but these findings may be a function of faulty memory self-efficacy operationalization and poor instrumentation. Other studies have not accurately operationalized memory self-efficacy and thus have produced confusing findings (Mcdonald-Misczak, Hertzog, & Hultsch, 1995). In four studies, however, the memory training course significantly increased memory self-efficacy and memory performance in the short-term, 4 weeks to 3 months (Best, Hamlett, & Davis, 1992; Dellefield & McDougall, 1996; Lachman, Steinberg, & Trotter, 1987; Lachman, Weaver, Bandura, Elliott, & Lewkowicz, 1992). Further, perceived self-efficacy predicted memory performance when self-efficacy was measured with questionnaires that ranged from simple to complex. Therefore, studies designed to improve self-efficacy (memory beliefs and confidence) may be as important as teaching mnemonic strategies (Bandura, 1989; Berry, 1989; Berry & West, 1993).

MAINTENANCE OF GAINS

The maintenance of gains is a concern for sustaining the effects of a cognitive intervention over time (Stigsdotter & Backman, 1989). Five previous studies reported conflicting findings of the long-term (1 + years) effects of memory training. Anschutz et al. (1987) reported on nine of ten original subjects and indicated that while these individuals used the method of loci for remembering a new word list, they did not use this mnemonic to enhance their recall in everyday situations. Scogin and Bienanias (1988) followed 27 of 43 original participants in a self-taught memory training program. The memory training group had a significant decrease in memory performance and a considerable decrease in mnemonic usage over time, but no change in memory complaints. Hayslip et al. (1995) reported on 108 of 358 original subjects. Assessment at 3 years post-training indicated that use of memory strategies was diminished. After one year, Oswald, Rupprecht, Gunzelmann, and Tritt (1996) found that elderly with a mean age of 79 years who participated in a combined memory improvement and psychomotor training program sustained their memory improvement and independent living ability. Willis and Schaie (1986) and Willis and Nesselroade (1990) found that with five booster sessions, elderly participants ($N = 25$) maintained their fluid ability training over a 7-year period. Since only one study provided booster sessions, or any additional training beyond the initial program, booster sessions may be necessary to reinforce previously learned material, and therefore influence functional ability.

Retention of Subjects

Previous memory improvement studies had varying levels of subject retention when followed longitudinally. Scogin, Storandt, and Lott (1985) followed 43 original participants from a self-taught memory training program and reported a 63% retention rate at 3 years. Anschutz et al. (1987) reported a 90% retention on 10 subjects after 3 years. Willis, Jay, Diehl, and Marsiske (1992) followed 237 members (*M* age = 76.9; *M* education = 12.08 years) of the Seattle Longitudinal Study for 7 years with a retention rate of 43%. Hayslip et al. (1995) study reported a 30% retention on 358 subjects after 3 years.

COMPREHENSIVE MEMORY IMPROVEMENT PROGRAM

Cognitive-Behavioral Model of Everyday Memory (CBMEM)

The Cognitive-Behavioral Model comprehensive model of stress inoculation, health promotion, memory self-efficacy, and memory strategy training was developed to improve, maintain, or prevent decline in the everyday memory of older adults. Although cognitive-behavioral interventions were originally developed and applied to emotionally based disorders (e.g., depression, phobias, impulse control, and evaluation anxiety), several trends in medicine have suggested that cognitive factors are likely to play an important role in all areas along the health-illness continuum. Therefore, cognitive-behavioral strategies are useful beyond their initial focus.

Memory programs for the older adults have usually emphasized two of the four components in the CBMEM model: mnemonic strategies and stress inoculation. Mnemonic strategies were discussed above; mnemonic training may also include visual imagery skills. Imagery procedures have been investigated under the following terms: mental practice, mental imagery practice, mental rehearsal, psyching-up, visuomotor behavior rehearsal, mental preparation, visual imagery, imagery procedures, and covert practice. Usually a visual image is associated with a mnemonic device. For example, individuals can be taught to increase the elaboration of processing of visual-image associations used in a mnemonic device.

Only recently have a few programs incorporated aspects of memory self-efficacy. The argument for using this aspect is that older adults lack a sense of mastery for memory abilities, either because they have observed changes in their own memory or because their culture teaches that memory declines are inevitable. As a result, older adults do not try as hard as younger adults to remember. They then remember less, experience reduced feelings of self-efficacy, and so on.

A comprehensive memory training program for older adults must include the four components of stress inoculation, health promotion, memory self-efficacy, and memory strategy training. The CBMEM Model is the first package to address all three of these. Based on Bandura's self-efficacy theory, the CBMEM program includes all four components. When delivered in the right dose, the program increases the individual's belief in their ability to use their memory and this improves their self-efficacy in memory-demanding situations.

Operationalization of Bandura's theoretical sources of self-efficacy. Bandura (1977, 1982, 1997) postulated four principal sources of self-efficacy information. First are enactive mastery experiences. The curriculum is organized so that the exercises increase gently from less difficult to more difficult. As people begin to feel more competent and comfortable, they will be encouraged to take more risks. Principles of adult learning will be used throughout the program, so that is no one will be embarrassed or intimidated in front of the group, and all relevant experience will be discussible. Second, vicarious experiences that alter efficacy beliefs through transmission of competencies and comparison with the attainments of others will be operationalized through the group format and group sharing of the experiences. Third, verbal persuasion and allied social influences, designed to reinforce that one possesses certain capabilities, are operationalized through continual feedback on performance accomplishments and encouragement for continued progress. Fourth are physiological and affective states. People tend to feel anxious in situations where competence is questioned. Stress inoculation taught in the pre-training session and practiced in subsequent sessions assists the participants in dealing with stressful situations. Participants are reminded to practice relaxation techniques such as taking a few deep breaths at stressful times to alleviate memory anxiety.

The phases of memory improvement may be differentiated as six distinct phases in which participants learn activities and content that is least challenging in the early phases and progress to most challenging during the final week as CBMEM moves to completion.

1. Modeling techniques. Participants take part in nonthreatening memory exercises that are fun, enjoyable, and constitute a level playing field for every individual. They utilize their crystallized intelligence acquired through experience and knowledge; no new learning is therefore required to participate. It is simply a rewarding combination of fun and games and the satisfaction of meeting a supported intellectual challenge. The goal of a typical exercise is to identify common names, nouns, and places beginning with different letters given by the instructor. The next more challenging section version is to identify these similar categories of objects when the last letter is given.

2. Observing their memory.   Group comfort level increases the support needed in this phase. Members of the group learn to realistically assess the strengths and weaknesses of their own memory abilities through vicarious experiences with their colleagues and friends as they watch others participate and perform. The participants are challenged in an easy interesting fashion. Participants use memory without being tested on new material.

3. Awareness.   Participants develop an awareness of attention and concentration and begin to use more complex memory strategies such as association and visualization. Memory exercises as a group allow all members of the class to offer their unique contributions and develop confidence in their abilities through enactment of personal mastery. The group models the ability to self-reflect.

4. Mastery coping.   Participants attend the class which builds their confidence and enjoyment through effective learning experience and overrides any anxiety about potential embarrassment or being called upon to perform beyond their level of confidence and comfort. The participants begin to spontaneously respond to the instructor's general request to participate directly; i.e., through recalling content discussed at a previous class.

5. Controlled handling.   The instructor calls on specific individuals to participate in memory-demanding tasks. Participants' use of the memory textbook allows controlled access to information since, even though an individual may occasionally miss a class, the content is available through reading the book. Participants speak with each other between the classes due to the common bonds that are formed from vicarious and enactive mastery experiences.

6. Suspension.   Participants relax their anxieties and defenses and develop the ability to observe themselves and neighbors as they experience memory problems and their solutions, practice relaxation, and use deep breathing in memory-demanding situations, thereby facilitating their out-of-the classroom confidence in their ability.

The CBMEM model was tested in three groups of elderly at risk for cognitive impairments: Hispanic community-residing, assisted living, and retirement village. The curriculum was based on a published memory training course entitled "Improving Your Memory: How to Remember What You're Starting to Forget" (see Fogler & Stearn, 1994). Each person, except the

Hispanic elders, received a copy of the book (English version). The same instruments were used across the three groups for consistency. Cognitive function was assessed with the Mini-Mental State Exam (MMSE). Depression was operationalized with the Geriatric Depression Scale. Health status was operationalized by the Health Scale, a subscale of the Multilevel Assessment Instrument (Lawton et al., 1982). Functional ability (IADLs) was operationalized with the Instrumental Activities of Daily Living Scale (Lawton, 1988; Lawton & Brody, 1969). The IADL scale contains a total of eight items: ability to use the telephone, shopping, food preparation, housekeeping, laundry, mode of transportation, medications, and finances. Metamemory with the MIA (Dixon et al., 1983), Memory Self-Efficacy with the Memory Efficacy Questionnaire (Lachman et al., 1987), and memory performance with the Rivermead Behavioral Memory Test (RBMT).

Hispanic elders. This study tested the effects of a 4-week, nine-session group intervention taught in Spanish to Hispanic older adults entitled "Quieres Mejorar Tu Memoria" (Do you wish to improve your memory?). The program was based on Bandura's self-efficacy theory and was designed to increase memory self-efficacy and strategy use (McDougall, 1998). A total of 33 older adults with an average age of 69 years, no cognitive impairment, and attending a senior center participated in the study. A booster session and a post-test were given at 3 months to the intervention group of 22 elders. At posttest, the intervention reported greater confidence in preventing decline in their memories, and in particular greater use of the internal strategy of elaboration and the external strategies of list and note. This pilot study provides evidence that elderly Hispanics with low education and poverty-level incomes can make gains in using memory strategies as well as confidence in their ability to prevent further decline in their memories. Even though participants' overall evaluation of their memories had not changed, they increased strategic behaviors, which boosted their memory self-efficacy and confidence in being able to prevent further decline with age.

Assisted living elders. This pilot study tested the effects of an eight-session, group intervention entitled "MEMORIES, MEMORIES, Can We Improve Ours?" A total of 18 older adults (13 female, 5 male) without cognitive impairment participated. Participants averaged 81 years of age and had some college. Males were significantly more depressed than females. At pretest the experimental group rated their overall memory higher than the control group. Posttests were completed 1 week following the CBMEM intervention. Pearson correlations at pretest were significant for memory performance and memory self-efficacy. Change scores from pretest to posttest were significant for memory performance, memory efficacy, use of internal memory strategies (elaboration and rehearsal), and use of external memory strategies. Since there were large differences in cell size between the experimental and control groups, statistical group comparisons were not possible. An issue of great importance is whether the participants are retaining their new learning. There was near-perfect attendance in class. The class had greater pre- and post-test scores than the average scores of older adults reported in established normative studies.

Retirement village.   This study tested the effects of a 4-week, eight-session group intervention, the Cognitive-Behavioral Model of Everyday Memory, derived from Bandura's Self-Efficacy Theory, in which older adults learned the skills necessary to improve, maintain, or prevent memory decline, and change negative or stereotypical beliefs about cognitive aging. A total of 78 older adults (58 females, 20 males) participated with an average MMSE score of 28. Dependent variables included memory performance measured by the Rivermead Behavioral Memory, memory self-efficacy by the Memory Efficacy Questionnaire, and Instrumental Activities of Daily Living scale. There were no differences between experimental and control groups on the demographic variables of age, education, depression, and health. Overall, males had significantly more years of education (16.34 vs. 14.58) than females, $p = .0538$. The experimental intervention was dismantled into two components: X 1 and X 2. Treatment 1 was the 8-session CBMEM course, with the published memory book given to each participant on the first day of the class. Treatment 2 was the book given to participants 4 weeks before completing the 8-session CBMEM program. There were 31 subjects in X 1, 19 in X 2, and 28 in the wait-list control group. Pretesting occurred over a 3-day period so that the three groups were separated. Posttests (T2) for X 1 were completed 4 1/2 weeks following the CBMEM intervention. Posttests (T2) for X 2 and control groups were completed within the week following the completion of the first CBMEM intervention over a 2-day period so that the three groups were temporally separated. Posttests (T3) for X 2 and wait-list control groups were completed within 1 week after completing the second CBMEM intervention. The control group scored significantly higher on memory achievement than experimental group 2. In the experimental groups there were 31 subjects in Treatment 1 and 19 subjects in Treatment 2 group; there were 28 subjects in the wait-list control group. Correlations between depression and memory performance scores were inversely related at pre- and post-testing. Correlations between memory efficacy and memory performance measures were nonsignificant. In the short term, the classes boosted memory performance scores, memory confidence, and beliefs about memory. There were no changes in instrumental activities of daily living from pre- to post-testing. The wait-list control group achieved significant gains on all outcome measures.

FUTURE STUDIES

Unfortunately, the Verhaeghen, VanRanst, and Marcoen (1993) study ignored several important aspects of memory training now known to influence outcomes, i.e., memory performance. First, follow-up instruction (booster sessions) facilitates the use of these newly learned memory strategies in elders' everyday lives. Second, elders' memory self-efficacy (beliefs and confidence) impacts performance. Third, the inclusion of subjective measures in memory training is recommended (Floyd & Scogin, 1997). Fourth, greater emphasis needs to be placed on the modification of participants' attitudes toward aging-related memory loss (Floyd & Scogin, 1997). Fifth, longitudinal studies designed to determine the long-term outcomes of the memory training will determine if retention occurred. Sixth, establishing a relationship between a memory intervention and functional ability (IADLs) is the next step in assisting older adults to remain independent. No study has provided a relationship between an older adult's ability to perform IADLs and the administration of a cognitive intervention designed to improve memory self-efficacy and everyday memory. Studies are needed to determine whether cognitive interventions affect an older adult's ability to perform IADLs. If failure in cognitive ability can be improved through intervention, perhaps early decline in functional independence, and the need for formal services, can be delayed. While previous memory training programs have provided strong evidence that older adults can improve their cognitive abilities, at least in the short term, they have not addressed elders' concerns with improving their ADLs and IADLs, nor followed them longitudinally to determine long-term outcomes of the memory training.

REFERENCES

Anschutz, L., Camp, C. J., Markley, R. P., & Kramer, J. J. (1987). Remembering mnemonics: A three-year follow-up on the effects of mnemonics training in elderly adults. *Experimental Aging Research, 13*, 141–143.

Baltes, P. B., & Danish, S. J. (1980). Intervention in life-span development and aging. In R. R. Turner & H. W. Reese (Eds.), *Life-span developmental psychology* (pp. 49–78). New York: Academic Press.

Baltes, P. B., Kliegel, R., & Dittman-Kohli, F. (1988). On the locus of training gains in research on the plasticity of fluid intelligence in old age. *Journal of Educational Psychology, 80*(3), 392–400.

Bandura, A. (1977). Self-efficacy: Toward a unifying theory of behavioral change. *Psychological Review, 84*(2), 191–215.

Bandura, A. (1982). Self-efficacy mechanism in human aging. *American Psychologist, 37*(2), 122–147.

Bandura, A. (1988). Self-efficacy conception of anxiety. *Anxiety Research, 1*, 77–98.

Bandura, A. (1989). Regulation of cognitive processes through perceived self-efficacy. *Developmental Psychology, 25*(5), 729–735.

Bandura, A. (1997). *Self-efficacy: The exercise of control.* New York: W. H. Freeman.

Bellezza, F. S. (1981). Mnemonic devices: Classification, characteristics, and criteria. *Review of Educational Research, 51*(2), 247–275.

Berry, J. M. (1989). Cognitive efficacy across the life span: Introduction of the special series. *Developmental Psychology, 25*(5), 683–686.

Berry, J. M., & West, R. L. (1993). Cognitive self-efficacy in relation to personal mastery and goal setting across the life span. *International Journal of Behavioral Development, 16*(2), 351–379.

Berry, J. M., West, R. L., & Dennehey, D. M. (1989). Reliability and validity of the memory self-efficacy questionnaire. *Developmental Psychology, 25*(5), 701–713.

Best, D. L., Hamlett, K. W., & Davis, S. W. (1992). Memory complaint and memory performance in the elderly: The effects of memory skills training and expectancy change. *Applied Cognitive Psychology, 6*, 405–416.

Blazer, D. G. (1990). Epidemiology of psychiatric disorders and cognitive problems in the elderly. In R. Michels (Ed.), *Psychiatry* (pp. 1–12). Philadelphia: J B Lippincott.

Brooks, J. O., Friedman, L., & Yesavage, J. A. (1993). A study of the problems older adults encounter when using a mnemonic technique. *International Psychogeriatrics, 5*(1), 57–65.

Brown, E., & Deffenbacher, K. (1975). Forgotten mnemonists. *Journal of the History of the Behavioral Sciences, 11*(4), 342–349.

Burt, D. B., Zembar, M. J., & Niederehe, G. (1995). Depression and memory impairment: A meta-analysis of the association, its pattern, and specificity. *Psychological Bulletin, 117*(2), 285–305.

Camp, C. J., Markley, R. P., & Kramer, J. J. (1983). Spontaneous use of mnemonics by elderly individuals. *Educational Gerontology, 9*, 57–71.

Cornelius, S. W., & Caspi, A. (1986). Self-perceptions of intellectual control and aging. *Educational Gerontology, 12*, 345–357.

Cronnin-Stubbs, D. (1996). Delirium intervention research in acute care settings. In J. J. Fitzpatrick & J. Norbeck (Eds.), *Annual Review of Nursing Research* (pp. 57–73). New York: Springer Publishing Company.

Dellefield, K. S., & McDougall, G. J. (1996). Increasing metamemory in community elderly. *Nursing Research, 45*, 284–290.

Dittmann-Kohli, F., Lachman, M. E., Kliegl, R., & Baltes, P. (1991). Effects of cognitive training and testing on intellectual efficacy beliefs in elderly adults. *Journal of Gerontology, 46*(4), 162–164.

Dixon, R. A., & Hultsch, D. (1983). Structure and development of metamemory in adulthood. *Journal of Gerontology, 38*(6), 682–688.

Fitz, A. G., & Teri, L. (1994). Depression, cognition, & functional ability in patients with AD. *Journal of the American Geriatrics Society, 42,* 186–191.

Floyd, M., & Scogin, F. (1997). Effects of memory training on the subjective memory functioning and mental health of older adults: A meta-analysis. *Psychology and Aging, 12*(1), 150–161.

Fogler, J., & Stern, L. (1994). *Teaching memory improvement to adults* (rev ed.). Baltimore: John Hopkins University Press.

Ford, A. B., Haug, M. R., Roy, A. W., Jones, P. K., & Folmar, S. J. (1992). New cohorts of urban elders: Are they in trouble? *Journal of Gerontology: Social Sciences, 47*(6), S297–S303.

Fratiglioni, L., Viitanen, M., von Strauss, E., Tontodonati, V., Herlitz, A., & Winblad, B. (1997). Very old women at highest risk of dementia and Alzheimer's disease: Incidence data from the Kungsholmen Project, Stockholm. *American Academy of Neurology, 48,* 132–138.

Gilewski, M. J., Zelinski, E. M., & Schaie, K. W. (1990). The memory functioning questionnaire for assessment of memory complaints in adulthood and old age. *Psychology and Aging, 5*(4), 482–490.

Hayslip, B., Kennelly, K. J., & Maloy, R. M. (1990). Fatigue, depression, and cognitive performance among aged person. *Experimental Aging Research, 16,* 111–115.

Hayslip, B., Maloy, R. M., & Kohl, R. (1995). Long-term efficacy of fluid ability interventions with older adults. *Journal of Gerontology: Psychological Sciences, 50B*(3), P141–P149.

Helkala, E. L., Koivisto, K., Hanninen, T., Vanhanen, M., Kuuisto, J., Mykkanen, L., Laakso, M., & Riekkinen, P. (1997). Stability of age-associated memory impairment during a longitudinal population-based study. *Journal of the American Geriatrics Society, 45*(1), 120–122.

Herrmann, D. J., & Petro, S. J. (1990). Commercial memory aids. *Applied Cognitive Psychology, 4,* 439–450.

Hertzog, C., Dixon, R. A., Schulenburg, J. E., & Hultsch, D. F. (1987). On the differentiation of memory beliefs from memory knowledge: The factor structure of the metamemory in adulthood scale. *Experimental Aging Research, 13*(2), 101–107.

Herzog, A. R., & Rodgers, W. L. (1989). Age difference in memory performance and memory ratings as measured in a sample survey. *Psychology and Aging, 4*(2), 173–182.

Hill, R. D., Sheikh, J. I., & Yesavage, J. (1988). The effect of mnemonic training on perceived recall confidence in the elderly. *Experimental Aging Research, 13*(4), 185–188.

Hoch, C. C., Reynolds, C. F., Buysse, D. J., Fasiczka, A. L., Houck, P. R., Mazumdar, S., & Kupfer, D. J. (1993). Two-year survival in patients with mixed symptoms of depression and primary degenerative dementia. *The American Journal of Geriatric Psychiatry, 1*(1), 59–66.

Kliegel, R., Smith, J., & Baltes, P. B. (1989). Testing the limits and the study of adult age differences in cognitive plasticity of a mnemonic skill. *Developmental Psychology, 25,* 247–256.

Kliegel, R., Smith, J., & Baltes, P. B. (1990). On the locus and process of magnification of age differences during mnemonic training. *Developmental Psychology, 26*(6), 894–904.

Lachman, M. E., & Jelalian, E. (1984). Self-efficacy and attributions for intellectual performance in young and elderly adults. *Journal of Gerontology, 39*(5), 577–582.

Lachman, M. E., Steinberg, E. S., & Trotter, S. D. (1987). Effects of control beliefs and attributions on memory self-assessments and performance. *Psychology and Aging, 2*(3), 266–271.

Lachman, M. E., Weaver, S. L., Bandura, M., Elliott, E., & Lewkowicz, C. J. (1992). Improving memory and control beliefs through cognitive restructuring and self-generated strategies. *Journal of Gerontology: Psychological Sciences, 47*(5), P293–P299.

Lawton, M. P. (1988). Scales to measure competence in everyday activities. *Pyschopharmacology Bulletin, 24*(4), 609–614.

Lawton, M. P., & Brody, E. M. (1969). Assessment of older people: Self-maintaining and instrumental activities of daily living. *Gerontologist, 9,* 179–186.

Lawton, M. P., Moss, M., Fulcomer, M., & Kleban, M. H. (1982). A research and service oriented multilevel assessment. *Journal of Gerontology, 37*(1), 91–99.

Lichtenberg, P. A., Ross, T., Millis, S. R., & Manning, C. A. (1995). The relationship between depression and cognition in older adults: A cross-validation study. *Journal of Gerontology: Psychological Sciences, 50B*(1), P25–P32.

Light, L. L. (1991). Memory and aging: Four hypotheses in search of data. *Annual Review of Psychology, 42,* 333–376.

Luszcz, M. A. (1993). When knowing is not enough: The role of memory beliefs in prose recall of older and younger adults. *Australian Psychologist, 28*(1), 16–20.

McDonald-Misczak, L., Hertzog, C., & Hultsch, D. F. (1995). Stability and accuracy of metamemory in adulthood and aging: A longitudinal analysis. *Psychology and Aging, 10*(4), 553–564.

McDougall, G. J. (1993). Older adults' metamemory: Coping, depression, and self-efficacy. *Applied Nursing Research, 6*(1), 28–30.

McDougall, G. J. (1994). Predictors of metamemory in older adults. *Nursing Research, 43*(4), 212–218.

McDougall, G. J. (1995a). Memory self-efficacy and strategy use in successful elders. *Educational Gerontology, 21,* 357–373.

McDougall, G. J. (1995b). Memory strategies used by cognitively intact and cognitively impaired older adults. *Journal of the Academy of Nurse Practitioners, 7*(8), 369–377.

McDougall, G. J. (1995c). Metamemory and depression in cognitively impaired older adults. *Nursing Research, 44*(5), 306–311.

McDougall, G. J. (1998). Increasing memory self-efficacy and memory strategy use in Hispanic elders. *Clinical Gerontologist, 19*(2), 57–76.

McDougall, G. J., & Balyer, J. L. (1998). Decreasing mental frailty, in at-risk elders. *Geriatric Nursing, 19*(4), 220–224.

McGuire, L. C. (1996). Remembering what the doctor said: Organization and adults' memory for medical information. *Experimental Aging Research, 22*(4), 403–428.

Mortimer, J. A. (1997). Brain reserve and the clinical expression of Alzheimer's disease. *Geriatrics, 52*(Suppl. 2), S50–S53.

Niederehe, G., & Yoder, C. (1989). Metamemory perceptions in depression of young and older adults. *The Journal of Nervous and Mental Disease, 177*(1), 4–14.

Nussbaum, P. D., & Sauer, L. (1993). Self-report of depression in elderly with and without progressive cognitive deterioration. *Clinical Gerontologist, 13*(1), 69–80.

Oswald, W. D., Rupprecht, R., Gunzelmann, T., & Tritt, K. (1996). The SIMA-project: Effects of 1 year cognitive and psychomotor training on cognitive abilities of elderly. *Behavioural Brain Research, 78*, 67–72.

Plemons, J. K., Willis, S. L., & Baltes, P. B. (1978). Modification of fluid intelligence in aging: A short-term longitudinal training approach. *Journal of Gerontology, 33*, 224–231.

Poon, L. W. (1985). Differences in human memory with aging: Nature, causes and clinical implications. In J. E. Birren & K. W. Schaie (Eds.), *Handbook of the psychology of aging* (2nd ed.) (pp. 427–462). New York: Van Nostrand Reinhold.

Poon, L. W. (1992). Toward an understanding of cognitive functioning in geriatric depression. *International Psychogeriatrics, 4*, 241–265.

Porter, R. J. (1991). *Maximizing human potential: Decade of the brain, 1990–2000.* Bethesda, MD (NTIS No. 91-133769).

Rebok, G. W., & Offerman, L. R. (1983). Behavioral competencies of older college students: A self-efficacy approach. *The Gerontologist, 32*, 428–432.

Rebok, G. W., & Balcerak, L. J. (1989). Memory self-efficacy and performance differences in young and old adults: The effect of mnemonic training. *Developmental Psychology, 25*(5), 714–721.

Riggs, K. M., Lachman, M. E., & Wingfield, A. (1997). Taking charge of remembering: Locus of control and older adults' memory for speech. *Experimental Aging Research, 23*(3), 237–256.

Rinn, W. E. (1988). Mental decline in normal aging: A review. *Journal of Geriatric Psychiatry and Neurology, 1*, 144–158.

Roberts, P. (1983). Memory strategy instruction with the elderly: What should memory training be the training of? In M. Pressley & J. R. Levin (Eds.), *Cognitive strategy research: Psychological foundations* (pp. 75–100). New York: Springer Verlag.

Rowe, J. W., & Kahn, R. L. (1987). Human aging: Usual and successful. *Science, 237*, 143–149.

Ryan, E. B., & See, S. K. (1993). Age-based beliefs about memory changes for self and others across adulthood. *Journal of Gerontology: Psychological Sciences, 48*(4), P199–P201.

Schaie, K. W. (1989). The hazards of cognitive aging. *The Gerontologist, 29*(4), 484–493.

Scogin, F., & Bienias, J. (1988). A three-year follow-up of older adult participants in a memory skill-skills training program. *Psychology and Aging, 3*, 334–337.

Scogin, F. R., Storandt, M., & Lott, L. (1985). Memory-skills training, memory complaints, and depression in older adults. *Journal of Gerontology, 40*, 562–586.

Seeman, T. E., Rodin, J., & Albert, M. (1993). Self-efficacy and cognitive performance in high-functioning older individuals. *Journal of Aging and Health, 5*(4), 455–476.

Stigsdotter, A., & Backman, L. (1989). Multifactorial memory training with older adults: How to foster maintenance of improved performance. *Gerontology, 35*, 260–267.

Stigsdotter Neely, A., & Backman, L. (1993a). Maintenance of gains following multifactorial and unifactorial memory training in late adulthood. *Educational Gerontology, 19*, 105–117.

Stigsdotter Neely, A., & Backman, L. (1993b). Long-term maintenance of gains from memory training in older adults: Two 31/2-year follow-up studies. *Journal of Gerontology: Psychological Sciences, 48B*(3), P233–237.

Stigsdotter Neely, A., & Backman, L. (1995). Effects of multifactorial memory training in old age: Generalability across tasks and individuals. *Journal of Gerontology: Psychological Sciences, 50B*(3), P134–140.

Turnure, J. E., & Lane, J. F. (1987). Special educational applications of mnemonics. In M. M. McDaniel & M. Pressley (Eds.), *Imagery and related mnemonic processes: Theories, individual differences, and applications* (pp. 329–357). New York: Springer Verlag.

Verhaegen, P., & Marcoen, A. (1992). On the mechanism of plasticity in young and older adults after instruction in the method of loci: Evidence for an amplification model. *Psychology and Aging, 11*(1), 164–178.

Verhaegen, P., Marcoen, A., & Goosens, L. (1992). Improving memory performance in the aged through mnemonic training: A meta-analytic study. *Psychology and Aging, 7*, 242–251.

Verhaegen, P., VanRanst, N., & Marcoen, A. (1993). Memory training in the community: Evaluations by participants and effects on metamemory. *Educational Gerontology, 19*, 525–534.

West, R. L. (1989). Planning practical memory training for the aged. In L. W. Poon, D. C. Rubin, & B. A. Wilson (Eds.), *Everyday cognition in adulthood and late life* (pp. 573–597). Cambridge, England: Cambridge University Press.

West, R. L., Boatwright, L. K., & Schleser, R. (1984). The link between memory performance, self-assessment, and affective status. *Experimental Aging Research, 10*(4), 197–200.

West, R. L., Crook, T. H., & Barron, K. L. (1992). Everyday memory performance across the life span: Effects of age and noncognitive individual differences. *Psychology and Aging, 7*(1), 72–82.

Williams, J. M., Little, M. M., Scates, S., & Blockman, N. (1987). Memory complaints and abilities among depressed older adults. *Journal of Consulting and Clinical Psychology, 55*(4), 595–598.

Willis, S. L., Blieszner, R., & Baltes, P. B. (1981). Intellectual training research in aging: Modification of performance on the fluid ability of figural relations. *Journal of Educational Psychology, 73*(1), 41–50.

Willis, S. L., Jay, G. M., Diehl, M., & Marsiske, M. (1992). Longitudinal change and prediction of everyday task competence in the elderly. *Research on Aging, 14*, 68–91.

Willis, S. L., & Nesselroade, C. S. (1990). Long-term effects of fluid ability training in old-old age. *Developmental Psychology, 26*(6), 905–910.

Willis, S. L., & Schaie, K. W. (1986). Training the elderly on the ability factors of spatial orientation and inductive reasoning. *Psychology and Aging, 3*, 239–247.

Willis, S. L., & Schaie, K. W. (1993). Everyday cognition: Taxonomic and methodological considerations. In J. M. Puckett & H. W. Reese (Eds.), *Lifespan developmental psychology: Mechanisms of everyday cognition* (pp. 33–53). Hillsdale, NJ: Erlbaum.

Woodruff-Pak, D. S. (1989). Aging and intelligence: Changing perspectives in the twentieth century. *Journal of Aging Studies, 3*(2), 91–118.

Yesavage, J. A. (1985). Nonpharmacological treatments for memory losses with normal aging. *American Journal of Psychiatry, 142*(5), 600–605.

Chapter 10

Primary Health Care

BEVERLY J. MCELMURRY
GWEN BRUMBAUGH KEENEY

ABSTRACT

Primary Health Care (PHC) has been promulgated for over two decades as a global strategy for ensuring basic health care for all people. PHC is characterized by equity, accessibility, availability of resources, social participation, intersectoral community action, and cultural sensitivity. While PHC can be discussed as philosophy or a process, it is critical that PHC be understood as a community focus in health care that differs from a primary care focus on individuals. Capturing PHC components in community-based interventions in order to advance the development of a rigorous research base requires a shift in thinking about what constitutes acceptable methods and evidence for evaluating changes in health care. To this end, the authors of this review discuss perspectives and available research that inform practice within multidisciplinary teams, highlight the importance of social discourse, and review participatory evaluation issues for achieving a working relationship with communities. Particular attention is focused on education for nurses' roles in PHC activities within implementation models fostering community mobilization and development. An action plan is suggested as a means for situating discrete research activity within a PHC framework.

Keywords: Primary Health Care, Social Discourse, Community Health, Participatory Evaluation, Nurses' Role, Multidisciplinary Practice

The International Conference on Primary Health Care, held in Alma-Ata, endorsed primary health care (PHC) as a framework for attaining Health for

All (HFA). Subsequently, United Nations' member states, including the United States (U.S.), have ratified the Declaration of Alma-Ata (1978) and begun incorporating primary health care principles into national health policies. International organizations, such as the International Council of Nurses (ICN) and the American Nurses Association (ANA), have promoted primary health care and advocated for policies and programs consistent with primary health care concepts and objectives ("ICN Statement," 1991; *Scope of Practice,* 1985).

> Within the Alma-Ata Declaration primary health care is explained and defined. Primary health care is essential health care based on practical, scientifically sound and socially acceptable methods and technology made universally accessible to individuals and families in the community and through their full participation and at a cost that the community and country can afford to maintain at every stage of their development in the spirit of self-reliance and self-determination. It forms an integral part both of the country's health system, of which it is the central function and main focus, and of the overall social and economic development of the community. It is the first level of contact of individuals, the family and community with the national health system bringing health care as close as possible to where people live and work, and constitutes the first element of a continuing health care process. (*Alma-Ata,* 1978, pp. 3–4)

Copious discourse pertaining to primary health care conceptualization, policy implications, and implementation issues has been propounded through professional publications and assemblies. The preponderance of primary health care literature continues to be in the form of commentary and anecdotal reports. As the first review of primary health care (PHC) to appear in an *Annual Review of Nursing Research,* the purpose of this chapter is to identify and describe the existing literature, relate what has been learned, and discuss directions for future PHC research and reviews.

Undertaking a literature review for primary health care is a challenging and complex task. PHC is comprised of multiple, interdependent concepts. Maintaining the integrity of PHC requires incorporation of all the PHC components. However, the totality is cumbersome to attend to in program development and dissemination efforts. Reviewing PHC literature is further complicated by the disparate understanding of PHC concepts and the inherent diversity of PHC applications. The following is a description of the literature review process that guided the formation of this review of PHC. To be congruous with PHC's multisectoral nature, multidisciplinary literature has been assimilated to enable a discussion of relevant PHC concepts and approaches. Multidisciplinary literature was gleaned from the WHO Collaborating Center for International Nursing Development in Primary Health Care at the University of Illinois at Chicago, nine anthologies prepared for PHC courses, and the extensive collections of the authors.

A systematic approach was devised to identify and retrieve nursing's contribution to PHC research. Nursing research literature was identified via a computerized search of the Cumulative Index of Nursing and Allied Health Literature (CINAHL) citations from 1982 to June 1997. "Primary health care" as adjacent words was used for a keyword search. The search was further limited by adding "research" as a keyword. The reviewers are aware of several articles matching the preceding criteria which have been published in CINAHL-indexed journals that were not retrieved in this search. In the interest of sampling clarity and replicability, only articles retrieved through the CINAHL search were considered for the nursing literature review. The CINAHL search identified 178 citations.

The citations and abstracts were examined manually to determine if primary health care was a component of the research. Literature was excluded when "primary health care" appeared in citations only as an alternate term for "primary care" or "general practice." Further winnowing was necessary due to the recent CINAHL subsumption of unrelated "primary care" literature into the "primary health care" subject heading. Citations were excluded only by consensus, when both reviewers were unable to identify a relationship to PHC as delineated in the Alma Ata Declaration (1978). Citations were accepted for full-text review if either reviewer identified any possible linkage with PHC. Fifty-five citations were identified for full-text inspection. Two articles from international journals were not included in the final sample after several unsuccessful attempts to obtain texts. Fifteen citations were dropped due to lack of PHC relevancy after full texts were perused by both reviewers. One research program was identified twice, once as a dissertation citation and once as a journal citation. Another research program appeared in two journals with different foci for reporting findings. Each pair was consolidated and dealt with as one research program. The final sample totaled 36 for this literature review.[1]

The intent of the investigators was to report a qualitative synthesis of the research literature to identify lessons learned. This was accepted as an appropriate strategy due to the predominance of qualitative designs within the sample literature (Patton, 1990). The review process was organized by utilizing a table format for each research report to document citation information, purpose, sample and sampling, research design, data collection methods, findings, and future research recommendations. The tables were designed to facilitate identification of research foci and cross-case comparisons. PHC categories were identified from the retrieved literature and provided a basis for sorting the literature. After extensive review, the small sample size in each category

---

[1]A complete listing of sample literature with citations and descriptions is available from the first author upon request.

was too disparate to identify coherent themes. Therefore, attempting to produce a synthesis was futile.

In the interest of moving nursing research forward, the investigators decided to proceed with the broader multisectoral literature review. A presentation of the state of primary health care provides a basis to enhance the formulation of future PHC research programs.

Five PHC categories were identified within the literature and are used to provide a framework for organizing this review. The five categories are (a) PHC concepts, (b) social discourse, (c) PHC implementation, (d) participatory evaluation, and (e) human resources.

PRIMARY HEALTH CARE CONCEPTS

Efforts to build understanding of PHC are evident in the proliferation of World Health Organization (WHO) publications (*Formulating Strategies*, 1979; *Global Strategy*, 1981; "Indicators," 1986; Mahler, 1981; *Meaning of Health*, 1985; *Ninth General Programme*, 1994; "Target 2000," 1987; Tarimo & Creese, 1990; WHO, 1987; "WHO in Action," 1987). Original case study research identified commonalities of successful community health programs that provided major premises for developing PHC (Djukanovic & Mach, 1975; Newell, 1975). PHC was conceived to address global inequities in basic health status through comprehensive, community-based, social action approaches. The Alma-Ata Declaration called for a reorientation of health policy at national and local levels, incorporating PHC principles of equitable distribution, community participation, multisectoral collaboration, prevention, and appropriate technology. Application of PHC principles has been championed as a basis for the development of sustainable health programs that are available, accessible, appropriate, affordable, and acceptable (*Evolution*, 1985).

Conceptual explication, reiteration, and interpretation continue in recent nursing literature (Berland, 1992; Blackburn, 1994; McElmurry, Swider, & Watanakij, 1992; Ntoane, 1993; Woods, 1992). Several authors have attempted to clarify the concept of primary health care by contrasting it with primary care or primary nursing (Barnes et al., 1995; Egwu, 1984; Powell, 1986; Smith, Forchuk, & Martin, 1985; St. John, 1993). Primary health care facilitates health and well-being within a socioeconomic, community-development context. Primary care is the provision of first contact, direct medical care, and health services for individuals and families. As an integral subset of primary health care, the development of primary care systems and practice should also reflect PHC principles (Goeppinger, 1984; Innes, 1987; Marion, 1996; National Institute of Nursing Research (NINR) Priority Expert Panel, 1995).

Constructing a scientific knowledge base for PHC is challenging. Conceptual complexity of PHC is inherent due to the symbiosis of PHC principles. Research and application often represent selective PHC, focusing on one or two principles within PHC. Selective PHC enables clarity for program planning and communication, but has also contributed to disparate and fragmented PHC perspectives. Baum and Sanders (1995) contend that the underlying principles of PHC can only be realized by returning to the unabridged tenets within the Alma Ata Declaration.

Conceptual discussion in multisectoral literature reflects the tendency towards selective PHC. Integrating traditional values and cultural practices with contemporary health care are highlighted as integral components of PHC (Bushy, 1992; Fendall, 1982; Hezekiah, 1990; Pilon, 1990–91; Sharma & Ross, 1990; Stone, 1992). Cultural congruence in program planning is also essential for sustainability and economic viability (Ager, 1990; van der Geest, 1992). Community lay workers, as part of a collaborative PHC team, have been recognized as crucial links for enhancing acceptability, appropriateness, and health care access (Fuller, 1995; Stewart, 1990). Community mobilization has been linked with a case management model as a strategy for community self-determination or self-care (Holzemer, 1992). Community empowerment and social change have been associated with community self-reliance, self-efficacy, and competency (Eng, Salmon, & Mullan, 1992; Jones & Meleis, 1993; S. Smith, 1991).

Community participation has been recognized as a cornerstone for actualizing PHC. The concept of community participation may be best understood along a continuum, with varying numbers of community members, diverse types of representation, and different degrees of community involvement (Al-Mazroa & Al-Shammari, 1991; Meleis, 1992; Rifkin, 1990, 1996; Sawyer, 1995). Watts (1990) interpreted community involvement as integrally connected to substantive democracy. A methodology for measuring processes related to community participation in PHC was developed. Measures of rank for five process indicators (needs assessment, leadership, organization, resource mobilization, and management) are intended to assess change over time and also reveal group difference in perceptions (Bichmann, Rifkin, & Shrestha, 1989).

SOCIAL DISCOURSE

One of the major themes that we find essential in reflecting about PHC is that of understanding the processes of social discourse in order to arrive at a social ethic. In discussing what needs to be done to reform health care, Caplan

(1996) urges us to provide a clear message on the values that guide health care. If we value the community focus of our work in PHC, then we are concerned about respect for others, sensitivity to the differences between cultural, racial, ethnic, and socioeconomic groups, and creating outcomes that reflect civic consensus about health for the community. Ensuring that varied stakeholders in health care have a place at the decision making table is a laudable goal and as we know, unattainable to date. Given what could be a pretty gloomy discussion of the deficits in the nursing research literature about social ethics or social discourse, we have chosen instead to try to make the case for a framework for participation based on the notion of the interdisciplinary work that is inherent in any mention of the multi-sectoral nature of PHC.

Chiu and Wilson (1996) provide a succinct overview of the ethical perspectives that guide nursing and identify ethical relativism, utilitarianism, and Kantian ethics as well as moral justice and caring as the basis for our actions. However, they rightfully note that most of us act on the basis of the integration of nursing viewpoints. Our behavior reflects a complex activity in which we seek to understand the situation of a given community and to respond according to the individuals and cultures found in that situation.

As we are writing to explicate a nursing contribution to the research on PHC, it is a premise that we expect nurses to be contributors to this discourse. To this extent, we seek the outcomes that Maher and Thompson-Tetreault (1994) identified when they examined classrooms that respected cultural diversity. In those classrooms that were most effective, students and teachers valued the construction of knowledge that meant a person had found mastery, voice, authority, and positionality on a given topic. To us, the construction of such knowledge is interwoven with the opportunity to reflect about experiences in order to arrive at expanding horizons. Thus, it is not surprising that many members of the nursing profession have expressed discontent with the lack of their instrumental participation in the current changes sweeping the health field. For health professionals, particularly nurses, PHC is an arena where care actions and social actions are interwoven (Davis, 1997). How then might nurses find ways to ensure their voice in the policy and practice arenas where decisions are being made, particularly about primary health care issues? In our experience, nurses can resonant with the advice of Kritek (1994) that focused on development of moral courage to resolve our conflicts. A major thesis of the Kritek position was that most nurses in leadership positions find themselves at uneven tables when it comes time to negotiate and/or resolve conflicts. One way to capture the type of leadership suggested by Kritek is to examine behavior that is socially active, person-centered, and articulate about what we hope to accomplish in our negotiations.

Richardson (1994), while ostensibly dealing with participatory research, does explain how a low-income, underserved community was consulted in planning for a new health resource center. While Richardson found little to guide their community consultation approach, their methodology focused on raising public awareness of the issues, meeting with local groups, conducting workshops to develop a vision for potential services, structuring to obtain feedback on possible center services, and field trips to observe other centers. He observed that when people are not accustomed to being consulted, there is a need to build in support for expressing their views and to allow sufficient time for community involvement to evolve. It was important to have designated staff assigned the role of developing community discourse and participation.

Given the desire to have nursing participation in the social discourse about community based health care, two questions come to mind: What are some of the major areas that need to be discussed by community members? And, can we identify nursing research that would guide our decisional processes and practices relative to those topics? An immediate concern is the issue of populations that are vulnerable and need special consideration for their health care. Another area of concern in thinking about the development of primary health care services is that of ensuring public participation in the decisions about how scarce health care resources will be used. Davis (1997) has raised some interesting questions about how nurses work with lay health workers. While the professional may make the case that unlicensed personnel represent a second-class system of care, particularly for low-income and vulnerable groups or populations, such ideas need to be challenged. Often the lay health worker can better understand and respect the values and cultures within their communities.

Generally, a cursory consideration of the areas above helps one realize that in social discourse one faces the need to take positions on different topics and options. To get to this point, feeling prepared to take positions, there is some literature that professionals have used that is at least scholarly, if not meeting the usual criteria of researched practices. For example, there is nursing ethics literature that covers the professional code, the nature or characteristics of the nurse-patient relationship, advocacy roles, respect for religious/spiritual dimensions in health care, and, increasingly, what it means to have empowered constituents. Most of that literature will be useful in shaping the depth and wisdom of the person that comes to the table to negotiate health care decisions, but it will not provide a research base for those decisions.

Nursing is but a microcosm of the struggle to understand how to achieve full participation in social discourse on health. The Council for International Organizations of Medical Sciences (Bankowski & Bryant, 1995) has urged that the health sector be guided by certain principles. One of the more important principles is that

> mechanisms should be developed to ensure that communities are enabled
> to meaningfully participate in the development of health policy and services,

and communities and individuals should be involved in determining the
nature and quality of health care. (p. viii)

PRIMARY HEALTH CARE IMPLEMENTATION

Within primary health care is the assumption that socioeconomic and cultural
contexts are essential for developing programs that are appropriate, acceptable,
and sustainable. Given that each community has its own unique set of circumstances, diversity of PHC program designs is expected. However, some common concepts and practices have been recognized and adapted for local
implementation.

Community participation is a fundamental component of PHC. However,
diverse interpretations of community participation exist. The continuum of
community participation extends from professionally driven, top-down models
seeking to respond to community input, via surveys or a community representative on an institutional board, to bottom-up approaches with full community
ownership of health programs, including decision-making and program implementation (Raymond & Patrick, 1988). Rifkin (1986, 1987, 1990) has documented originating rationales for community participation in PHC,
operationalized strategies, difficulties encountered, and experiential lessons
learned. Rifkin's (1996) recent writing speaks cogently for a shift from a
linear, causal scientific paradigm to a relativistic, flexible approach that attends
to the dynamic nature of community participation processes. A new paradigm
is proposed for analysis of adaptive change through interpretation of existing
relationships and events. Several methods and tools have been designed to
evaluate community participation (Bichmann et al., 1989; Kelly & Van Vlaenderen, 1996; La Forgia, 1985; Ugalde, 1985). One tool for assessing incorporation of community participation in program planning was developed by Kroutil
and Eng (1989). Their 14-item instrument builds on the body of work of
Cohen and Uphoff which focuses on three dimensions for participation: (a)
who, (b) what, and (c) how.

In addition to determining the intended scope of community participation,
PHC program planners need to identify the parameters of the community.
Defining a community in the midst of social change and increasingly diverse
populations requires consideration of self-defined community alliances. Geo-
graphic location and ethnic or cultural heritage provide a context for identifying
some communities. However, individuals and families may feel connected to
different community configurations based on interests, values, or family origins
(Meleis, 1992).

Many PHC programs have been designed to mobilize communities to
assess, manage, and resolve their health needs using strategies that are appro-

priate for the unique context of their community (Fox & Komchum, 1992; Freeman, 1993; Morris, 1992; Tamsang & Anderson, 1990). Schorr's (1997) writing is congruent with appropriate technology concepts, using non-dramatic, low-tech activities that can be accomplished within community contexts. Mobilization and participation are recognized as methods for achieving health for all, and occur in conjunction with social change and empowerment (Eng et al., 1992; Jones & Meleis, 1993; McMurray, 1991; Smith, 1991).

Common models for implementing PHC have relied on lay community members to provide a bridge between formal health care programs and the local community (Bender & Pitkin, 1989). A frequent strategy has been to identify individuals from local communities to serve as lay or community health workers (CHWs). Varying forms of health education programs have been designed to prepare CHWs for such roles. Other common strategies have included developing child-to-child programs (Hawes, 1988; Jabre, 1986; Onyejiaku & Rogers, 1989; Tay, 1989) or interacting with women's groups (Arole, 1988; Chamberlain, 1993; Quigley & Ebrahim, 1994a, 1994b; Wong & Chen, 1991). All three lay community member models assume that

(a) basic health information can be learned by individuals from within the community;
(b) lay helpers can understand local culture, values, and practices;
(c) lay workers can communicate basic health information to their communities; and
(d) communities are more likely to accept new information from people they know and trust (*Alma-Ata,* 1978; Bender & Pitkin, 1987; Berman, 1984; Eng & Young, 1992; Giblin, 1989; Swider & McElmurry, 1990; Werner & Bower, 1982).

Effective small-scale PHC programs are widely recognized in the international literature (Berman, Gwatkin, & Burger, 1987; *Strengthening the Performance,* 1989). In particular, CHW programs have been credited with improvements in health knowledge, coverage and equity of health services, prenatal care attendance, prevalence of breastfeeding, nutritional status, immunization rates, infant mortality rates, incidence of diarrheal diseases, and malaria morbidity (Bender & Pitkin, 1987; Berman, 1984; Chabot & Waddington, 1987; Curtale, Siwakoti, Lagrosa, LaRaja, & Guerra, 1995; Menon, Snow, Greenwood, Hayes, & N'Jie, 1990; Stock-Iwamoto & Korte, 1993; Van Norren, Boerma, & Sempebwa, 1989; Watkins et al., 1994; World Bank, 1993).

In contrast, large PHC programs persistently have encountered implementation difficulties. Vertical programs, which develop strategies and objectives centrally, tend to inhibit community innovations based on local priorities and issues. A sense of community ownership or commitment is diminished when community members and local personnel are not fully included in formulating program foci and determining their own method for implementation (*Strengthening the Performance*, 1989).

PARTICIPATORY EVALUATION

A goal in primary health care is to ensure communication and collaboration between community members and health professionals. Thus, one of the areas that continues to challenge those interested in evaluating PHC services is how to engage community members in the evaluation process. In organizing the literature retrieved on participatory evaluation, the natural groups for the literature were those authors dealing with general ideas on the topic, those with special interest in research perspectives such as naturalistic evaluation and participatory research, and those with a concern for stakeholders, particularly minority issues and/or feminist perspectives in evaluation. Another way to look at the literature identified was whether it sorted into mainstream perspectives or represented less traditional ideas.

A useful article for sorting the participatory evaluation literatures is the framework for planning that Kinsey (1981) authored almost two decades ago. The framework represents a pragmatic process that leads one through

(a) consideration of the objectives, limits purpose and methods for participatory evaluation;
(b) the context in which the valuation will occur and including content, input, process and results;
(c) the desired participants in the evaluation; and
(d) the phases in program implementation such as planning, design, implementation, and analysis.

While a pragmatic focus, it would also be useful in negotiating with communities regarding proposed PHC programs. A common criticism of those approaching community partnerships is whether the idea came from the community or whether the community was involved in particular aspects of the partnership. Reviewing Kinsey's process with the intended community partners in the planning phases would be a means of avoiding later reproach.

Evaluation of community-based health care initiatives or programs are complicated by the confusion between outcomes from evaluation and whether those outcomes are actually used and/or become part of a changed or evolved system of care. Good outcomes do not necessarily ensure a changed system

(Weiss, 1988). Cousins and Edell (1992) pick up this idea in their discussion of the case for participatory evaluation. A particularly useful aspect of their discussion highlights the linkage concept. In essence, the linkage concept translates into that which connects what is learned from evaluation/research with the users of such information (Laurell, Noriega, Martinez, & Villegas, 1992). These authors emphasize that linkage occurs more often when investigators and community partners and/or practitioners connect or interact. Like the social construction of knowledge, the use of new understandings and information by communities/agencies/organizations means we must think of them as learning environments and then attend to what enhances learning in those contexts (Dawson & D'Amico, 1985; Mathisen, 1990). The Cousins and Edell (1992) work with organizations and organizational learning can be paraphrased as a question guiding future community-based research: To achieve a learning community, what inquiry processes, interpretive frameworks, and perceptual lenses need to be installed to simplify the complexity and management of information that a community needs to achieve its health goals?

We recognize the use of participatory evaluation to establish the research base for PHC. However, some authors have discussed whether process evaluation is less worthy than outcomes evaluation (Digman, Tillgren, & Michielutte, 1994), and/or whether responsiveness to participants and users of research findings diminishes the technical quality of the research conducted (Greene, 1990). Process and responsiveness are crucial aspects of participatory evaluation. If such aspects do introduce limitations in a study, that can be acknowledged, but it need not impede moving forward with the participatory evaluation of PHC.

For Whitmore (1988), the evaluation process can have three phases: (a) individual, (b) group, and (c) environmental or action-oriented. We add to this the idea that in our efforts to understand participatory evaluation, an important emphasis is the identification of the stakeholders in the process and the expected outcomes.

The Center for Community Education and Action (CCEA) in Massachusetts represents a broad perspective on evaluation when it urges participatory research. Their definition of such research covers the initial definition of the problems to be solved and actions or interventions to be taken to solve those problems (Center for Community Education and Action (CCEA) and Center for International Education (CIE), 1991). The over 180 references reviewed in the CCEA document represent the alternative or fugitive literature to some extent, as many of the references are difficult to retrieve or out of print. While useful, the extensive listing of references included in the CCEA materials often describe small case studies, or illustrate programs tried in a variety of countries to launch a media campaign or create public awareness of a health policy that needs to be changed. Many terms are mentioned in discussing participatory research, such as community education, community research, participatory education, community planning, community development, and community organizing. The authors included in the CCEA material on participatory research are those associated with liberatory or emancipatory goals and valuing critical theory, action research, and popular education. Such themes represent a common focus in much of the primary health care literature, particularly that originating from authors/scholars outside of the U.S.

Unlike the CCEA references, almost all of the computerized information retrieval systems located more traditional evaluation references. By traditional, we mean professionally driven evaluation plans, often plans derived without consultation with those most affected by the services evaluated. This criticism is not meant to negate the evaluation, but it is meant to raise question about the comprehensiveness of the evaluation strategies used to date.

There is an increasing literature about quality of care and patient satisfaction that could be interpreted as movement toward participatory concerns (Attree, 1996; Mansour & Al-Osimy, 1993) and primary health care goals (Dykeman, 1998). However, the quality-of-care literature may be driven by goals other than ensuring the participatory behavior of the community members, e.g., risk aversion or marketing services.

Various means have been used by authors to deal with the issue of obtaining the "objective" data they need and to engage the participation of the community. Rovers (1986) proposed a dual method to meet agency needs for information and a participatory approach to recognize the community's ability to judge responsiveness of services to their need. Participatory evaluation models as mechanisms for community input and community self-assessment have been developed by Feuerstein (1978, 1980) and Nichter (1984). In some cases, investigators have developed tools/instruments based on the extant literature and conducted focus meetings with targeted evaluation participants for the dual purpose of obtaining a measure and teaching the community what factors to examine in making judgments about the existing conditions or services (Conrad, Balch, Reichelt, Muran, & Oh, 1994; Watanakij & McElmurry, 1995).

The concern for community participation in evaluation must, of course, consider the skills and abilities of the participants in the evaluation and the purpose for the evaluation. In many respects the simpler the tool, the better. For this reason, Feuerstein (1986) remains an excellent example of selecting a measure that relates to the behavior desired of the community member. Thus, if monitoring of child growth and development, as well as maternal self-sufficiency, is desired, an important measure will be the parent's ability to accurately weigh and monitor the child. In a similar theme, Scrimshaw and

Hurtado (1987) propose rapid assessment procedures for primary health care that are identified as practical anthropological fieldwork and draw upon observation, field notes, interviews, focus groups, etc. What is useful in the rapid assessment methods identified is that they are related to the essential elements of primary health care, such as safe water or nutrition, and then linked to relatively efficient sources or means for obtaining the relevant data that document health-seeking behavior.

 A useful overview and illustration of participatory research is Narayan's (1996) description of water and sanitation projects throughout many parts of the world. The emphases underlying the use of such a method was capacity building, use of results, short-cut methods, multiple methods, and capturing the expertise of the nonexpert. Two particularly useful chapters are the innovative data collection methods that work in the field and the training of lay field workers. Narayan's reference serves as both an overview of this form of evaluation and a useful handbook regardless of the focus of one's evaluation. While we favor the term "participatory research" to capture the importance of community involvement in primary health care, related concepts are those of community participation, coalitions, partnerships, and mobilization.

HUMAN RESOURCES

The international nursing literature reflects ongoing efforts to understand the roles for nurses within a PHC framework. PHC has required new or expanded roles for nurses in policy formation, community mobilization and development, intersectoral collaboration, professional and community teaching, and research. For the purposes of this review, our discussion will focus on the two predominant role topics in the nursing literature: (a) educational reorientation to prepare nurses for work within a PHC framework, and (b) nurses' roles in relation to PHC teams.

NURSING EDUCATION FOR PRIMARY HEALTH CARE

WHO has repeatedly called for reorientation of health education programs to prepare health professionals to work within a primary health care framework. In 1979, the ICN proclaimed that nursing education needed to be more conducive to primary health care implementation (Swann, 1984). Nurses need to be prepared to promote and facilitate primary health care approaches within communities, educational systems, and policy formulation. Curricula designs should be oriented to communities, technologically and socially appropriate, learner centered, and emphasize problem-solving approaches (*Education and Training*, 1984).

The WHO summarized objectives for health education training for primary health care as:

1. Adopt a new outlook and be concerned not only with disease prevention and control but also with development in general and with people oriented technologies;
2. Act as "facilitators" of action by the people;
3. Promote the two-way transfer of technologies between the health system and community;
4. Assume an advocacy role for the cause of health vis-a-vis both the people and the decision-makers; and
5. Recognize the contribution that professionals in other sectors can make to the promotion of health (*New Approaches*, 1983, p. 32).

Since that time, numerous WHO documents have presented recommendations for educational approaches to prepare health professionals, including nurses, for primary health care (J. P. Ben-Dov, Bin-Nun, & Levi, 1988; *Community-Based Education*, 1987; *Health Manpower*, 1985; *Increasing the Relevance*, 1993; *Nursing Beyond*, 1994; *Regulatory Mechanisms*, 1986; Storey, Roemer, Maglacas, & Riccard, 1988).

The process of reorienting nursing education to prepare nurses for primary health care has been progressing very slowly (J. P. Smith, 1989). However, several countries have incorporated primary health care concepts into nursing curricula during the last decade. Pakistan developed a core nursing course to teach PHC as a philosophy and guide to action (Edwards & Tompkins, 1988). In Canada, primary health care axioms were used to provide the foundation for the development of a conceptual framework for nursing education (Stewart, 1990). Davis and Deitrick (1987) describe a collaborative U.S. curriculum process designed to convey PHC concepts through combined didactic and experiential learning opportunities. Eight Latin American countries integrated PHC into all four student levels with an emphasis on the development of student's process skills for interpersonal interactions and community motivation (Manfredi, 1983). A one-year intensive post-basic training program for primary health care nurses was instituted in South Africa to promote respectful, caring attitudes towards communities and traditional beliefs; develop positive, interactive learning/teaching strategies; and cooperation rather than competition (Schneider, Malumane, Ngwenya, & Blackett-Sliep, 1989). In Papua New Guinea, a continuing education program was created to develop skills in community relations and communication, problem identification and problem solving, and project implementation so that nurses could be redirected from curative, clinic-based roles to preventive, community-based roles (Spear, Oddi, Vor der Bruegge, & Hamilton, 1990).

As the U.S. moves toward sweeping health care reform, nurses have been in the forefront of promoting primary health care strategies. The National League for Nursing's (NLN) Nursing's Agenda for Health Care Reform and the American Association of Colleges of Nursing (AACN) forecast the movement of nursing towards primary health care within community-based systems (cited in Oermann, 1994). Nursing leaders have called for the reformation of nursing education to emphasize experiential learning, critical thinking, ethical issues, community interactions (Oermann, 1994), health policy, and political activism (Flynn, Ray, & Selmanoff, 1987; Williams, 1993). Laffrey and Page (1989) recommend master's degree curricula with courses in epidemiology, health planning and evaluation, leadership, community organization and development, political and legislative nursing roles, to prepare community health nurse specialists to meet community health needs. Flynn (1984) provided examples of baccalaureate, master's and doctoral course content and community learning experiences which integrated cultural and political relevancy, community health needs, community assessment, essential services, intersectoral interaction, participation and self-reliance, appropriate technology, and multiprofessional teamwork.

Evaluation of international nursing educational experience with primary health care curricula could provide a valuable contribution to U.S. nurse educators as curricula incorporating primary health care concepts are being developed. The World Health Organization has prepared an evaluation tool for nursing curriculum that is primarily designed for internal institutional assessment for curriculum content relevant to primary health care (*Guide to Curriculum*, 1985). Primary health care training should be designed to prepare health workers to respond to the felt needs of communities. Therefore, the education of nurses needs to prepare nurses for practice that is relevant to the expectations and health needs of the communities. However, a 1988 WHO/ICN joint report recognized that nursing course content is often

> . . . "more of the same" because teachers themselves know no more, and it does not provide preparation for community activities such as policy-formulation, community mobilization, priority-setting, managing health centers, budgeting and working with other health-related sectors. (*Nursing in Primary Health Care*, 1989, p. 9)

Evaluation and research activities are recommended as part of primary health care curriculum development and implementation (*Guide to Curriculum*, 1985; Yu, 1992). To date, the emphasis has been placed on assessment of curriculum content within the training programs (*Community-Based Education*, 1987; *Guide to Curriculum*, 1985).

If curricula are intended to be responsive and relevant to community needs, then community members and nurses in community practice can provide essential evaluation and input for the development and revision of community-oriented primary health care curricula. A case study, with interviews and observation, identified inadequate gender sensitivity and lack of social awareness among Soweto PHC nurses (Walker, 1995). Using data from interviews and questionnaires, Anderson's (1987) combined quantitative and qualitative methods to analyze community health nurses' satisfaction with their educational preparation for primary health care roles and their actual experiences in practice. The majority of nurses felt their educational program had prepared them for their community PHC practice. However, 55% reported that there were few occasions to contribute to health care in accord with their educational preparation. In response to their own frustrations, the PHC nurses identified suggestions for resolution. A suggestion to teach character development was directed back to the educational programs.

PRIMARY HEALTH CARE TEAMS

Nurses and community representatives are often identified as vital members of PHC teams ("Cities in Distress," 1991). Multidisciplinary or multi-sectoral teams facilitate coordinated and comprehensive PHC endeavors. PHC teams interact with community members to develop and sustain health programs and services. Collaboration, respecting the expertise of each PHC team member, is promoted. The constituency of PHC teams is determined by the needs, resources, and priorities associated with each setting's unique context. WHO has recognized that nurses should have a key role in primary health care, since nurses are the most numerous and widely dispersed health professionals and work closely with people in communities (Storey et al., 1988). Lay workers, often called community health workers (CHWs), serve as representatives of their communities and provide a bridge between health professionals and community members (Bender & Pitkin, 1987).

Community health professionals represent a broad spectrum of interests and understandings. Part of community health nursing has focused on individuals or families in community settings. Other community health nurses identify the aggregate community as the client (Goeppinger, 1984). The community perspective of PHC programs provides the framework for discussion about role differentiation and community interaction with the PHC team. Brown (1994) examined how general practitioners and community nurses viewed the concepts of community and participation. Like many authors, Brown does not differentiate primary care from primary health care, and uses the terms interchangeably. However, his qualitative study found that the key dimensions in the practitioners views centered about individual versus collective ethics and professional versus lay control tensions. It is not likely that such a finding surprises community-based practitioners.

Nursing literature related to PHC personnel has been focused on role development of nurses within PHC. Rogers (1989) analyzed Nigerian nurses' activities to identify content of nursing practice in PHC programs. Interviews, questionnaires, nursing record review, and participant observation revealed that nurses' main roles were as sources of support, and providing connections for services and information. Nursing interventions associated with these roles were building intersectoral linkages, recruitment of influence, and community mobilization and education. Wiles and Robison (1994) employed semistructured interviews with British nurses, health visitors, and midwives to discover issues related to their experiences as PHC team members: leadership; team identity; understanding of team members' roles and responsibilities; disagreement regarding roles and responsibilities; access to general practitioners; and philosophies of care.

Descriptive literature identifies an active nursing role in new program planning, implementation, evaluation, and policy changes (Orpaz & Korenblit, 1994). Labelle (1986) contends that nurses have historically been involved in social action to address environmental, economic, and social issues that affect health, and should continue to be proponents for social change towards PHC.

Nursing role development literature has also investigated the relationship of nurses with lay workers. Bless, Murphy, and Vinson (1995) provide an in-depth description of nurses' roles in primary health care programs. Underlying PHC tenets are woven into practical application through partnership with CHWs to address broad health concerns of community members. Identified PHC nursing roles with CHWs are teacher, mediator, friend, collaborator, liaison, planner, organizer, coordinator, case manager, and public health crusader. Ethnic health workers are endorsed to serve as intermediaries between nurses and communities, providing essential expert cultural knowledge for meeting the needs of culturally diverse groups (Fuller, 1995). Examination of concepts within PHC and professionalism, in association with cultural diversity issues, provides a basis for recommendations that foster effective teamwork between nurses and ethnic workers. Nurses have promoted lay health workers and participated in training programs for appropriate community peers, such as traditional birth attendants (Ross, 1988; Singh, 1994; Smit, 1994), traditional healers (Blackett-Sliep, 1989), children (Onyejiaku & Rogers, 1989), and lady health visitors (Hezekiah, 1993).

CONCLUSION

The development of a chapter on primary health care has been a challenge. At the outset, we wish to emphasize that PHC can not be understood by analysis of the research conducted by only one discipline, nursing. By definition, primary health care requires multidisciplinary participants working in consort with members of the community that wish health services. This means that we can not appreciate the concept, process, and/or philosophy of primary health care without reading widely and integrating from many disciplines that which indicates the state of the research base for primary health care at this point in time. Therefore, while we seek to explicate that knowledge advanced by nurse investigators, it is an insufficient source of knowledge for the scope of primary health care.

In some ways, this state of affairs is as it should be for this topic. PHC as a conceptual arena for practice and research is only a few decades old. Within the domain of concepts and theories, developing ideas may be unwieldy, ambiguous, and understood in context of the historical situation and in comparison to alternative ideas. "Knowledge so conceived . . . forces our mind to make imaginative choices and thus makes it grow, It makes our mind capable of choosing, imagining, criticizing" (Feyerabend, 1981, p. 159). Facing this issue highlights many of the current concerns in health care generally.

Our frustration with the effort to make sense of the literature led to the development of a map for evaluating primary health care (Figure 10.1). It is a useful heuristic, particularly when investigators wish to place their study within a PHC context. As we reviewed our notes, the existing literature had bits and pieces that often did not convey the "worldview" of the author(s) or the PHC "big picture." Therefore, the figure is constructed to bridge individual, family, and community elements, with areas of concern in health system research as well as traditional evaluation perspectives and the crucial perspectives in PHC such as participatory evaluation. Locating one's research within the figure can start by clarifying what objectives are desired in terms of health and social policy outcomes relevant to nursing practice. Then, specify whether your work places a main emphasis on planning, monitoring an ongoing activity, or evaluating the outcomes from a specific program. From there, one can determine whether the study focuses on program design, components, operational processes, or outputs. A final area for reflection about one's research is the decision on what criteria are of particular concern in that research, and what types of evaluation design(s) are the best means for tying the focus and criteria together. In a sense, the figure presents a discussion guide for identifying a conceptual map to guide your PHC research. We suggest that the figure is best used as a point of departure for discussion of proposed research.

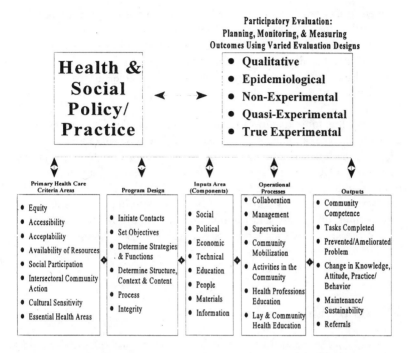

Figure 10.1.   Mapping a Primary Health Care Action Plan.

Note. From McElmurry, Buseh, & Keeney, July 1988.

There are sweeping changes in health care as corporatization of facilities management and health insurance occurs. Some have indicated that the deprofessionalization of nursing has occurred and medicine is undergoing the same process (Young, 1996). Hopefully, the health consumer movement will be useful in restoring some balance to what is rapidly becoming one of the most disgraceful health situations for any country, let alone one as wealthy as the U.S.

Primary health care is not a topic that can be addressed without recognition of the values that undergird its conceptualization. Thus, it is useful to examine what we mean when we use the term PHC. A variety of sources can be cited beginning with the original Alma-Ata (1978) document. Of particular concern is the importance of:

- defining minimum or essential health services that should be available to all regardless of income;

- ensuring community participation in the formation of health policy as well as the implementation of health services;
- working to achieve collaboration across the various sectors seeking to advance health and health care; and
- addressing the community's need for accessible, affordable, appropriate, and acceptable health care.

Most of all, this topic requires that nurses shift their thinking to concern for the health care of communities, how that care should be structured and evaluated, and what it means in terms of nursing leadership. For nursing to provide leadership in PHC, it will be necessary to become instrumental and active in shaping health policies, partnerships, and services. As G. Smith (1997) has noted, when communities partner with institutions to improve health, people begin to think differently and respond creatively. Any fundamental shift in how a profession views its work and world view takes time. That shift or transition is occurring, and primary health care is a framework for helping us envision the desired future.

REFERENCES

Ager, A. (1990). The importance of sustainability in the design of culturally appropriate programmes of early intervention. *International Disability Studies, 12*(2), 89–92.

Alma-Ata 1978: Primary health care. (1978). *Report of the International Conference on Primary Health Care, Alma-Ata, USSR, 6-12 September 1978 (Health For All Series, No. 1)*. Geneva: World Health Organization.

Al-Mazroa, Y., & Al-Shammari, S. (1991). Community participation and attitudes of decision-makers towards community involvement in health development. *Bulletin of the World Health Organization, 69*(1), 43–50.

Anderson, S. V. (1987). Response of nursing education to primary health care: The training and practice of post basic community health nurses in Botswana. *International Nursing Review, 34*, 17–25.

Arole, M. (1988). A comprehensive approach to community welfare: Growth monitoring and the role of women in Jamkhed. *India Journal of Pediatrics, 55*(Suppl.), S100–S105.

Attree, M. (1996). Towards a conceptual model of "quality care." *International Journal of Nursing Studies, 33*(1), 13–28.

Bankowski, Z., & Bryant, J. H. (Eds.). (1995). *Poverty, vulnerability, and the value of human life: A global agenda for bioethics*. Geneva: Council for International Organizations of Medical Sciences.

Barnes, D., Eribes, C., Juarbe, T., Nelson, M., Proctor, S., Sawyer, L., Shaul, M., & Meleis, A. I. (1995). Primary health care and primary care: A confusion of philosophies. *Nursing Outlook, 43*, 7–16.

Baum, F., & Sanders, D. (1995). Can health promotion and primary health care achieve health for all without a return to their more radical agenda? *Health Promotion International, 10,* 149–160.

Bender, D. E., & Pitkin, K. (1987). Bridging the gap: The village health worker as the cornerstone of the primary health care model. *Social Science & Medicine, 24,* 515–528.

Ben-Dov, N., Bin-Nun, G., & Levi, B. (1988). *Megatrends affecting the reorientation of nursing in Europe.* Vienna, Austria: WHO, Regional Office for Europe.

Berland, A. (1992). Primary health care: What does it mean for nurses? *International Nursing Review, 39,* 47–48, 52.

Berman, P. A. (1984). Village health workers in Java, Indonesia: Coverage and equity. *Social Science & Medicine, 19,* 411–422.

Berman, P. A., Gwatkin, D. R., & Burger, S. E. (1987). Community-based health workers: Head start or false start towards health for all. *Social Science & Medicine, 25,* 443–459.

Bichmann, W., Rifkin, S. B., & Shrestha, M. (1989). Towards the measurement of community participation. *World Health Forum, 10,* 467–472.

Blackburn, K. (1994). Primary health care: A Darling Downs focus. *Australian Journal of Rural Health, 2*(3), 17–24.

Blackett-Sliep, Y. (1989). Traditional healers and the primary health care nurse. *Nursing RSA Verpleging, 4*(11), 42–44.

Bless, C., Murphy, D., & Vinson, N. (1995). Nurses' role in primary health care. *N& HC: Perspectives on Community, 16,* 70–76.

Brown, I. (1994). Community and participation for general practice: Perceptions of general practitioners and community nurses. *Social Science & Medicine, 39,* 335–344.

Bushy, A. (1992). Cultural considerations for primary health care: Where do self-care and folk medicine fit? *Holistic Nursing Practice, 6*(3), 10–18.

Caplan, A. (1996). Do ethics and money mix? The moral implications of the corporatization of health care. In E. D. Baer, C. M. Fagin, & S. Gordon (Eds.), *Abandonment of the patient* (pp. 87–99). New York: Springer Publishing.

Center for Community Education & Action, & Center for International Education. (1991). *Participatory research: An annotated bibliography.* Amherst, MA: University of Massachusetts.

Chabot, J., & Waddington, C. (1987). Primary health care is not cheap: A case study from Guinea Bissau. *International Journal of Health Services, 17,* 387–409.

Chamberlain, A. (1993). Learning from each other: Inspiration and example from Nicaragua. *Community Development Journal, 28*(1), 31–37.

Chiu, W., & Wilson, D. (1996). Resolving the ethical dilemma of nurse managers over chemically-dependent colleagues. *Nursing Ethics, 3*(4), 285–293.

Cities in distress: A rescue strategy. (1991). *International Nursing Review, 38,* 105–110, 117.

Community-based education of health personnel. (1987). (Technical Report Series #746). Geneva: WHO.

Conrad, K. M, Balch, G. I., Reichelt, P. A., Muran, S., & Oh, K. (1994). Musculoskeletal injuries in the fire service. *American Association of Occupational Health Nurses Journal, 42*(1), 572–581.

Cousins, J. B., & Edell, L. M. (1992). The case for participatory evaluation. *Educational Evaluation and Policy Analysis, 14,* 397–418.

Curtale, F., Siwakoti, B., Lagrosa, C., LaRaja, M., & Guerra, R. (1995). Improving skills and utilization of community health volunteers in Nepal. *Social Science & Medicine, 40,* 1117–1125.

Davis, A. J. (1997). Selected ethical issues in planned social change and primary health care. *Nursing Ethics, 4*(3), 239–243.

Davis, J. H., & Deitrick, E. P. (1987). Unifying the strategies of primary health care education. *International Nursing Review, 34,* 102–106.

Dawson, J. A., & D'Amico, J. J. (1985). Involving program staff in evaluation studies: A strategy for increasing information use and enriching the database. *Evaluation Review, 9*(2), 173–188.

Digman, M., Tillgren, P. F., & Michielutte, R. (1994). Developing process evaluation for community-based health education and research and practice: A role for the diffusion model. *Health Values, 18*(5), 56–59.

Djukanovic, V., & Mach, E. P. (1975). Alternative approaches to meeting basic health needs in developing countries: A joint UNICEF/WHO study. Geneva: WHO.

Dykeman, M. C. (1998). Patient satisfaction in an HIV positive community: A secondary analysis. Unpublished doctoral dissertation, University of Illinois at Chicago.

Education and training of nurse teachers and managers with special regard to primary health care. (1984). (Technical Rep. Series #708). Geneva: WHO.

Edwards, N. C., & Tompkins, C. H. (1988). An approach to international education in primary health care. *Nurse Educator, 13*(2), 31–36.

Egwu, I. N. (1984). Update: Primary care is not the same as primary health care, or is it? *Family and Community Health, 7*(3), 83–88.

Eng, E., Salmon, M. E., & Mullan, F. (1992). Community empowerment: The critical base for primary health care. *Journal of Family and Community Health, 15,* 1–12.

Eng, E., & Young, R. (1992). Lay health advisors as community change agents. *Family & Community Health, 15*(1), 24–40.

Evolution of primary health care. (1985). (HFA Leadership/IM.1). Geneva: World Health Organization.

Fendall, R. (1982). Ayurvedic medicine and primary health care. *World Health Forum, 3*(1), 90–94.

Feuerstein, M. T. (1978). The educative approach in evaluation: An appropriate technology for a rural health programme. *International Journal of Health Education, 21*(1), 56–64.

Feuerstein, M. T. (1980). Community participation in evaluation: Problems and potentials. *International Nursing Review, 27,* 187–190.

Feuerstein, M. T. (1986). *Partners in evaluation: Evaluating development and community programmes with participants.* London: Macmillan.

Feyerabend, P. (1981). How to defend society against science. In I. Hacking (Ed.), *Scientific revolutions* (pp. 156–167). Oxford: Oxford University Press.

Flynn, B. C. (1984). Public health nursing education for primary health care. *Public Health Nursing, 1*(1), 36–44.

Flynn, B. C., Ray, D. W., & Selmanoff, E. D. (1987). Preparation of community health nursing leaders for social action. *International Journal of Nursing Studies, 24,* 239–248.

Formulating strategies for Health for All by the year 2000. (1979). (Health for All Series, No. 2). Geneva: WHO.

Fox, P. G., & Komchum, S. (1992). Primary health care in an unsettled area of northern Thailand. *International Nursing Review, 39,* 49–51.

Freeman, P. (1993). A culturally orientated curriculum for Aboriginal health workers. *World Health Forum, 14,* 262–266.

Fuller, J. (1995). Challenging old notions of professionalism: How can nurses work with paraprofessional ethnic health workers? *Journal of Advanced Nursing, 22,* 465–472.

Giblin, P. T. (1989). Effective utilization and evaluation of indigenous health care workers. *Public Health Reports, 104,* 361–368.

Global strategy for Health for All by the year 2000. (1981). (Health for All Series, No. 3). Geneva: WHO.

Goeppinger, J. (1984). Primary health care: An answer to the dilemmas of community nursing? *Public Health Nursing, 1*(3), 129–140.

Greene, J. C. (1990). Technical quality versus user responsiveness in evaluation practice. *Evaluation and Program Planning, 13,* 267–274.

Guide to curriculum review for basic nursing education: Orientation to primary health care and community health. (1985). Geneva: WHO.

Hawes, H. (1988). *Child-to-Child: Another path to learning* (UIE Monographs 13). Hamburg, West Germany: United Nations Educational, Scientific, and Cultural Organization, Institute for Education.

Health manpower requirements for the achievement of health for all by the year 2000 through primary health care. (1985). (Technical Report Series #717). Geneva: WHO.

Hezekiah, J. (1993). The pioneers of rural Pakistan: the lady health visitors. *Health Care for Women International, 14,* 493–502.

Holzemer, W. L. (1992). Linking primary health care and self-care through case management. *International Nursing Review, 39,* 83–89.

ICN statement for WHA Technical discussions on strategies for Health for All in the face of rapid urbanization. (1991). *International Nursing Review, 38,* 108.

Increasing the relevance of education for health professionals. (1993). (Technical Report Series #838). Geneva: WHO.

Indicators for health for all strategies. (1986). *World Health Statistics Quarterly, 39*(4). Geneva: World Health Organization.

Innes, J. (1987). Primary health care in perspective. *Canadian Nurse, 83*(8), 17–18.

Jabre, B. (1986). *Education and primary health care* (Digest No. 17). Paris, France: UNESCO-UNICEF Co-operative Programme.

Jones, P. S., & Meleis, A. I. (1993). Health is empowerment. *Advances in Nursing Science, 15*(3), 1–14.

Kelly, K., & Van Vlaenderen, H. (1995). Evaluating participation processes in community development. *Evaluation & Program Planning, 18,* 371–383.

Kinsey, D. C. (1981). Participatory evaluation in adult and non-formal education. *Adult Education, 51*(5), 155–168.

Kritek, P. B. (1994). *Negotiating at an uneven table: Developing moral courage in resolving our conflicts.* San Francisco, CA: Jossey-Bass.

Kroutil, L. A., & Eng, E. (1989). Conceptualizing and assessing potential for community participation: A planning method. *Health Education Research, 4,* 305–319.

Labelle, H. (1986). Nurses as a social force. *Journal of Advanced Nursing, 11,* 247–253.

Laffrey, S. C., & Page, G. (1989). Primary health care in public health nursing. *Journal of Advanced Nursing, 14,* 1044–1050.

La Forgia, G. M. (1985). 15 years of community organizing for health in Panama. *Social Science & Medicine, 21,* 55–65.

Laurell, A. C., Noriega, M., Martinez, S., & Villegas, J. (1992). Participatory research on workers' health. *Social Science and Medicine, 34,* 603–613.

Maher, F. A., & Thompson-Tetreault, M. K. (1994). *The feminist classroom.* New York: Basic Books.

Mahler, H. (1981). The meaning of "Health For All by the Year 2000." *World Health Forum, 2*(1), pp. 5–22.

Manfredi, M. (1983). Primary health care and nursing education in Latin America. *Nursing Outlook, 31,* 105–108.

Mansour, A. A., & Al-Osimy, M. H. (1993). A study of satisfaction among primary health care patients in Saudi Arabia. *Journal of Community Health, 18*(3), 163–173.

Marion, L. N. (1996). Nursing's vision for primary health care in the 21st century. Washington, DC: American Nurses Publishing.

Mathisen, W. C. (1990). The problem-solving community: A valuable alternative to disciplinary communities? *Knowledge: Creation, Diffusion, Utilization, 2,* 410–427.

McElmurry, B. J., Swider, S. M., & Watanakij, P. (1992). Primary health care. In M. Stanhope & J. Lancaster (Eds.), *Community health nursing: Processes and practices for promoting health* (3rd ed., pp. 34–44). St. Louis, MO: Mosby.

McMurray, A. (1991). Advocacy for community self-empowerment. *International Nursing Review, 38,* 19–21.

Meaning of Health for All. (1985). (HFA Leadership/MC.3). Geneva: WHO.

Meleis, A. I. (1992). Community participation and involvement: Theoretical and empirical issues. *Health Services Management Research, 5,* 5–16.

Menon, A., Snow, R. W., Greenwood, B. M., Hayes, R. J., & N'Jie, B. H. (1990). Sustained protection against mortality and morbidity in rural Gambian children by chemoprophylaxis given by village health workers. *Transactions of the Royal Society of Tropical Medicine and Hygiene, 84,* 768–772.

Morris, R. I. (1992). People's Community Clinic: Collaboration in the Third World. *Nursing Connections, 5*(4), 2938.

Narayan, D. (1996). *Toward participatory research.* (World Bank Technical Paper Number 307). Washington, DC: World Bank.

National Institute of Nursing Research Priority Expert Panel. (1995). *Community-based health care: Nursing strategies* (NIH Publication No. 95-3917). Bethesda, MD: U.S. Department of Health and Human Services.

New approaches to health education in primary health care. (1983). (Technical Report Series #690). Geneva, Switzerland: WHO.

Newell, K. W. (1975). Health by the people. *WHO Chronicle, 29,* 161–167.

Nichter, M. (1984). Project community diagnosis: Participatory research as a first step toward community involvement in primary health care. *Social Science and Medicine, 19,* 237–252.

Ninth general programme of work: Covering the period 1996–2001. (1994). HFA Series No. 11. Geneva, Switzerland: WHO.

Ntoane, C. (1993). The challenge of primary health care. *Nursing RSA Verspleging, 8*(10), 35–39, 43.

Nursing beyond the year 2000. (1994). (Technical Report Series #842). Geneva, Switzerland: WHO.

Nursing in primary health care: Ten years after Alma-Ata and perspectives for the future. (1989). Report of the Joint WHO/ICN Consultation, August 1–3, 1988, Ferney-Voltaire.

Oermann, M. (1994). Reforming nursing education for future practice. *Journal of Nursing Education, 33,* 215–219.

Onyejiaku, E. E., & Rogers, S. (1989). The child: A pragmatic instrument in primary health care. *International Nursing Review, 36,* 185–187.

Orpaz, R., & Korenblit, M. (1994). Family nursing in community-oriented primary health care. *International Nursing Review, 41,* 155–159.

Patton, M. Q. (1990). *Qualitative evaluation and research methods* (2nd ed.). Newbury Park, CA: Sage.

Pilon, A. F. (1990–1991). Health for all by the year 2000: Cultural handicaps and possible solutions. *International Quarterly of Community Health Education, 11*(1), 79–83.

Powell, G. (1986). Primary health care: What is it? *The New Zealand Nursing Journal, 79*(12), 20–23.

Quigley, P., & Ebrahim, G. J. (1994a). Can women's organizations bring about health development? *Journal of Tropical Pediatrics, 40,* 294–298.

Quigley, P., & Ebrahim, G. J. (1994b). Women and community health workers promoting community health and development. *Journal of Tropical Pediatrics, 40,* 66–71.

Raymond, J. S., & Patrick, W. (1988). Empowerment for primary health care and child survival: Escalating community participation, community competence, and self-reliance in the Pacific. *Asia-Pacific Journal of Public Health, 2*(2), 90–95.

Regulatory mechanisms for nursing training and practice: Meeting primary health care needs. (1986). (Technical Report Series #738). Geneva, Switzerland: WHO.

Richardson, K. (1994). Consultation for primary health care. *Health & Social Care in the Community, 2,* 317–321.

Rifkin, S. B. (1986). Lessons from community participation in health programmes. *Health Policy and Planning, 1*(3), 240–249.

Rifkin, S. B. (1987). Primary health care, community participation, and the urban poor: A review of the problems and solutions. *Asia-Pacific Journal of Public Health, 1*(2), 57–63.

Rifkin, S. B. (1990). *Community participation in maternal and child health/family planning programmes.* Geneva, Switzerland: World Health Organization.

Rifkin, S. B. (1996). Paradigms lost: Toward a new understanding of community participation in health programmes. *Acta Tropica, 61,* 79–92.

Rogers, S. (1989). *"Since the nurses came": Primary health care nursing in a Nigerian village.* Unpublished doctoral dissertation, University of California, San Francisco.

Ross, J. (1988). Upgrading traditional midwifery in Sierra Leone: An overview with special reference to Koinadugu district. *Midwifery, 4*(2), 58–69.

Rovers, R. (1986). The merging of participatory and analytical approaches to evaluation: Implications for nurses in primary health care programs. *International Journal of Nursing Studies, 23,* 211–119.

Sawyer, L. M. (1995). Community participation: Lip service? *Nursing Outlook, 43*(1), 17–22.

Schneider, H., Malumane, L., Ngwenya, S., & Blackett-Sliep, V. (1989). The training of primary health care nurses. *Nursing RSA, 4*(11), 37–38.

Schorr, L. B. (1997). *Common purpose: Strengthening families and neighborhoods to rebuild America.* New York: Anchor Books.

Scope of practice of the primary health care nurse practitioner. (1985). Kansas City, MO: American Nurses Association.

Scrimshaw, S. C. M., & Hurtado, E. (1987). *Rapid assessment procedures for nutrition and primary health care: Anthropological approaches to improving programme effectiveness.* Los Angeles: UCLA Latin American Center Publications.

Sharma, A., & Ross, J. (1990). Nepal: Integrating traditional and modern health services in the remote area of Bashkharka. *International Journal of Nursing Studies, 27,* 343–353.

Singh, A. (1994). Profile of traditional birth attendants in a rural area of North India. *Journal of Nurse-Midwifery, 39,* 119–123.

Smit, J. J. M. (1994). Traditional birth attendants in Malawi. *Curationis: South African Journal of Nursing, 17*(2), 25–28.

Smith, G. (1997). *Health care partnerships: Meeting the heads of underserved communities around the world.* Battle Creek, MI: W. K. Kellogg Foundation.

Smith, J. P. (1989). Guidelines for regulatory changes in nursing education and practice to promote primary health care [editorial]. *Journal of Advanced Nursing, 14,* 603–605.

Smith, R. H., Forchuk, C., & Martin, M. (1985). Primary what? *International Nursing Review, 32,* 174–175, 180.

Smith, S. (1991). "Why no egg?" Building competency and self-reliance: A primary health care principle. *Canadian Journal of Public Health, 82,* 16–18.

Spear, S. F., Oddi, L. F., Vor der Bruegge, E., & Hamilton, C. B. (1990). Nurses as a key PHC link in Papua New Guinea. *International Nursing Review, 37,* 207–210.

St. John, W. (1993). Primary health care: A clarification of the concept and the nursing role. *Contemporary Nurse, 2,* 73–78.

Stewart, M. J. (1990). From provider to partner: A conceptual framework for nursing education based on primary health care premises. *Advances in Nursing Science, 12*(2), 9–27.

Stock-Iwamoto, C., & Korte, R. (1993). Primary health workers in north east Brazil. *Social Science & Medicine, 36,* 775–782.

Stone, L. (1992). Cultural influences in community participation in health. *Social Science & Medicine, 35,* 409–417.

Storey, M., Roemer, R., Maglacas, A. M., & Riccard, E. A. P. (1988). *Guidelines for regulatory changes in nursing education and practice to promote primary health care.* Geneva, Switzerland: Division of Health Manpower Development, World Health Organization (WHO/EDUC/88.194).

Strengthening the performance of community health workers in primary health care. (1989). Report of a WHO Study Group on Community Health Workers (Technical Report Series No. 780). Geneva, Switzerland: World Health Organization.

Swann, R. L. (1984). Nursing in PHC: Challenges and responses. *The Nursing Journal of India, 75*(1), 13–16, 18.

Swider, S. M., & McElmurry, B. J. (1990). A women's health perspective in primary health care: A nursing and community health worker demonstration project in urban America. *Journal of Family and Community Health, 13*(3), 1–17.

Tamsang, J., & Anderson, S. (1990). Inspiring nursing students to mobilize communities in Nepal. *International Nursing Review, 37,* 345–347.

Target 2000: Health for all from words to deeds. (1987). *World Health Forum, 8,* 164–183.

Tarimo, E., & Creese, A. (Eds.). (1990). *Achieving health for all by the year 2000: Midway reports of country experiences.* Geneva, Switzerland: World Health Organization.

Tay, A. K. B. (1989). *"Child-to-Child" in Africa: Towards an open learning strategy* (Digest No. 29). Paris, France: UNESCO-UNICEF Co-operative Programme.

Ugalde, A. (1985). Ideological dimensions of community participation in Latin American health programs. *Social Science & Medicine, 21,* 41–53.

van der Geest, S. (1992). Is paying for health care culturally acceptable in Sub-Sahara Africa? Money and tradition. *Social Science and Medicine, 34,* 667–673.

Van Norren, B., Boerma, J. T., & Sempebwa, E. K. N. (1989). Simplifying the evaluation of primary health care programmes. *Social Science & Medicine, 29,* 1091–1097.

Walker, L. (1995). The practice of primary health care: A case study. *Social Science & Medicine, 40,* 815–824.

Watanakij, P., & McElmurry, B. J. (1995). Measuring quality of life in Thai and US communities. *International Nursing Review, 42,* 121–123.

Watkins, E. L., Harlan, C., Eng, E., Gansky, S. A., Gehan, D., & Larson, K. (1994). Assessing the effectiveness of lay health advisors with migrant farmworkers. *Family & Community Health, 16*(4), 72–87.

Watts, R. J. (1990). Democratization of health care: challenge for nursing. *Advances in Nursing Science, 12*(2), 37–46.

Weiss, C. H. (1988). If program decisions hinged only on information: A response to Patton. *Evaluation Practice, 9*(3), 15–28.

Werner, D., & Bower, B. (1982). *Helping health workers learn.* Palo Alto, CA: Hesperian Foundation.

Whitmore, E. (1988). *Participatory evaluation approaches: Side effects and empowerment.* Doctoral dissertation, Cornell University.

Wiles, R., & Robison, J. (1994). Teamwork in primary care: The views and experiences of nurses, midwives and health visitors. *Journal of Advanced Nursing, 20,* 324–330.

Williams, A. (1993). Community health learning experiences and political activism: A model for baccalaureate curriculum revolution content. *Journal of Nursing Education, 32,* 352–356.

Wong, M. L., & Chen, P. C. Y. (1991). Self-reliance in health among village women. *World Health Forum, 12,* 43–48.

Woods, M. (1992). Philosophical issues in primary health care delivery in New Zealand. *Nursing Praxis in New Zealand, 7*(1), 22–27.

World Bank. (1993). *World Development Report 1993: Investing in health.* Oxford: Oxford University Press.

World Health Organization. (1987). Distribution of resources for health for all. *World Health Statistics Quarterly, 40*(4) [Special issue].

WHO in action: Primary health care in practice. (1987). *World Health Forum, 8,* 56–66.

Young, Q. (1996). The case against profit-driven managed care. In E.D. Baer, C. M. Fagin, & S. Gordon (Eds.), *Abandonment of the patient* (pp. 65–70). New York: Springer Publishing.

Yu, M. (1992). The role of nurse educators in the reorientation of nursing education towards primary health care. *Hong Kong Nursing Journal, 5,* 23–26.

Chapter 11

Uncertainty in Chronic Illness

ABSTRACT

In this chapter, the research on uncertainty in chronic illness is reviewed and critiqued. Two theoretical perspectives of uncertainty that can be applied across the range of chronic illness are presented. Research on the causes and consequences of uncertainty in chronic illness are considered and critiqued. The review addresses research on adults and on parents of chronically ill children. Conclusions include the areas requiring further investigation.

Keywords: Uncertainty, Chronic Illness, Management of Uncertainty, Hope, Life Transitions

Uncertainty is a constant experience of chronic illness due to the unpredictable and inconsistent symptom onset, continual questions about recurrence or exacerbation, and unknown future due to living with debilitating conditions. In conditions that have received the full range of treatment, uncertainty about the chance for recurrence is a major theme (Hilton, 1988), although in conditions characterized by remissions and exacerbations, the uncertainty about the next attack is a constant companion (Becker, Janson-Bjerklie, Benner, Slobin, & Ferketich, 1993; Wiener, 1975). For persons who receive treatment such as transplants, what the future holds becomes uncertain (Mishel & Murdaugh, 1987). Unlike uncertainty in acute illness—where the uncertainty is somewhat localized in the issues of diagnosis, treatment, and recovery—the uncertainty in chronic illness involves more areas of life and influences daily routines and activities (Cohen, 1993a; Weitz, 1989).

This chapter is limited to research with a chronically ill population. It includes research on persons with illnesses that had an acute phase, such as cancer and coronary artery disease, but who now are considered in a chronic illness or condition. Other populations included are those with illnesses known for stabilization and then destabilization, such as diabetes, asthma, or chronic obstructive pulmonary disease, and illnesses with remissions and exacerbations, such as systemic lupus erythematosus, arthritis, multiple sclerosis, and AIDS. Areas of research on uncertainty such as uncertainty in pregnancy, training of physicians to manage uncertainty, and environmental or workplace uncertainty are not included. Articles were selected if the investigator focused on illness, and uncertainty was: (a) the major topic, (b) one of the major topics under study, (c) measured in quantitative studies, or (d) a major theme from qualitative work. If uncertainty was mentioned, but not treated as a distinct topic, the research was not included. This chapter differs from the chapter on uncertainty in acute illness (Mishel, 1997) by focusing on the major conceptualizations of uncertainty in chronic illness by Mishel (1990) and Selder (1989). The reconceptualization of uncertainty offered by Mishel (1990) extends uncertainty theory from the 1988 work which applies to acute illness to a reformulation applying to the experience of chronic illness. Finally, the literature on uncertainty in chronic illness emphasizes antecedents of uncertainty that differ from those in acute illness, and uncertainty management methods that are broader than those reported in acute illness.

Information was retrieved through computerized databases including Medline (1976–1997), Cumulative Index to Nursing and Allied Health Literature (CINAHL) (1982–1997), and PsychLIT (1984–1997), along with use of the "invisible college" approach (Cooper, 1982). The work of investigators known to the authors was tracked along with a search for publications from users of the Mishel Uncertainty in Illness Scales (MUIS). Since all users of the MUIS are located in a data bank, names were taken from this list to check for publications. The ancestry approach of tracking citations from published studies also was employed. The personal library of the chapter author was culled for relevant publications on uncertainty in illness.

The result of the literature search netted 24 qualitative and 27 quantitative studies on adults with chronic illness and 10 qualitative and 5 quantitative studies on parents of children or children themselves with chronic illness. Two articles present conceptualizations of uncertainty in chronic illness and two articles present reviews that address uncertainty in chronic illness.

CONCEPTUALIZATION OF UNCERTAINTY IN ILLNESS

Two major conceptualizations of uncertainty can be applied across the range of chronic illness: Selder's (1989) life transition theory and Mishel's (1990) reformulated uncertainty in illness theory. Selder (1989) addressed the process of going through a major life transition with the goal of resolving uncertainty. Selder presented a life transition theory that described how people restructured their lives and resolved uncertainty after a major experiential transition. The theory was described as applicable to events that qualified as disrupting one's view of reality. Such events may include illness, but are not limited to illness experiences, and may include acute loss as well as other individually defined events. According to this theory, the disruption creates uncertainty about beliefs and behavior. Selder described a period of transition culminating in a restructuring of reality that involved incorporating past identity into a new meaning to events. Recognizing the permanence of the change was reported to reduce uncertainty. The goal of the life transition is to restructure reality and resolve uncertainty in order to regain the integrity of the self. The individual goes through a period of transition in which reality as it once was is seen as permanently altered. Selder identified a number of behaviors that were used to reduce uncertainty and to reform the sense of self so that a constancy between the past and present views of self was maintained.

Although Selder did not address chronic illness specifically, she addressed all situations in which present reality is shattered. The components of the theory include a sudden disruption of reality which may limit its applicability to chronic illness in which there is a slow eroding of the prior identity. Also, Selder proposed that all persons who experience a sudden disruption of reality will go through this process, and that the uncertainty can be reduced. Since the goal of the transition is to accommodate the new reality into the past sense of self, priority is given to assimilation of changes into a person's sense of self. A number of studies conducted by Selder and colleagues support the theory, but there are no published studies by independent investigations that do so (Kachoyeanos & Selder, 1993; Van Riper & Selder, 1989).

In contrast to Selder's view's, Mishel (1990) offered an extension of her earlier work on uncertainty to accommodate chronic illness. Although Mishel labeled the new theory as the reconceptualization of uncertainty, it does not replace the original theory presented in 1988. Instead, it is an expansion of the theory, that addresses living with continual uncertainty as found in chronic illness. The focus of the theory was not on management of uncertainty in order to eliminate it, as in the earlier theory, or as proposed by Selder (1989), but, on the integration of uncertainty into one's life and one's life view. Mishel's expanded view of uncertainty shares some similar themes about uncertainty with Selder's ideas, but is targeted specifically to persons with the experience of living with continual, constant uncertainty, either from a chronic illness or a treated acute illness with possible recurrence and extension. Mishel's theory also differs from Selder's work in that Mishel described the process as occurring gradually, beginning as the illness insidiously invades the person's life, whereas Selder focused on an acute event as the start of a change process. Also, the theories differ on the emphasis given to growth and increasing complexity. Selder emphasized the interplay of the self and the coherence between the new views of reality and the past whereas Mishel focused more on growth to altered values and changed paradigm for reality which enables more options and choices.

Building on the tenets of chaos theory, uncertainty from an illness was described by Mishel as spreading into many areas of a person's life, dismantling the meaning given to everyday events and being the stimulant for disorder. As the uncertainty spreads into major life areas, the person is not able to eliminate it, and it functions to dismantle the person's view of self and of reality. This results in a period of great disorganization, and slowly a new view of reality is formed. Uncertainty is viewed as the force leading to a new perspective on life where a new value system is constructed. The new orientation toward life is viewed as a growth experience, where a mechanistic orientation is discarded in favor of a probabilistic paradigm. Uncertainty is accepted as a reality of life, and because of this new value system, the person sees that many options are possible, and is not limited to a cause-and-effect paradigm. The person emerges with a more complex view of life and a more complex level of functioning. This is a gradual process and not presented as attainable by all. In order for uncertainty to be a growth experience, support for this transition is needed from one's closest relationships and often from the health care providers. The person needs time to focus on self, and if this time is not available, the process of integrating the uncertainty into one's view of life will not occur.

The theories offered by Mishel and by Selder differ from the substantive theory generated from qualitative investigations in that Mishel and Selder's theories are not focused on one population, one age group, or one type of chronic illness. Also, substantive theory generated from one investigation was not studied further by other investigators. The substantive theories are limited in their scope, may not be applicable to all chronic illnesses and all populations, and are not considered as conceptualizations of uncertainty in this review. Such work includes the substantive theory offered by Mishel and Murdaugh (1987) on redesigning the dream in patients and family members who had a heart transplantation; the work by Charmaz (1994) on identifying dilemmas of chronically ill men; Wiener's (1975) early work on tolerating the uncertainty in rheumatoid arthritis, and Cohen's (1993b, 1995) work on living with sustained uncertainty for families with a child experiencing a chronic life-threatening illness.

On the other hand, a number of studies are finding a process similar to that described by Mishel (1990). Findings are beginning to be reported from qualitative investigations in support of this theory. Since the theory depicts a nonlinear process, it is best suited to qualitative studies, where multiple interviews of the same individuals can be done to elicit the movement in the process. Nelson's (1996) hermeneutic phenomenologic investigation with women 2 and 6 years post-treatment for breast cancer described the growth-producing aspects of uncertainty. Women reported a new found freedom of expression that evolved from uncertainty. They also noted that they needed their support system as they grew through the ebb and flow of uncertainty throughout the survival trajectory. Pelusi (1997), without reference to Mishel's theory, describes a journey for breast cancer survivors into growth and enlightenment in the midst of uncertainty. Facing a future of uncertainty, women found new meaning in ever-changing roles. Similarly, Brown and Powell-Cope (1991) reported that the findings from their grounded theory methodology supported that AIDS family caregivers went through a process of transition through uncertainty. They noted that transitions involve a period of major change in life, accompanied by uncertainty, in which one questions basic assumptions and plans for living in the world which results in a transformed self-identity. They acknowledged the parallels between their findings and the Mishel theory of uncertainty, and they note that their findings support an expanded perspective on the acceptance of uncertainty. Likewise, Fleury, Kimbrell, and Kruszewski (1995) in a grounded theory study of women following a cardiac event, reported that psychological healing involved a struggle through the uncertainty surrounding the cardiac event. Women grew through the uncertainty to focus on multiple alternatives, possibilities, and an appreciation for the impermanence of life situations. On the other hand, Baier (1995) found that the reconceptualization of uncertainty theory fit some of the people and not others among the interview sample of people with schizophrenia. Baier noted this may be due to the use of single interviews with each person which limited the depth of the data. Currently, there is emerging support for the reconceptualized view of uncertainty.

THE NATURE OF UNCERTAINTY IN CHRONICALLY ILL ADULTS

Of the 47 studies on uncertainty in chronic illness included in this review, 24 were qualitative investigations, with the majority using a grounded theory approach. The narrative data from the qualitative investigations and the statistical findings from the quantitative studies are presented together in order to address the antecedents, nature, and management of uncertainty and the adjustment to uncertainty. Only the major themes are presented from qualitative data.

Causes of Uncertainty

Nature of the illness.   Three aspects of the illness seem to cause uncertainty: (1) severity of the illness; (2) erratic nature of symptomatology; and (3) ambiguity of symptoms. Support for severity of the illness as a significant predictor of uncertainty was reported by Braden (1990) in a study of patients with rheumatoid arthritis who found that severity of rheumatoid arthritis was a major predictor of uncertainty. Likewise, Janson-Bjerklie, Ferketich, and Benner (1993) reported that dyspnea intensity, perceived illness severity, episode distress, and nocturnal dyspnea were all significantly associated with uncertainty among 95 asthmatic adults. Other studies, specifically with persons with multiple sclerosis or rheumatoid arthritis, where illness severity was defined as functional ability, reported contrary evidence (Bailey & Nielsen, 1993; Wineman, 1990).

It seems to be the erratic nature of symptom onset and disease progression that is the major antecedent to uncertainty in chronic illness, particularly among the collagen- and respiratory-related conditions. Symptom onset, duration, intensity, and location are unforeseeable and the attack is capricious, disturbing the person's lifestyle. With each attack, the boundaries placed around the disease to control its impact on life are disrupted (Gaskins & Brown, 1992; Wiener, 1975). Many chronic diseases are characterized by periods of stability that are abruptly severed by erratic flares of disease exacerbation (Becker et al., 1993; Brown & Powell-Cope, 1991). Although one may have past experience with erratic symptom display, prior history with illness attack does not decrease the uncertainty about how to manage the assault (Becker et al., 1993). Among asthma patients, a new rule about the attack is created out of each sudden severe episode. This new rule falls with the next sudden illness episode (Becker et al., 1993). In women with interstitial cystitis, Webster and Brennan (1995) reported that these women experienced uncertainty about the changing course of the illness, inability to predict pain severity, and unpredictability of symptoms. Similar uncertainties existed whether the women were in remission or having minimal, moderate, or severe symptoms.

Closely related to the erratic nature of the symptoms, the inability to distinguish symptoms of the chronic illness from other bodily changes or the development of a new symptom were sources of uncertainty for pregnant women with multiple sclerosis (Smeltzer, 1994), persons living with AIDS (Weitz, 1989), and women surviving breast cancer (Hilton, 1988). For illnesses that can reoccur, any change in bodily function can function to trigger uncertainty about disease recurrence, particularly when the symptom is similar to the original symptom of illness onset (Hilton, 1988; Mishel & Murdaugh, 1987; Nelson, 1996; Pelusi, 1997). On the other hand, Regan-Kubinski and Sharts-Hopko (1995) noted that HIV-positive mothers did not report their symptoms or the up-and-down course of their illness as sources of uncertainty, but the progression of HIV was a cause for uncertainty.

Generally, the findings supported symptom unpredictability in occurrence, intensity, and duration as a major issue in chronic illness. This differs from an acute illness situation where, once a diagnosis is made, symptoms are tracked to treatment and associated with a trajectory.

Unknown future.   Concerns about the future are seldom studied in quantitative studies, but do emerge in qualitative studies, where a broader scope of issues can emerge. From qualitative studies, short- and long-range future plans have been identified as sources of uncertainty. Care providers of persons with AIDS reported that plans for any future time were difficult to structure, and that life took on the aspect of living one day at a time (Brown & Powell-Cope, 1991). Likewise, pregnant women with multiple sclerosis expressed uncertainties about future parenting issues (Smeltzer, 1994). Breast cancer survivors also experienced uncertainty due to ever-changing social and interpersonal roles (Pelusi, 1997). Women surviving breast cancer, where the disease was under control but the possibility of recurrence continually existed, reported intense uncertainty about their ability to plan for their future (Nelson, 1996).

Concept of self.   The impact of the illness on regular life routines has been found to initiate changes in the person's concept of self. Questioning one's identity is a source of uncertainty. Charmaz (1994) reported that the realization that their bodies have changed caused chronically ill men to move into a phase of questioning who they are and what changes they will undergo. This led them to become aware of how the uncertainty was spreading throughout their life. Similarly, caregivers of persons with AIDS described a chaotic period where they were being managed and overwhelmed by the illness—an experience that generated incredible uncertainty (Brown & Powell-Cope, 1991). Comparable experiences were described by Fleury et al. (1995) when women recovering from an acute cardiac event viewed the illness as changing their identity of self, thus thrusting them into uncertainty about what they believed or valued. Further support is provided by Mishel and Murdaugh (1987) who found that changes in their spouse post-heart transplant led the healthy spouse to consider uncertainties about their interpersonal relationship. In contrast to the causes of uncertainty in an acute illness, the experience and realization of chronicity generates questions about life that promotes existential uncertainty. Fluctuation in the view of self was a consistent finding across studies, and documents one of the changes described by Mishel (1990) in moving from uncertainty as an aversive event to uncertainty as an opportunity for growth.

Lack of information.   Lack of information has been identified as a cause of uncertainty in acute and chronic illness, but it has a different twist when applied to chronic illness. Chronic illness differs from acute illness in that chronic illness requires extensive management by the patient, while acute illness is treated primarily by the expert. Lack of information was reported by Mason (1985) as a major source of uncertainty among persons with diabetes. Lack of information about management of the illness, outcome, causation, and severity were identified as the origin of the uncertainty. For patients awaiting transplantation, the lack of information generating uncertainty resides in not knowing when they will get the organ or if they ever will (Weems & Patterson, 1989). Among COPD patients about to be discharged on home oxygen, limited understanding of the treatment was a major cause of uncertainty (Small & Graydon, 1993). Similarly, as new complications arouse in patients with diabetes, lack of knowledge about how to prevent or manage these contributed to the uncertainty (Nyhlin, 1990). Since knowledge about how to manage a chronic illness evolves over time, those most recently diagnosed with an illness demonstrated significantly more illness-related uncertainty then those who have lived with the illness for over 10 years (Moser, Clements, Brecht, & Weiner, 1993). Similarly, not knowing what they can do to prevent disease recurrence caused uncertainty in women who were about 4 years post-breast cancer diagnosis (Hilton, 1988). At this time, findings for lack of information as a cause of uncertainty are consistent across a number of studies. More work is needed to identify the point in the trajectory of living with a chronic illness where lack of information is most paramount in causing uncertainty. Questions still remain whether it is at diagnosis, recurrence, exacerbation or during daily living where this factor is preeminent.

Social support.   Social support, a frequently studied antecedent of uncertainty in acute illness, has not received the same attention in chronic illness. Although the topic of social relationships is embedded in many of the descriptive reports, it is not frequently targeted as a major theme tied clearly to uncertainty. For chronic illness where stigma is a major issue (Weitz, 1989), the questions of whom to tell, how others will respond to their HIV status, how to get care for the child, and what will happen to the child, were sources of uncertainty among HIV-positive mothers (Regan-Kubinski & Sharts-Hopko,

1995). These issues are clearly related to social network and interpersonal relationships. Likewise, caregivers of persons with AIDS experienced the issue of "going public" and the questionable acceptance of others as a basis for uncertainty concerning the reaction of others (Brown & Powell-Cope, 1991). Although not directly citing the relationship between support and uncertainty, Charmaz (1994) discussed the importance of family members in helping the chronically ill remove the uncertainty surrounding the sense of self. On the other hand, Fleury et al. (1995) noted that perceived loss of role in the family contributed to the uncertainty concerning a personal future in women recovering from a cardiac event.

In two quantitative investigations on the role of social support and uncertainty, Moser et al. (1993) found no relationship between social support and uncertainty in a sample of patients with systematic sclerosis. In a well-designed study, Wineman (1990) reported that unsupportiveness of interactions was a significant predictor of higher uncertainty, although there was no confirmation of a relationship between support and uncertainty among persons with multiple sclerosis. It may be that separating the positive and negative dimensions of social support enable its effect to be clearer. Since the family shares many of the residuals of chronic illness, the unsupportive element may enhance the patient's sense of being alone to manage the unpredictability of the disease, while the supportive nature of interactions may not have any impact on this aspect of uncertainty. In support of those findings, Smeltzer (1994) reported that women with MS who are pregnant fear negative reactions from others, and so present the pregnancy as an "accident" or agree to Caesarean delivery to avoid negative attributions from others.

In a number of investigations on family members' response to the chronic illness, uncertainty has been a prominent negative experience (Brown & Powell-Cope, 1991; Hilton, 1993; Mishel & Murdaugh, 1987; Rowat & Knafl, 1985; Wineman, O'Brien, Nealon, & Kaskel, 1993). Although this does not tie social support directly to uncertainty for the patient, it does indicate that uncertainty is an issue for the family member as well as for the patient. A care provider dealing with uncertainty may not be available as a source for support for the patient. Family members of chronic pain patients identified the uncertainty as the worst feature of the well spouse's experience. The uncertainty involved the nature of the pain, parameters of day-to-day living, and methods to manage the pain (Rowat & Knafl, 1985). Similarly, caretakers of AIDS patients felt that their life was monitored by the uncertainty about what the patient's symptoms meant, plus the uncertainty about how to provide sufficient care (Brown & Powell-Cope, 1991). Among spousal caregivers of persons with multiple sclerosis, higher levels of subjective burden was significant related to more uncertainty (O'Brien, Wineman, & Nealon, 1995). Wineman et al. (1993) investigated the differences in the perception of illness uncertainty between husbands and wives where one spouse had multiple sclerosis. For both spouses, those with high uncertainty were more dissatisfied with family life. For the well partner, the congruence between each partner's perception of uncertainty was the crucial factor determining the well spouse's family satisfaction. Congruence or shared understanding and expectations seems to be very important for the well spouse, and may be necessary in order for the well spouse, to be a supportive presence (Wineman et al., 1993).

Absence of support appears to be due to either questionable acceptance from others of the illness, or to the behavior of the ill person or supportive person's, in the caretaking role, experiencing their own uncertainty. Further work is needed to identify the contingencies that influence when family members and others function to reduce uncertainty.

Health care providers.   Although there are not a large number of studies in which health care providers are discussed, they are particularly important in three areas: getting a diagnosis, self-management, and the interaction between the illness and normal role function. For a number of chronic illnesses, diagnosis is a matter of eliminating other alternatives. Stewart and Sullivan (1982) reported that the inability to determine a diagnosis heightened uncertainty. They reported that 60 persons with multiple sclerosis described contact with 227 physicians for a total of 420 diagnostic tests and treatments. A variety of diagnoses are given to persons with lupus, multiple sclerosis, and other collagen-related conditions. As each diagnosis fails, uncertainty increases, along with erosion of faith in the physician's judgement (Mishel, 1993). Support for the physicians role in reducing diagnostic uncertainty was reported by Mushlin, Mooney, Grow, and Phelps (1994). These investigators found that uncertainty fell significantly after receiving a diagnosis of multiple sclerosis among a group of patients measured prior to and after diagnostic testing. Those who received a specific diagnosis, even if their future outlook was worse because of having the disease, felt less uncertain and had improved well-being, as compared with those who had a non-decisional outcome (Mushlin et al., 1994).

A few investigations addressed the patient's perception of medical control over the illness in relation to uncertainty. In one study comparing psychological characteristics of patients with multiple sclerosis who did and did not participate in a treatment regimen, perceived medical control of illness was explored. Higher levels of perceived medical control of illness was associated with less uncertainty among those who chose to participate in the treatment (Armor, McDermott, & Schiffer, 1996). This relationship was not found in those who refused the treatment. However, the study is flawed by the small number of subjects in each group, which compromised the power to detect meaningful differences between acceptors and refusers, and by an inappropriate sample size for the selected data analysis. The relationship between perceived control and uncertainty received stronger support from a related study of 92 patients with rheumatoid arthritis. Affleck, Tennen, Pfeiffer, and Fifield (1987), using items from the Mishel Uncertainty in Illness Scale, reported that patients with rheumatoid arthritis perceived their illness as more predictable when they perceived that their health care provider had control over their illness. These are the only two studies that look at perceived medical control, and it is an area worthy of further investigation, since the findings support some role for perceived medical control in managing uncertainty.

The role of the health care provider in modifying uncertainty surrounding self-management was not supported in two investigations. Mason (1985) reported that diabetic patients with a self-management regime often had uncertainty concerning the disease label, how to manage the disease, cure, and causation. The patient's understanding of the diabetes was reported to be at variance with that of the physician. Mason concluded that the doctor-centered style of communication was not conducive to resolving the patient's uncertainties. Furthermore, Becker et al. (1993) reported that asthmatics were reluctant to seek emergency medical care during a breathing crisis for fear of inadequate treatment. These patients had learned self-management, and were afraid that health care workers were not as knowledgeable as the themselves. Even when physicians are expert on the disease, they may not be knowledgeable or helpful when the issue is the interaction of the disease with normal roles such as pregnancy. In a study of pregnant women with multiple sclerosis, women questioned whether the health care provider could distinguish the symptoms of multiple sclerosis from changes of normal pregnancy (Smeltzer, 1994). These women reported that questions and concerns were not answered to their satisfaction. The health care provider was often noncommittal or uninformative concerning the effect of their illness on pregnancy. This heightened the women's sense of uncertainty (Smeltzer, 1994). Although the health care provider has been reported to have a major role in reducing uncertainty in persons who have an acute illness (Mishel, 1997), the findings reported to date show less support for the role of the health care provider in helping the chronically ill manage uncertainty. The process of receiving a diagnosis has been found to consistently erode confidence in the physician. Similarly, inability to fully control chronic illness and the development of patient self-management strategies has been found to reduce the importance of the health care provider's role in managing uncertainty in chronic illness.

Uncertainty and personality dispositions. All of the studies addressing personality dispositions are quantitative in design. Due to the emphasis on cognitive variables in the psychology literature, a number of measures have been developed that facilitate exploration of these factors. Investigations in this area have produced findings for a number of cognitive-oriented dispositions that are associated with uncertainty. Braden (1991), using an investigator-developed measure of uncertainty, tested the benefit of a self-management intervention for persons with lupus. The author reported that the relationship between uncertainty and enabling skills changed over time. The magnitude of the relationship increased over time with enabling skills and self-efficacy related to less uncertainty following the last class session and 2 months after class completion. In an earlier study, Braden (1990) found that monitoring, and obtaining the personally desired level of information, decreased illness uncertainty in patients with rheumatoid arthritis. Further support for the role of cognitive dispositions and uncertainty was offered by Affleck et al. (1987). The investigators reported that patients with rheumatoid arthritis perceived their illness as more predictable when they felt they had greater personal control over symptoms and over the course of the disease. Similarly, Armor et al. (1996) reported perceived personal control of illness was strongly related to less uncertainty in multiple sclerosis patients who had accepted treatment, In a somewhat similar study, health-related hardiness was associated with less uncertainty among patients with systemic sclerosis (Moser et al., 1993).

Considering spirituality and its dimensions as personality factors, two studies have addressed spiritual well-being and uncertainty. Crigger (1996), testing an uncertainty model for women with multiple sclerosis, reported that in the model with the best fit for the data, spiritual well-being predicted a lower level of uncertainty. Landis (1996) explored the role of spiritual well-being as a buffer in the relationship between uncertainty and psychosocial adjustment. In a sample of 94 people with diabetes mellitus, the existential well-being component of the spiritual well-being scale was significantly inversely related to uncertainty. In the regression analyses, existential well-being mediated the relationship between uncertainty and psychosocial adjustment. Findings from two studies support that spiritual well-being, or a component of the concept, may play a role in modifying uncertainty and positively affecting overall psychosocial adjustment. Further studies in the area would help to clarify the effective components of spiritual well-being in modifying uncertainty.

Management of uncertainty.   Study of methods to cope with uncertainty differ across quantitative versus qualitative studies. In studies using the MUIS as the measure of uncertainty, Janson-Bjerklie et al. (1993) found no relationship between uncertainty and coping in persons with asthma, while Braden (1990) found a weak relationship between uncertainty and self-help among persons with rheumatoid arthritis. Other investigations of chronically ill samples, using the MUIS as the measure of uncertainty, have reported a significant association between higher uncertainty and strategies to control emotion, with lower uncertainty associated with more action strategies (McCain & Cella, 1995; Viney & Westbrook, 1984; Wineman, Durand, & Steiner, 1994). Lack of consistent findings may be due to issues in measuring uncertainty in chronic illness. The MUIS was not developed as a measure of chronic illness. The community form of the MUIS was modified from the original MUIS for use with chronically ill samples, but the question exists as to whether it is an accurate reflection of enduring uncertainty (Mast, 1995). Similarly, Mishel (1997) has noted the problems with existing scales to measure coping. With issues surrounding the measurement of uncertainty and the measurement of coping in chronic illness, it is not surprising that the findings of the relationship between uncertainty and coping are neither consistent nor very informative.

While methods to manage uncertainty in quantitative studies are limited to what can be measured by existing scales (Mishel, 1997), in qualitative investigations, a number of strategies to manage uncertainty have been identified. In these studies, it is impossible to determine the level of uncertainty, since measurement is not relevant to the methods. Also, it is difficult to determine which coping methods are specific to management of uncertainty, since such linkages are not clear in the narrative. We can assume that these coping methods exist, but the link to uncertainty remains to be specified. As noted by Mast (1995), the study of coping with uncertainty could benefit from triangulated studies.

Whereas McCain and Cella (1995) in a quantitative study of persons with AIDS, noted that strategies to control emotion were the predominant methods to manage uncertainty. Allan (1990), Gaskins and Brown (1992), and Weitz (1989), from their qualitative investigations, reported on a number of strategies used by AIDS patients to manage uncertainty. These included obtaining information from similar others who are doing well, engaging in health maintenance activities, maintaining everyday living patterns, creating cognitive explanations for symptoms, and restructuring one's commitments to incorporate a sudden change in health status.

The major management method used to manage uncertainty across a number of chronic illnesses was to restructure life to incorporate the unpredictable onset of symptoms (Baier, 1995; Becker et al., 1993; Loveys, 1990; Nyhlin, 1990; Price, 1993; Small & Graydon, 1993; Weitz, 1989; Wiener, 1975). In order to do this, some specific strategies were: to live one day at a time, to pace activities according to remissions and flares, and to assume a cautious approach to life (Baier, 1995; Johnson & Morse, 1990; Mason, 1985; Wiener, 1975). Other methods are to identify the markers of danger or to delineate the boundaries of control over the illness (Becker et al., 1993; Mishel & Murdaugh, 1987; Weiner, 1975). Similarly, Charmaz (1994) discussed the bracketing used by chronically ill men to control the uncertain event and wall it off from spreading into other areas of life. Smeltzer (1994) discussed how pregnant women with multiple sclerosis develop contingency plans to handle disease flares and rehearsed caring for the baby during an exacerbation of the disease. The focus was on normalizing life so that the unpredictable attack could be incorporated into life without major disruption or social embarrassment.

Another strategy for managing the uncertainty associated with an illness characterized by erratic onset and duration is getting to know the illness. This involves structuring a program for self-management which incorporates markers and other known triggers for the onset of illness attacks and the trial and error activities to find a point for self-regulation. It is similar to restructuring life, except that there is more emphasis on self-management (Baier, 1995; Becker et al., 1993; Price, 1993; Weiner, 1975). Pacing, a strategy identified by Weiner (1975), illustrated the self-management aspect of these strategies. She defined pacing as identifying what activities one is able to do and under what circumstances. This is done along with monitoring physical status so that one can try to foresee what activities exacerbate an attack of the illness and what activities can safely be completed.

For those with a stable condition that can reoccur and progress, managing uncertainty to gain a sense of control involves some strategies similar to those mentioned such as health maintenance, talking and comparing with similar others, gauging progress, seeking information along with emotion control strategies found in quantitative investigations (Hilton, 1988; Johnson & Morse, 1990).

Mishel (1993) offered a review of the major management methods and included many of those mentioned here plus the method of forming illness schema. This involves constructing a personal scenario for the illness which includes why or how the illness began, how it will progress, and how the individual will recover. This enables the person to integrate unseemingly incongruent events into a framework that makes sense for the individual. Weitz (1989) described a variant of this method found in men at risk for AIDS to explain why they were not vulnerable. Other methods include setting limits, which involves rules for avoiding events that threaten the person's ability. Such a method was used by patients following heart transplantation to decrease the risk of infection (Mishel & Murdaugh, 1987). Other methods involve the use of rituals or belief in a higher power. Rituals have been used throughout history to try to gain predictability over random events. A variety of these methods have been seen in cancer patients who believe that certain behaviors will prevent recurrence. Turning the uncertainty over to a higher power is likely to emerge in future studies as spirituality becomes a focus as an uncertainty management method.

Lastly, incorporating the uncertainty is an approach where there is a change in the person's and family's perspective in life, away from an orientation to control and predictability toward an acceptance of unpredictability and uncertainty as normal. Uncertainty becomes the rhythm of life (Mishel, 1990).

Uncertainty and adjustment. Although most of the studies of adjustment have been quantitative in methodology and have considered a variety of outcomes, emotional state is a frequent measure of adjustment. McCain and Cella (1995) found that uncertainty was significantly associated with a poorer mood state. Likewise, Wineman, Schwetz, Goodkin, and Rudick (1996) found that uncertainty was a significant predictor of poorer mood and less hopefulness in multiple sclerosis patients at their time of entry into a clinical drug trial. Mullins et al. (1995) in a study of adaptation in persons with post-polio syndrome reported that illness uncertainty, along with a measure of causal attributions, was the strongest predictor of psychological distress. Inconsistent with these findings is the report by Small and Graydon (1992) that uncertainty was not a significant predictor of negative mood in patients hospitalized for COPD, although the findings are questionable due to small sample size for the number of variables considered in the analysis. Fewer studies have addressed other outcomes as components of adjustment. Although there have been many studies of uncertainty and adjustment in acutely ill individuals, there is less study using the same measures in chronically ill populations. Work by Failla, Kuper, Nick, and Lee (1996) on adjustment of women with Systemic Lupus Erythematosus using the Psychosocial Adjustment to Illness Scale (Morrow, Chiarello, & Derogatis, 1978), a measure used frequently in studies of the acutely ill, found that uncertainty was significantly related to worse psychosocial adjustment. Although most of the studies have included a sufficient sample size to determine the role of uncertainty in adjustment, some of the research findings are questionable due to small subject to variable ratio, inclusion of self-selected sample, and inclusion of those with the most severe state of the illness. A few studies have been conducted on the relationship between uncertainty and adjustment among spousal care providers. Investigators of the caretaker or spousal experience reported that spouses of chronic pain patients found the uncertainty unbearable, felt trapped, and suicidal (Rowat & Knafl, 1985). Less severe findings were reported by Wineman et al. (1993) who found that congruence in uncertainty was a major predictor of family satisfaction. Spouses where incongruence existed had lower levels of family satisfaction. Among spousal caregivers of multiple sclerosis patients,

O'Brien et al. (1995) found that uncertainty along with perceived burden were the strongest predictors of caregivers' health impairment and mood, although the authors express caution concerning the findings due to low subject-to-variable ratio.

In contrast, there are a number of investigations, qualitative in design, that support a transition through uncertainty to a new orientation toward life, with acceptance of uncertainty as a part of life. The samples include diabetic patients facing long-term complications (Nyhlin, 1990); men with a chronic illness with an uncertain course (Charmaz, 1994); AIDS family caregivers (Brown & Powell-Cope, 1991); persons with HIV infection (Katz, 1996); persons with schizophrenia (Baier, 1995); spouses of heart transplant patients (Mishel & Murdaugh, 1987); women recovering from a cardiac event (Fleury et al., 1995); and women surviving treatment for breast cancer (Nelson, 1996; Pelusi, 1997). However, in many of these studies uncertainty is not defined, and the clarity of the link between uncertainty and a new perspective on life varies across studies (Charmaz, 1994; Katz, 1996). Other investigators noted that patients learned to live with uncertainty, but there was no discussion of the process by which this occurred. Nyhlin (1990) described the process used by diabetics to cope with enduring uncertainty and described that a new normal is created which involves finding personal meaning in the illness and its consequences. Similarly, Mishel and Murdaugh (1987) proposed a substantive theory about the new orientation to life among spouses of heart transplant patients living with the uncertainty of life after transplantation. In support of the changes brought by the uncertainty of chronic illness, Fleury et al. (1995) proposed healing as the basic social process explaining women's struggle through the uncertainty surrounding recovery after a cardiac event. Baier (1995) reported that uncertainty may be a source of hope for some and a danger for others, but all of the people with schizophrenia interviewed in the study claimed that their view of life had changed. Similarly, Nelson (1996) found that breast cancer patients' search for meaning was based on a growth-producing experience through uncertainty.

Although the process of change through uncertainty is closely aligned to the theories posited by Mishel (1990) and Selder (1989), few of these investigators refer to the theoretical work to support their findings. This limits the support for current theories and reduces the opportunities for new investigations to build on prior work in the area. However, all investigators described the gradual acknowledgement made by the person that the uncertainty and its consequences were lasting. The uncertainty spread into many areas of life and in accommodating to it, basic ideas about the self began to change. In all of the substantive theories developed to explain living with continual uncertainty, emphasis is placed on the restructuring of reality as a major component of the process. The person emerges from the reappraisal with a new view of self and a new value system (Brown & Powell-Cope, 1991; Charmaz, 1994; Fleury et al., 1995; Mishel & Murdaugh, 1987; Nyhlin, 1990; Nelson, 1996).

CAUSES AND CONSEQUENCES OF UNCERTAINTY IN PARENTS OF CHRONICALLY ILL CHILDREN

In the literature on chronic illness and uncertainty in children included in this review, there are only three studies in which the child's perception of uncertainty was investigated. As in the acute illness studies, the majority of the work is on the parents of the ill child. Very few of the studies to be reviewed identify the ages of the children, the length of time since diagnosis, or present a definition of chronic illness that guided subject selection. Some investigators used the same sample for more then one study and did not refer to the literature as a cut of the data from a larger study. Most of the studies contained a grounded theory methodology, but few present any information on the procedures used to analyze the data.

Causes of Uncertainty

The unknowns about current illness status and prognosis are frequently cited as a cause of uncertainty (Burkhart, 1993; Cohen, 1993a; MacDonald, 1996; Murray, 1993). Cohen reports that questions about survival are answered by physicians with generalizations or statistical probabilities. Further findings from this study were that searching for information about prognosis is not profitable since definitive answers may not exist. Comaroff and Maguire (1981) in their study of 60 children with leukemia note that the question of long-term or permanent remission is continually evaluated against available evidence. They report that parents attempt to formulate timetables and statements of probabilities for themselves concerning the course of the illness. Similarly, Murray (1993) reports from her interviews with ten parents of children with epilepsy that uncertainty about the cause of the disease was related to uncertainty about prognosis. Inability to determine a seizure pattern was a component of the uncertainty about the current state of the illness. Murray described how parents reported temporal uncertainty about when seizures will occur and what will be good and bad phases, and event uncertainty about what is and is not a seizure. Similarly, MacDonald (1996) reported from her interviews with eight mothers of children with asthma that they were unable to determine good from bad times because they were uncertain about cues of impending danger.

Comaroff and Maguire (1981) made the point that the phase of remission entails learning to live with the uncertain status of the illness. They noted that remission disorients the parents and raises problems of uncertainty about planning for a more regular life and daring to hope. Jessop and Stein (1985), from a study of 209 mothers of chronically ill children aged birth to 11, remarked that stability in chronic illness may encourage the child to strive as a normal child, thus creating more uncertainty about the future. Clarke-Steffen (1993) noted that day-to-day uncertainty lessened, but uncertainty about ultimate survival continued. In this regard, Cohen (1995b) identified selected events labeled as "triggers" that increased the parents' uncertainty about their child's survival. Such triggers included routine medical visits, bodily changes such as energy or appetite, changes in treatment regime, negative events with other children, and new developmental demands. Similarly, in one of the rare investigations of the child's perspective, Koocher (1985) reported that children in remission from cancer have triggers that remind them of the residual risk. These are similar to those identified by Cohen (1995) and include the anniversary of the diagnosis, passage of significant life events, and the recent diagnosis or death of a known child.

A number of the qualitative investigations of parents of a chronically ill child referred to the parents' interactions with health care providers as a precipitant of uncertainty. Sharkey (1995), using a grounded theory methodology on interview data from four families, reported that concerns about professional caregivers were a cause for uncertainty in all four families. Specifically, it was the presence of home care nurses who were unfamiliar with the child and the family that raised concerns about safety and leaving the child alone. It was noted by a number of investigators that physicians were not a source of clear information (Cohen, 1993b; Comaroff & Maguire, 1981). Cohen reported that treatment uncertainty was generated from information overload and deficit under which parents are expected to make treatment decisions for their child. In this regard, Comaroff and Maguire (1981) cite a number of physician behaviors that increase uncertainty which include over simplistic and over optimistic models and lack of clear biomedical guidelines for parents. MacDonald (1996) reported that mothers of children with asthma often received conflicting information and instructions and eventually had to assume an advocacy role as the expert. Again, as in the research on health care providers for acutely ill children, there is little evidence among the data to support that health care providers function to reduce parental uncertainty.

Uncertainty Management and Adjustment to Uncertainty

The literature is quite scant and limited to a few studies on each topic. Only one quantitative study of parental coping with uncertainty has been published.

Sterken (1996) reported on a correlational analysis of uncertainly and coping in fathers of children with cancer. Uncertainty was significantly associated with emotion-oriented coping and with less confrontive coping. These findings are similar to those reported for coping with uncertainty among ill adults, but they should be viewed with caution, since only 31 of 150 eligible fathers completed the study, raising a question about the representativeness of the sample. In the qualitative studies on management of uncertainty, a number of strategies that parents use to manage uncertainty have been identified. MacDonald (1996) described a process through which mothers of children with asthma began to master uncertainty through learning to trust their assessment of the situation, gaining knowledge, and asserting in the health care environment. Comoraff and Maguire (1981) noted that parents compared their child to similar others who appeared to be doing well. This method of social comparison was similar to the management method used by both acutely ill and chronically ill adults. They also found that parents gathered multiple types of data to systematize it in a way to remain optimistic. Further support for these findings is provided by Cohen (1993b) who reported that parents try to find positive meaning in verbal and nonverbal communication from health professionals and look for positive messages in a variety of actions or events. Other methods of managing information to reduce uncertainty included discounting information or transforming or reframing it into more positive message (Cohen, 1993a). Gaining control over unpredictable seizure activity in children with epilepsy was managed by parents keeping a diary in order to identify some patterns and consistency (Murray, 1993). Brett and Davies (1988) described vigilance as a method to manage uncertainties during remission. The authors found that siblings and parents both were vigilant and that this vigilance relaxed when the family members felt more certain about the ill sibling's survival. Similarly, Cohen (1993a) described constant vigilance and eventually periodic monitoring as methods to manage uncertainty. Other investigators noted management methods, such as preserving usual family life, while others used opposite methods, such as living day to day (Burkhart, 1993; Cohen, 1993a, 1993b).

In the studies on children's responses to uncertainty, Koocher (1985) reported that children cured of cancer managed uncertainty by either being preoccupied that the cancer would return, believing that treatment made them immune to cancer, or not worrying about it at all. In a study of adolescents with cystic fibrosis, adolescents with high scores on the unpredictability factor of the MUIS had a longer future time perspective (Yarcheski, 1988). Such a finding may indicate that such children do not see their illness as having a negative downward trajectory. Their sense of unpredictability may imply hope.

The primary work on adjustment to uncertainty by parents with a chronically ill child is the work done by Clarke-Steffen (1993) and Cohen (1993b). These investigators have independently proposed substantive theory generated from a grounded theory methodology for how families integrate uncertainty into their life and change their orientation to their world. Cohen noted that the strategies used to manage uncertainty were not only to reduce uncertainty, but to maintain uncertainty where it serves to reduce distress. This implies a positive role for uncertainty over time which is similar to the orientation provided by Mishel (1990). Both investigators described that parents changed their beliefs, values, relationships, and routines. Cohen (1993b) proposed that very little was expected to be predictable and the view of the future was circumspect. Both investigators found that the change was viewed as permanent by the parents. The change in view of the world is similar to that proposed by Selder (1989) and Mishel (1990) and the change in behavior and values reported by subjects in studies with chronically ill adults (Brown & Powell-Cope, 1991; Charmaz, 1994; Fleury et al., 1995; Mishel & Murdaugh, 1987; Nyhlin, 1990).

CONCLUDING COMMENTS AND RESEARCH DIRECTIONS

Conceptualizations of uncertainty are frequent in studies of chronic illness. Both substantive theory specific to a population or diagnostic group and the two main theories by Mishel and Selder have produced a rich field of theory. Furthermore, a number of studies are being published that confirm the theory presented by Mishel (1990). However, in most of the current work, there is limited effort to integrate the substantive theories or to tie the inductive work to either overarching theory by Mishel or Selder. Without such effort, the building of a knowledge base for uncertainty in chronic illness is limited.

Major differences in the findings on uncertainty in chronic illness can be traced to the design of the study as either qualitative or quantitative. Concerning the causes of uncertainty, the findings from qualitative data have provided a rich description of the causes of uncertainty across a variety of chronic illnesses. The findings concerning the nature of the symptoms are consistent, even if the specific symptoms differ across illnesses. Also from the qualitative work, symptom unpredictability, an unknown future, and the possibility of disease recurrence and extension have been identified as causes of uncertainty. Lack of information to make the future more predictable has also emerged from qualitative studies as an antecedent of uncertainty. The identification of these antecedents has come from many qualitative investigations where these same themes emerged. This literature is rich with descriptions of each of these causes of uncertainty, especially the unpredictability of symptoms. The uncertainty resulting from the erratic symptom display that is characteristic of some chronic illnesses has been fully described in the research done to date.

There is some early work on the evolving sense of self in chronic illness that is fueled by the uncertainty surrounding the future. Although there have been three or four studies that have explored this sense of self, more work is needed, especially in looking at the process across gender. The work by Charmaz (1994) and by Fleury et al. (1995) raise some questions about differences in the process among men and women.

The qualitative and quantitative findings on social support and health care providers are not consistent. More work is needed using triangulated studies where both measurement and interview might help clarify the role of these variables in influencing uncertainty. Since self-management is a major component of living with chronic illness, there is some evidence that health care providers tend to destroy patient self-management, thus generating uncertainty. Further investigations are needed to explore these relationships.

Interesting findings are emerging from quantitative studies of perceived personal control as a personality disposition for influencing uncertainty and the relationship between uncertainty and mood state. Likewise, spirituality is also being studied for its potential in modifying the impact of uncertainty in mood. Both of these avenues of study are important and point out that in a long-term illness, personality dimensions may come into play for their ability to reduce uncertainty or to reduce the negative impact of uncertainty.

The work on management of uncertainty has been enriched by the qualitative investigations where a variety of management methods have been found across a number of chronic illnesses. In contrast to the limited and ineffective coping strategies reported from the use of standardized scales, the findings from qualitative studies indicate that people are very resourceful in finding approaches for living with enduring uncertainty. More research is needed in this area with an attempt to replicate findings across studies so that support for particular strategies can emerge. At the present time, the findings are scattered, with no attempt to relate findings from one study to another.

Research on adjusting to uncertainty is divided into two camps. There are quantitative studies, where uncertainty results in a poorer psychosocial adjustment, and there are the qualitative studies, where uncertainty changes over time and leads to new views of the world and a growth experience for the subjects. This disparity related to research paradigm is likely due to the ability of qualitative studies to reflect a process that occurs, while quantitative studies index a slice of time using a specific measure that may not reflect a process, even if such could be measured. Yet, among the qualitative work, there is little attempt to unify the findings and to relate current results to what is known in the field. Furthermore, qualitative studies often are methodologically vague. The procedure for analysis of the data is often sparse and there is no definition or discussion of the concept of uncertainty. In the current research on uncertainty, the focus has been on the ill adult, with less attention to the family or parent of the child or the ill child. There is a need for more research on the family's experience of uncertainty. Of absolute importance is more study of the child's experience of uncertainty in both acute and chronic illness. The findings on the child's experience of uncertainty are negligible.

Lastly, the work on interventions to manage uncertainty were reviewed by Mishel (1997), and there is very little work done on interventions to manage uncertainty in chronic illness. Use of the theory on uncertainty in chronic illness could be a starting point for developing and testing such interventions.

ACKNOWLEDGMENT

I gratefully acknowledge the assistance of Donald Bailey, Graduate Research Assistant, for his skill in searching for articles and for his critical assessment of the materials for this review.

REFERENCES

Affleck, G., Tennen, H., Pfeiffer, C., & Fifield, J. (1987). Appraisals of control and predictability in adapting to a chronic disease. *Journal of Personality and Social Psychology, 53,* 273–279.

Allan, J. D. (1990). Focusing on living, not dying: A naturalistic study of self-care among seropositive gay men. *Holistic Nursing Practice, 4*(2), 56–63.

Armor, J. M., McDermott, M. P., & Schiffer, R. B. (1996). Psychological characteristics of MS patients: Determining differences based upon participation in a therapy regimen. *Rehabilitation Nursing Research, 8,* 102–111.

Baier, M. (1995). Uncertainty of illness for persons with schizophrenia. *Issues in Mental Health Nursing, 16,* 201–212.

Bailey, J. M., & Nielsen, B. I. (1993). Uncertainty and appraisal of uncertainty in women with rheumatoid arthritis. *Orthopaedic Nursing, 12*(2), 63–67.

Becker, G., Janson-Bjerklie, S., Benner, P., Slobin, K., & Ferketich, S. (1993). The dilemma of seeking urgent care: Asthma episodes and emergency service use. *Social Science and Medicine, 37,* 305–313.

Braden, C. J. (1990). A test of the self-help model learned response to chronic illness experience. *Nursing Research, 39,* 42–47.

Braden, C. J. (1991). Patterns of change over time in learned response to chronic illness among participants in a systemic lupus erythematosus self-help course. *Arthritis Care & Research, 4,* 158–167.

Brett, K. M., & Davies, E. M. B. (1988). "What does it mean?": Sibling and parental appraisals of childhood leukemia. *Cancer Nursing, 11,* 329–338.

Brown, M. A., & Powell-Cope, G. M. (1991). AIDS family caregiving: Transitions through uncertainty. *Nursing Research, 40,* 337–345.

Burkhart, P. V. (1993). Health perceptions of mothers of children with chronic conditions. *Maternal-Child Nursing Journal, 21,* 122–129.

Charmaz, K. (1994). Identity dilemmas of chronically ill men. *The Sociological Quarterly, 35*(2), 269–288.

Clarke-Steffen, L. (1993). A model of the family transition to living with childhood cancer. *Cancer Practice: A Multidisciplinary Journal of Cancer Care, 1,* 285–292.

Cohen, M. H. (1993a). Diagnostic closure and the spread of uncertainty. *Issues in Comprehensive Pediatric Nursing, 16,* 135–146.

Cohen, M. H. (1993b). The unknown and the unknowable: Managing sustained uncertainty. *Western Journal of Nursing Research, 15*(1), 77–96.

Cohen, M. H. (1995). The triggers of heightened parental uncertainty in chronic, life-threatening childhood illness. *Qualitative Health Research, 5*(1), 63–77.

Comaroff, J., & Maguire, P. (1981). Ambiguity and the search for meaning: Childhood leukaemia in the modern clinical context. *Society, Science & Medicine, 15B,* 115–123.

Cooper, H. M. (1982). Scientific guidelines for conducting integrative research reviews. *Review of Educational Research, 52,* 291–302.

Crigger, N. J. (1996). Testing an uncertainty model for women with multiple sclerosis. *Advances in Nursing Science, 18*(3), 37–47.

Failla, S., Kuper, B. C., Nick, T. G., & Lee, F. A. (1996). Adjustment of women with systemic lupus erythematosus. *Applied Nursing Research, 9,* 87–96.

Fleury, J., Kimbrell, L. C., & Kruszewski, M. A. (1995). Life after a cardiac event: Women's experience in healing. *Heart and Lung, 24,* 474–482.

Gaskins, S., & Brown, K. (1992). Psychosocial responses among individuals with human immunodeficiency virus infection. *Applied Nursing Research, 5,* 111–121.

Hilton, B. A. (1988). The phenomenon of uncertainty in women with breast cancer. *Issues in Mental Health Nursing, 9,* 217–238.

Hilton, B. A. (1993). Issues, problems, and challenges for families coping with breast cancer. *Seminars in Oncology Nursing, 9,* 88–100.

Janson-Bjerklie, S., Ferketich, S., & Benner, P. (1993). Predicting the outcomes of living with asthma. *Research in Nursing & Health, 16,* 241–250.

Jessop, D. J., & Stein, R. E. K. (1985). Uncertainty and its relation to the psychological and social correlates of chronic illness in children. *Society, Science & Medicine, 20,* 993–999.

Johnson, J. L., & Morse, J. M. (1990). Regaining control: The process of adjustment after myocardial infarction. *Heart and Lung, 19,* 126–135.

Kachoyeanos, M. K., & Selder, F. E. (1993). Life transitions of parents at the unexpected death of a school-age and older child. *Journal of Pediatric Nursing, 8,* 41–49.

Katz, A. (1996). Gaining a new perspective on life as a consequence of uncertainty in HIV infection. *Journal of the Association of Nurses in AIDS Care, 7*(4), 51–60.

292 OTHER RESEARCH

Koocher, G. P. (1985). Psychosocial care of the child cured of cancer. *Pediatric Nursing, 11,* 91–93.

Landis, B. J. (1996). Uncertainty, spirituality, well-being, and psychosocial adjustment to chronic illness. *Issues in Mental Health Nursing, 17,* 217–231.

Loveys, B. (1990). Transitions in chronic illness: The at-risk role. *Holistic Nursing Practice, 4,* 56–64.

MacDonald, H. (1996). "Mastering uncertainty": Mothering the child with asthma. *Pediatric Nursing, 22,* 55–59.

Mason, C. (1985). The production and effects of uncertainty with special reference to diabetes mellitus. *Society, Science, and Medicine, 21,* 1329–1334.

Mast, M. E. (1995). Adult uncertainty in illness: A critical review of research. *Scholarly Inquiry for Nursing Practice: An International Journal, 9,* 3–24.

McCain, N. L., & Cella, D. F. (1995). Correlates of stress in HIV disease. *Western Journal of Nursing Research, 17,* 141–155.

Mishel, M. H. (1990). Reconceptualization of the Uncertainty in Illness Theory. *Image: Journal of Nursing Scholarship, 22,* 256–262.

Mishel, M. H. (1993). Living with chronic illness: Living with uncertainty. In S. G. Funk, E. M. Tornquist, M. T. Champagne, & R. A. Wiese (Eds.), *Key aspects of caring for the chronically ill: Hospital and home* (pp. 46–58). New York: Springer Publishing Company.

Mishel, M. H. (1997). Uncertainty in acute illness. In J. Fitzpatrick & J. Norbeck (Eds.), *Annual review of nursing research* (pp. 57–80). New York: Springer Publishing.

Mishel, M. H., & Murdaugh, C. L. (1987). Family adjustment to heart transplantation: Redesigning the dream. *Nursing Research, 36,* 332–336.

Morrow, Y. Y., Chiarello, R. J., & Derogatis, L. R. (1978). A new scale for assessing patients' psychosocial adjustment to medical illness. *Medicine, 8,* 605–610.

Moser, D. K., Clements, P. J., Brecht, M. L., & Weiner, S. R. (1993). Predictors of psychosocial adjustment in systemic sclerosis: The influence of formal education level, functional ability, hardiness, uncertainty, and social support. *Arthritis and Rheumatism, 36,* 1398–1405.

Mullins, L. L., Cheney, J. M., Hartman, V. L., Albin, K., Miles, B., & Roberson, S. (1995). Cognitive and affective features of postpolio syndrome: Illness uncertainty, attributional style, and adaptation. *International Journal of Rehabilitation and Health, 1,* 211–222.

Murray, J. (1993). Coping with the uncertainty of uncontrolled epilepsy. *Seizure, 2,* 167–178.

Mushlin, A. I., Mooney, C., Grow, V., & Phelps, C. E. (1994). The value of diagnostic information to patients with suspected multiple sclerosis. *Archives of Neurology, 51,* 67–72.

Nelson, J. P. (1996). Struggling to gain meaning: Living with the uncertainty of breast cancer. *Advances in Nursing Science, 18*(3), 59–76.

Nyhlin, K. T. (1990). Diabetic patients facing long-term complications: Coping with uncertainty. *Journal of Advanced Nursing, 15,* 1021–1029.

O'Brien, R. A., Wineman, N. M., & Nealon, N. R. (1995). Correlates of the caregiving process in multiple sclerosis. *Scholarly Inquiry for Nursing Practice, 9,* 323–342.

Pelusi, J. (1997). The lived experience of surviving breast cancer. *Oncology Nursing Forum, 24, 8,* 1343–1353.

Price, M. J. (1993). An experiential model of learning diabetes self-management. *Qualitative Health Research, 3*(3), 29–54.

Regan-Kubinski, M. J., & Sharts-Hopko, N. (1995). Illness cognition of HIV-infected mothers. *Issues in Mental Health Nursing, 16,* 327–344.

Rowat, K. M., & Knafl, K. A. (1985). Living with chronic pain: The spouse's perspective. *Pain, 23,* 259–271.

Selder, F. (1989). Life transition theory: The resolution of uncertainty. *Nursing & Health Care, 10,* 437–451.

Sharkey, T. (1995). The effects of uncertainty in families with children who are chronically ill. *Home Health Care Nurse, 13*(4), 37–42.

Small, S. P., & Graydon, J. E. (1992). Perceived uncertainty, physical symptoms, and negative mood in hospitalized patients with chronic obstructive pulmonary disease. *Heart and Lung, 21,* 568–574.

Small, S. P., & Graydon, J. E. (1993). Uncertainty in hospitalized patients with chronic obstructive pulmonary disease. *International Journal of Nursing Studies, 30,* 239–246.

Smeltzer, S. C. (1994). The concerns of pregnant women with multiple sclerosis. *Qualitative Health Research, 4,* 497–501.

Sterken, D. J. (1996). Uncertainty and coping of fathers of children with cancer. *Journal of Pediatric Oncology Nursing, 13,* 81–90.

Stewart, D. C., & Sullivan, T. J. (1982). Illness behavior and the sick role in chronic disease: The case of multiple sclerosis. *Society, Science, and Medicine, 16,* 1397–1404.

Van Riper, M., & Selder, F. E. (1989). Parental responses to birth of a child with Down Syndrome. *Loss, Grief and Care: A Journal of Professional Practice, 3*(3–4), 59–76.

Viney, L. L., & Westbrook, M. T. (1984). Coping with chronic illness: Strategy preferences, changes in preferences and associated emotional reactions. *Journal of Chronic Diseases, 37,* 489–502.

Webster, D. C., & Brennan, T. (1995). Use and effectiveness of psychological self-care strategies for interstitial cystitis. *Health Care for Women International, 16,* 463–475.

Weems, J., & Patterson, E. T. (1989). Coping with uncertainty and ambivalence while awaiting a cadaveric renal transplant. *ANNA Journal, 16,* 27–32.

Weitz, R. (1989). Uncertainty and the lives of persons with AIDS. *Journal of Health and Social Behavior, 30,* 270–281.

Wiener, C. L. (1975). The burden of rheumatoid arthritis: Tolerating the uncertainty. *Social Science and Medicine, 9,* 97–104.

Wineman, N. M. (1990). Adaptation to multiple sclerosis: The role of social support, functional disability, and perceived uncertainty. *Nursing Research, 39,* 294–299.

Wineman, N. M., Durand, E. J., & Steiner, R. P. (1994). A comparative analysis of coping behaviors in persons with multiple sclerosis or a spinal cord injury. *Research in Nursing and Health, 17,* 185–194.

Wineman, N. M., O'Brien, R. A., Nealon, N. R., & Kaskel, B. (1993). Congruence in uncertainty between individuals with multiple sclerosis and their spouses. *Journal of Neuroscience Nursing, 25,* 356–361.

Wineman, N. M., Schwetz, K. M., Goodkin, D. E., & Rudick, R. A. (1996). Relationships among illness uncertainty, stress, coping, and emotional well-being at entry into a clinical drug trial. *Applied Nursing Research, 9,* 53–60.

Yarcheski, A. (1988). Uncertainty in illness and the future. *Western Journal of Nursing Research, 10,* 401–413.

Chapter 12

Nursing Research in Italy

RENZO ZANOTTI

ABSTRACT

Nursing in Italy is achieving a higher academic status as a result of decades of efforts in scientific knowledge development. Beginning in the 1980s, Italian nurses, supported by researchers from allied disciplines, have begun to design and implement research at the local, regional, and national level. This study is the first effort ever made to identify the main characteristics of Italian nursing research published in Italian journals. The review covers 14 years (1983–1997). Overall, 240 studies from 11 journals, research reports from books, and several conference proceedings have been considered. Inclusion criteria were based on quality of research design, considering components such as sampling, sample size, and method of data analysis. Each article was analyzed according to an interpretive scheme focusing on method of analysis, scientific merit, and authorship.

Of the 240 studies reviewed, journal articles selected from ten Italian journals accounted for 175 (73%), or the majority, of reviewed sources. Sixty-five (26%) research reports complete the remaining number. The major areas of research identified include nursing practice (43%), nursing education (6%), nursing administration and professional issues (34%), and knowledge and perceptions in society and nursing (17%). The majority of the research studies utilized survey models (47%), including several retrospective and longitudinal studies, followed by exploratory or descriptive (36%) and quasi-experimental (17%) designs. Many reports failed to identify the method of sampling used in the research design. However, of those that did, convenience samples were most often used. Random sampling was rarely reported. The majority of studies employed only descriptive statistics (i.e., frequency distribution, central tendency, variability, contingency tables, and correlation). Only few studies made use of advanced statistics for testing hypotheses (parametric and non-parametric tests) among which only a low percentage cited reliability testing. In 42% of the studies, the authors were represented by a group of nurses. Nurses and physicians worked together to author another 30% of the studies. The remaining studies were authored by either individual nurses (24%) or nurses and nonmedical professionals (4%). Much of the reviewed research has been carried out by nurses who have little or no research training.

Keywords: Nursing Research, Italian Nursing Research, Research in Italy

As a result of both internal and external changes, Italian nursing has undergone a profound evolution over the past 15 years. The most noticeable results of this continuing evolution include the shift of nursing education into the university and a new law which recognizes nursing as an independent and autonomous profession contributing to the Italian health system.

A recent and very important achievement in the Italian nursing community is the recognition of research as an important tool for the development of the discipline and the profession. Supported by researchers and statisticians, nurses have begun to design and implement regional projects. The 2-year university-based program created especially for teachers and administrators has provided a strong impulse toward this end. Students in these classes are encouraged to develop their own research projects. Undergraduate programs are also requiring students to carry out research projects in order to aid them in acquiring a basic understanding of the research process. The results of these efforts to facilitate the growth of nursing research in Italy are evidenced by the burgeoning body of literature being produced by Italian nurses.

This chapter represents the broadest and most current attempt to review the present-day body of Italian nursing research literature. It covers the past 14 years (1983–1997) and incorporates 240 studies from 11 different journals (see Table 12.1) and research reports from books and conference proceedings. It is representative of both the strides that Italian nursing research has made and the efforts it must continue to make in order to verify and develop its scientific knowledge.

THE REVIEW PROCEDURE

For the purpose of this review, studies published in Italian nursing journals between 1983 and 1997, as well as reports of research from national conferences and congresses, were reviewed. Inclusion criteria was based on quality

TABLE 12.1   Journals Reviewed for Research Review

Journals Reviewed	N = 175
La Rivista dell'Infermiere [*The Nurse's Journal*]	77
Infermiere Informazione [*Nurse Information*]	13
Professioni Infermieristiche [*Nursing Professions*]	31
QA [*Quality Assurance*]	12
Salute e Territorio [*Health and Territory*]	3
Nursing Oggi [*Nursing Today*]	14
L'Operatore Sanitario [*The Health Professional*]	1
Scenarious [Scenario]	10
Prospettive Socialie Sanitare [*Social and Health Perspectives*]	6
L'Infermiere [*The Nurse*]	4
Il Diabete & L'Infermiere [*Diabetes and Nursing*]	4

of research design considering components such as sampling, sample size, control, and method of data analysis. Each article was analyzed according to an interpretive scheme focusing on method of analysis, scientific merit, and authorship, in order to classify the studies into different areas of research. If the study lacked a coherent design, a literature review (or some equivalent thereof), a description of the actual research, or was not yet completed, it was not included in the analysis.

Of the 240 studies reviewed, journal articles selected from ten Italian journals accounted for 175 (73%), or the majority, of reviewed sources. Sixty-five (26%) research reports make up the remaining number. The major areas of research identified include nursing practice (43%), nursing education (6%), nursing administration and professional issues (34%), and knowledge and perceptions in society and nursing (17%). The majority of the research studies utilized survey models (47%), including several retrospective and longitudinal studies, followed by exploratory or descriptive (36%) and quasi-experimental [lacked random sampling] or pre-experimental [lacked random sampling, no control group] designs (17%). (See Table 12.2.)

Many reports failed to identify the method of sampling used in the research design. However, of those that did, convenience samples were most often used. Random sampling was rarely reported. The majority of studies employed only descriptive statistics (i.e., frequency distribution, central tendency, variability, contingency tables, and correlation). Several studies tested hypotheses (parametric and non-parametric tests) among which only a low percentage cited reliability testing. Very few studies made use of advanced statistics.

In 42% of the studies, the authors were represented by a group of nurses. Nurses and physicians worked together to author another 30% of the studies. The remaining studies were authored by either individual nurses (24%) or other (4%).

TABLE 12.2   Characteristics of the Research Reviewed

Sources	$N = 240$	
Journals	175	(72.9%)
Research reports	65	(27.1%)
Areas of research		
Nursing practice	103	(42.9%)
Nursing education	15	(6.3%)
Nursing administration and professional issues	81	(33.8%)
Knowledge and perceptions in nursing and society	41	(17.1%)
Research designs		
Survey models	113	(47.1%)
Exploratory/Descriptive	86	(35.8%)
Quasi- or pre-experimental	41	(17.1%)

ANALYSIS OF ITALIAN NURSING RESEARCH

Nursing Practice

This category includes 103 (43%) of the studies reviewed. Specific areas of research included critical care (12 studies), medical-surgical nursing (15), home and hospice care, geriatric, and psychiatric nursing (19), maternal and child and pediatric nursing (9), infectious diseases and chronic illness nursing (19), and the evaluation of quality of care (29). The majority of the studies were surveys, including a limited number of retrospective and longitudinal studies. The remaining were either pre-experimental, quasi-experimental, exploratory, or descriptive design.

Critical care.   Critical care in Italy is a large area, inclusive of several clinical settings, ranging from resuscitation units through transplant, intensive, and post-op care units. This section shows how the studies in critical care focus on different phenomena, from very specific technical activities such as intravenous therapy administration, to the patient's perceived psychological needs, and the epidemiology of some deadly events like traffic accidents. Intravenous therapy has been and still is a very much studied activity. In Intensive Coronary Care Unit (UCIC) critical care nurses, after being trained to administer and monitor heparin therapy according to clinical guidelines, autonomously provided heparin therapy to patients who had experienced a myocardial infarction. Moro and Spangaro (1994) using a quasi-experimental design in order to compare the outcomes, utilized both an experimental group, cared for by the nurses, and a control group, receiving the typical management of heparin therapy from physicians. No differences were observed between control and experimental groups. The authors concluded that nurses are able to safely and autonomously administer and monitor intravenous heparin therapy.

A cross sectional study (Biancoli et al., 1989) was conducted by a group of nurses and physicians with 103 intensive care unit (ICU) patients. The aim of the study was to evaluate the current procedure(s) being used to prevent the infection of intravascular canulae sites and develop a "best practices" care protocol based on the findings of the study. Martini and Pigato (1987) have observed and analyzed the quality and utilization of parenteral therapy in the ICUs of a hospital in Verona. In both surveys, authors found some but only minor potential risks in the procedures used at that time. Indications about how to improve the quality have been provided in the studies' discussions.

Marchini et al. (1989) did a retrospective study of 242 ICU patients who were post-acute myocardial infarction. This study demonstrated the value of a patient's relative at the bedside in decreasing the incidence of mental alterations during hospitalization. Addressing a related concern, Bertolotto, Biagi, Burlando, and Olcese (1996) looked at nurses' attitudes towards patients' relatives' visiting hours, and rights to information. Preiata (1986) conducted a survey of psychosocial and emotional problems of patients in critical care environments. The study results show that room noises, detachment from family relationship, impersonal relationship with formal caregivers, and lack of privacy are the most important causes of discomfort for patients. Interestingly, the author did not make any comment on data showing patients' negative perception of nurses versus a positive perception of doctors.

A regional survey on extra-hospital emergencies was conducted by Roggi (1987). The study focused on the development of an operative protocol for nursing activity for the improvement of caring during first-aid circumstances. There were also two pre-experimental studies. The first examined the use of a transfer device for patients who are confined to bed (Deana et al., 1993) and the second, on a device used to prevent obstructions of oro/nasotracheal tubes (Torre, 1994). Sposito, Ringo, and Villani (1989) conducted an epidemiological study about death due to cranial trauma in motorcyclists' accidents, in order to evaluate the impact of a new law making mandatory the use of helmets. The study results show a significant reduction of cranial trauma, but also a sharp increase of mortality, after the new law came in effect. However, the authors did not frame the phenomenon in a proper manner, and the results are questionable.

Medical-surgical nursing.   Among the 15 studies identified in this practice area, almost 35% of the studies concerned bedsores. Few of the other studies have addressed topics like pain management, infection rate, and a predictive model validation. One study (Apostoli et al., 1988) found the incidence rate ($n = 157$) of first cues of risk for developing bedsores to be 19%, with one-half of those occurring sometime after the first week of hospitalization. Another study (Brosolo et al., 1989) reported the results of a 2-year monitoring program focused on patients ($n = 679$) at risk of and with bedsores. The results suggested that a positive effect may be obtained through sustained attention and careful definition of the interventions planned. Rasero, Erico, Puccetti, and Tellarini (1996) conducted a prospective randomized trial of bone marrow transplant patients ($n = 30$) comparing infection rates in two groups ($n = 15$ each) using different hygiene protocols for heating, dressing, and nursing care. Results showed no significant differences between the two groups. This study was followed in the literature by a retrospective analysis of 295 bone marrow transplant patients with the same care protocols for rates of infection and infection vectors (Rasero, Errico, & Bertelli, 1997). The authors found positive 22% of the subjects (that is below the national average) white Gram + bacteria as main cause of infection.

Finally, Sabbadin et al. (1991) conducted a quasi-experimental study in the neurological units of two hospitals testing patterns of signs and symptoms predictive of some patient's needs in order to validate a diagnostic model based on Zanotti's framework.

Home and hospice care, geriatric, and psychiatric nursing.   Care for the elderly is a growing field throughout the world secondary to the graying of the world's population. In Italy, this is the direct result of a higher standard of living. This phenomena has led to changes in social perspectives as well as new stresses on the health care system. However, only 19 studies, or 8% of the total studies, could have been included in this area. Several qualitative studies have addressed a number of topics, including the experience of being terminally ill in hospital. Arciero et al. (1993) addressed the problem of terminal oncological patients' privacy and patients' needs as perceived by nurses. The study results indicate these patients' needs are minimally perceived. Milan and Targa (1992) evaluated questionnaires given to second and third year nursing students caring for terminally ill patients over a 3-month period, designed to elicit the inner emotions experienced by students when taking readings from dying persons. Brivio and Gamba (1989) and Delli (1994) conducted cross-sectional studies to evaluate the efficacy and the difficulties involved in a home care program for advanced cancer and terminal patients.

Bianchet et al. (1993), Nebuloni (1986), Boccagni, Prencipe, Ravelli, and Trecate (1991), and Caron, Florianello, and Oltolina (1992) have studied the situation of the hospitalized elderly in a number of hospitals. Specifically, Ambrogio and Gori (1997) have tested a "needs evolution tool" designed to predict the changing care needs of the elderly; Piras and Sansoni (1997) have used a nursing home sample to identify the unaddressed sexuality issues of the elderly; and Cecchetto (1995) has produced an epidemiological profile of elderly patients in a region of Italy.

Mother and child nursing and pediatric nursing.   Traditionally, in Italy, pediatric care has been an area of concern for the pediatric nurse, who is in some ways but not in all similar to the registered nurse. In the last decade, the schools for pediatric nurses have been closed (only two surviving) resulting in a massive move of registered nurses into pediatric and maternal clinical settings. The turnover seems correlated to the increasing number of nursing studies in these areas.

Fourteen studies were included in this area where quality of care, psychological relationships between newborns and parents, pre-surgery anxiety, eating habits, and education are the aspects more explored. The quality of care of pregnant women, and more specifically, the extension of and criteria for the use of drugs, were the subjects of an epidemiological study conducted by a group of Health Visitors (Work Group, 1990). Mele (1987), in a descriptive-explorative study, looked at the psychological implications of a forced separation between parents and newborns, and examined the parents' consequent need of information and the degree to which the nurse became involved in the fulfillment of that need. Cosi (1997) examined the fear and anxiety components in 7–14-year-old children and their parents when faced with a surgical procedure. The same questionnaire was used to assess both parent and child.

Di Cristofano (1989a) conducted an experimental study on children ($n = 21$) with an egg allergy to evaluate their allergic reactions to the measles vaccine. The results suggested that the anti-measles vaccine is not contraindicated in children with egg allergies. A longitudinal study was done by the same author (1989b) on the prevention of allergic illnesses in 172 newborns at risk for atopic syndrome.

A survey on the need for more educational intervention on eating habits in 460 elementary-school-aged children and their parents was implemented by a group of nurses (Colli & Mazzitelli, 1987). Data were collected from questionnaires completed by parents and children. Results evidenced the existence of high-risk habits that could be related to the actual incidence of obesity in the range of 6–10 year-old children. The study results have been used to implement educational interventions to educate both parents and children about the risks of obesity. A similar study was done with nursing students in an attempt to correlate body mass and eating habits (Dellai & Zampieron, 1996). In this study, knowledge of good eating habits was found to have no correlation with being overweight.

Infectious disease and chronic care nursing.   Care for HIV-infected persons is an international concern. In Italy, there is increasing concern about the social and economic costs involved in caring for this population. An exploratory study has been conducted by Salmaso, Scaggiante, Cadrobbi, Orsini, and Favaretti (1992) which estimates the care demand of patients with HIV or related pathologies and determines a rational and responsible use of both material and human resources in order to achieve a better quality of life for the patients.

Persons with diabetes have been studied by Italian nursing research literature. Milan et al. (1989) who examined the knowledge of diabetic patients about their condition, used a random sample ($n = 60$) divided into two groups.

The first group had previously taken an educational course in the day hospital, while the second group had not. The aim of the study was to evaluate patients' performance in managing their own disease and the problems occurring in the communication between nurses and patients. Results were suggestive of relationships between intensive course participation and the development of better skills in the management of diabetes. Monesi et al. (1992), evaluated the impact of training interventions (n = 100) while implementing a new method of diabetic foot care. Bedendo, Marchetto, and Stievano's (1986) exploratory study on the organization of a diabetic center found that clients were lacking knowledge in various aspects of their disease. As a result, a number of educational interventions were organized to enable patients to be more autonomous. Collareda, Gomitolo, Pellizzari, Corradin, and Erle (1995) have surveyed patients to elicit their perceptions of what their own greatest needs are related to diabetes care. Effects on blood sugar of an alternative sugar source for the making of traditional Italian pastries was examined in diabetic patients (Bonannini et al., 1996).

Grazia and Pozzi (1990), nurses in a nephrologic intensive care ward, studied the care and social aspects in a group of uremic (n = 65) patients who had undergone continuous ambulatory peritoneal dialysis (CAPD) treatments, while Andreoli et al. (1997), studied the characteristics of tuberculosis rehabilitation in the hospital through the analysis of hospital databases. The aim of the study was to forecast the needs of patients with tuberculosis. Finally, Bagnis et al. (1996) used self-administered questionnaires to assess patients' reactions to automated peritoneal dialysis (where they are more independent) versus the traditional method. Results showed a good patient acceptance of the automated peritoneal dialysis.

Quality of care.   Optimum care has become a concern throughout all of the health care industry. New standards of care are requiring that the competence of health care professionals, consumer satisfaction, and job satisfaction all be measured. Twenty-eight quality-of-care evaluation studies were found in which standards of care were a major focus.

Nine out of the 28 studies included in this section are consumer interviews determining satisfaction with the quality and care of the hospital personnel. A number of authors (D'Andrea et al., 1988; Fiorni et al., 1994; Masera et al., 1996; Pegoraro & Bertarelli, 1996; Sacco and Renis, 1997) studied the quality of care given in the hospitals. The variables observed were the frequency and epidemiology of infections, errors in pharmacological therapies, and the frequency of patient falls in the hospital. The aim of all these studies was to determine where care was lacking and formulate evaluation protocols to promote a positive change in nursing performance.

D'Andrea et al. (1988) surveyed the parents (n = 187) of children in the pediatric ward with the aim of evaluating the organization of the ward, the continuity of care, and the relationship with the personnel. Pegoraro and Bertarelli (1995, 1996) surveyed liver transplant patients in order to assess the quality and depth of care. Masera et al. (1996) asked parents to evaluate the quality of care they received following the diagnosis of acute lymphatic leukemia, revealing need for more support and education. Finally, Sacco and Renis (1997) interviewed patients receiving emergency psychiatric care at Bari Polyclinic that identified the value of skilled nurses from patient's perspective.

Other areas in which quality was assessed include Fiorni et al.'s (1994) work in determining the nurses' efficacy and efficiency during the endoscopy procedure as perceived by patients; frequency of falls in hospitals (Buzzai, Gasparini, Glavina, Lenhard, & Sema, 1991; Mariotto et al., 1992); and infections in intensive care units (Rolando et al., 1992). Brandi (1990) considered strategies and methodologies for evaluating quality in a study that looked at urinary infections in patients with vesical catheters.

Nursing Education

Two subsections are included in this area, undergraduate/university-based nursing education (10 studies) and continuing nursing education (5 studies). Three of the 15 were quasi-experimental in design, while the remaining were explorative or cross-sectional. In the area of continuing education, one cross-sectional study examined the continuing education of nurses who are teachers.

Undergraduate nursing education.　The evolution of nursing education system in Italy is still an undergoing process, where the turning point was the inclusion of nursing education into university in 1994. Ghizzoni and Agostino (1996) studied the educational background and professional references of nurses teaching at undergraduate university programs throughout a national mail survey (n = 120). The results revealed that the majority of nurse teachers have the 2-year special university school for teaching nursing and at least 2 years of clinical experience.

The development of diagnostic competency skills is generally overlooked in nursing schools; this is in part due to the lack of applied and experimental educational models in teaching and training. A didactic teaching intervention to assist students in the acquisition of diagnostic skills was tested by Zanotti and Bini (1994) and Fanton and Zanotti (1992). Samples included all third year nursing students. The purpose of the researchers was to test the validity and reliability of a new needs analysis model and the effectiveness of a didactic method in teaching the model.

Other authors have analyzed students' educational needs with regard to various matters such as death (Bertoni & Coato, 1994), health education (Mislej, 1984), and the English language (Nicastri, Poletti, Torsello, & Vian, 1991).

Continuing education. Using a quasi-experimental design introducing the use of new planning procedures, nursing activities, and psychological techniques in a hospital ward, Poletti, Vian, and Zanotti (1991) demonstrated the effectiveness of intensive, short-term education on the field in order to change traditional activities and attitudes in hospital nursing care.

Poletti, Vian, Vittadello, and Zanotti (1994a, 1994b) published the results of a 3-year quasi-experimental study for the development of skills in research using particular teaching methodologies in six schools in Veneto. In another article, Poletti and Zanotti (1992) introduced an exhaustive profile of empirically tested educational contents for preparing skilled nurse educators. The article, grounded on several years of empirical observations, analyzes the personal and professional skills that make good educators and the main problems they have to face when implementing innovative teaching in traditional settings.

Nursing Administration and Professional Issues

The main themes emerging from the 81 studies analyzed were systems analysis (42 studies) work environment (20), and nursing roles (19). Most of the research was exploratory and descriptive in nature, however, there were eight pre-experimental or quasi-experimental studies. One study employed a multivariate analysis, factor analysis, and cluster analysis (Poletti & Vian, 1992). Another study registered Cronbach's index calculation in order to evaluate the data reliability (Proli, 1997).

Systems analysis. Bedin et al. (1988) gathered information through a questionnaire administered in 322 intensive care units in Italy. Spada, Bonfoco, Bonzi, Boscolo, and Giroletti (1991) studied the structure of the critical care area (first aid, operating ward, and reanimation unit) in an Italian region. Day hospitals (Cossu et al., 1988; Di Giulio, 1988), and dialysis centers (Geatti, 1993) have been the focus of other studies. Evaluation of care levels (Acquafredda et al., 1987), work loads (Group of Nurses, 1990; Mannocci, 1987; Tosco, 1997), and organizational analysis of care services (Borsarelli, Galizio,

Pastorutti, Schirru, & Vittone, 1994; Brandi, 1991; Deriu, 1997; Paschini, 1985) were among the principal factors considered in analysis models. "Anomalous employment" is when a professional nurse is employed to perform activities which do not belong specifically to the nursing profession and which can be performed by other components of the care staff (physicians, ward secretaries, clerks, and socio-sanitary auxiliaries). Lombardo's (1991) research in this area provided information for planning the development of the nursing profession's future strategies and to facilitate its introduction into the sanitary services system.

Cavestri et al. (1996) examined the system by which stroke patients were assessed and admitted to rehabilitation programs. It was found that only 50% of eligible patients actually receive services. Proli (1997) evaluated the system by which an emergency room triaged its patients and compared the assessments of nurses and physicians with post-treatment evaluations. Another study implemented an innovative system for organic waste disposal after performing a cost-benefit analysis of the current and proposed systems (Ricci, Suzzi, Bassi, Corazza, & Rainaldi, 1996).

A study that was done by Poletti and Vian (1992) represented a novelty in Italy and abroad. The aim of the research was to produce basic knowledge on the nursing system in the Veneto region and to develop strategic proposals for the system's positive development in a medium-term perspective. The study obtained information and data on various aspects of the nursing system, such as clients' needs, satisfaction for received care and care results, the productivity of the system, living and working conditions of nursing staff, health workers' attitudes, and so on. This research played an important role in the development of the nursing system in the Veneto region for the year 2000.

Nurses frequently act as the managers for the convergence of data from several different sources from medicine to social work to physical therapy. A survey done by Bovino and Zanotti (1985) analyzed the nurse's role in the gathering and use of data. This was done by examining the paperwork produced in large hospitals and community services and determining the actual contribution and responsibility of each professional in the information process. The results indicated that nurses gather the great majority of data, but utilized it less than any other health professional. Poletti and Vian (1986) carried out a survey on the attitudes of Italian nurses (n = 1,439) towards the use of information in their activity. The results clearly indicated that nurses' attitudes toward information and the potential for its use are generally positive.

Equally interesting are the results of a study conducted by Pasquot (1986). This research examined the effect of a new computerized nursing schedule on nurses' practice. Another study was carried out by a group of nurses (Cossu et al., 1988) in which a Day Hospital was studied using an integrated computerized method of analysis named DAFNE. Using DAFNE, it has been possible to obtain a graphic representation of the different activities that took place and analyze the key links that play a major role in the organization's functioning. Finally, Zanotti (1992) demonstrated the utility of an innovative approach to the current level of home care and hospital nursing practice in Italy by identifying the strengths and limitations of a practice driven by theory in the current health system.

Work environment. The link between activity and professional autonomy has been the focus for several studies. ISIRI researchers (International Institute of Nursing Research, 1991b) using an exploratory design with a sample of 978 hospital-based nurses, found a predominance of routine activities characterized by a low level of autonomy, difficulties in relationships between nurses and clients, and willingness to participate ever more in the actual organization of work. Cornaglia, Mecca, and Miglioranza (1990), Molinaro et al. (1991), and Mammarella, Mennilli, and Di Renzo (1992) obtained the same results from a surveys of nurses on nephrology and dialysis wards.

In Italy the discussion on "burnout" began in the mid-eighties, but only recently has started to have scientific relevance and basis. Researchers have tried to identify the most frequent causes of such phenomena through analyzing work characteristics, patient/client typology, and demographic and personality characteristics of health workers. Kaldor, Deconi, and Pitacco (1994) and Gattolin, Marangon, Martini, Santinello, and Zannoto (1992) examined the relationship between burnout and job satisfaction, using the Metthews Burnout Scale (Metthews, 1986). Kaldor et al. verified the influence that these factors had on the burnout level of 217 nurses in a pediatric hospital, while Gattolin et al. compared the staff of two intensive care units and one surgical unit.

The consideration of professional risks in a hospital is a recent issue in Italy. In the last few years a number of national and international studies on this subject have been carried out. Buttan et al. (1985) did a retrospective survey between 1972 and 1984 in order to obtain the number and typology of accidents at work, classified by category of health worker. Caspani, Lattarulo, and Mantegazza (1989) examined the causes and the frequency of accidental needlesticks with used needles in a hospital in Legnano between 1984 and 1988. Piccini and Hoffer (1997) evaluated the effects of an educational intervention on the incidence of needlesticks. Viganò, Villa, and Corvi (1994) demonstrated the extent of the risks associated with work in units that use anesthetic gasses. This research led to the introduction of a new preventive model of sanitary supervision which operates according to defined protocols. Randi (1997) surveyed the smoking habits of hospital personnel. The results suggest a larger extension and depth of smoking habits in hospitals then it has been thought. Farina, Morra, and Bruziches-Bruziches (1997) and Capodaglio, Capodaglio, and Bazzini (1997) have both looked into the job risks presented by lifting and positioning. The latter study uses charts, interviews, and video-tapes of nurses to classify and analyze nursing manual activity.

Nursing Roles

In recent years, the Italian nursing profession has made great strides in developing as both a profession and a discipline. One product of these changes is the presence of a university level faculty for a Bachelor's of Nursing Science degree. However, for most nurses in Italy, their professional identity is still strongly linked to the traditional model which gives a dim image of the profession's worth in the schema of health care. A number of researchers have aimed to depict various roles of the nurse, the professional nurse, the nurse-educator, and the nurse-manager.

Sansoni (1991) and Chiari (1982) examined the functions and activities of nurse-educators. Alborghetti (1992), Lolli (1987), and Brandi (1992), through correlational models, analyzed the nurse's professional identity in relation to the organization of care models, basic and continuing education, and current laws governing the profession. Paschini (1985) and Borsarelli (1994) focused their attention on the head nurse's managerial roles, such as direction of personnel, coping with managerial problems, and finding organizational solutions.

Knowledge and Attitudes in Nursing and Society

Of 41 studies, 28 of the samples were nurses and the remaining 13 dealt with the general populace. The majority of studies used convenience sample; only two were experimental. The analysis of data, gathered mainly from anonymous and self-administered questionnaires, generally consists of a description of variables or of a simple calculation of correlation or contingency indexes. Only in the quasi/pre-experimental studies were techniques of inferential data analysis used or reliability of the instruments determined.

Nursing.   Ceroni, Di Furia, Giovanni, Notari, and Orsini (1989) carried out two studies, one on nurses' perception of patients' needs and difficulties encountered in nurse-patient relationships, and the other on patients' perceptions of care received and difficulties encountered in the patient-nurse relationship. Maccari, Ricci, and Valeri (1995) have surveyed nurses' opinions about visitation privileges for parents in UCIC (Intensive Coronary Care Unit) and

ICU wards. They found that, on average, patients are allowed visitors approximately 1.35 hours/day. Their work also revealed that 25% of the nurses surveyed will not give any information out to the family because they believe this to be the doctor's job. Zucchetti (1996), in efforts to evaluate the effects of change on education, utilized a sample of nursing students. The results of this study indicated that student nurses today believe the focus of nursing to be helping relationships, the nursing process, and the increased autonomy of the nurse.

The management of organizational conflicts is one of the most relevant skills for head nurses. Two explorative surveys analyze the frequency of conflictual relations experienced by head nurses and the strategies used to cope with them (Bettiolo et al., 1993; ISIRI, 1991a).

One-quarter of the studies included in this area dealt with the evaluation of nursing staff's knowledge of specific themes and of the existing care situation. Demichelis, Gruppo, and Marchisone (1990) conducted a survey about the sexual abuse of minors and the appropriate intervention of the professional nurse. Vignali et al. (1990) studied the levels of nursing students' knowledge about the rules of hygiene and prevention. Di Mauro (1991) compared knowledge of thalassemia major in newborns in third-year nursing students with that of students of a public secondary school.

Three thousand questionnaires were used to evaluate health care providers' knowledge about general preventive behaviors to adopt and the risks of direct contact with patients' blood (Arduini et al., 1989). Another survey was made of 241 students of nursing in a Milano school to test their knowledge about infections seen concurrently with HIV and to evaluate their direct experience with HIV patients in noninfectious disease wards (Villa et al., 1994). Ferrari, Di Giulio, Franchi, Fiorica, and Tognoni (1982) and Gruppo di Ricerca di Matera (1996) studied the process through which the relationship between therapeutic drugs and nurses is organized and concretely expressed in the profession.

Longhitano, Cavicchioli, and Petrillo (1991) evaluated care processes in the prevention of bedsores. The explorative survey of nurses ($n = 182$) revealed that not all wards applied specific preventive norms. Poletti et al. (1991) conducted a preliminary survey of physicians and nursing staff regarding possible changes in nursing activities in hospital wards and in home care service in Veneto. The statistical indexes obtained suggested that average attitudes toward change were generally positive, although remarkably more so in the community than in hospitals. Physicians, in particular those who were hospital-based, were generally more open to change than nursing staff.

Society.   Two studies have looked further into the issue of how Italian society views transplant issues. Gerbino and Frascotti (1995) assessed the general level of knowledge in the population (*n* = 700) concerning legal ethical, and other aspects of organ donation and transplant. The authors concluded from their information that the lack of correct information in society contributed to an insufficient number of organ donations. Casati, Nicoli, Fiocchi, and Milesi (1994) explored the issue "anonymity" of cardiac transplant donors and their recipients. The aim of this survey was to explore how many cardiac transplant recipients are aware of the identity of their donor, if they had any kind of contact with the family of the donor, and their overall opinion of the law that protects anonymity.

There are two studies that verify clients' knowledge. The first study was conducted by Cirillo et al. (1987), who, noticing the low birthrate of recent years, wanted to test the actual knowledge of a sample population in the city of Milan about contraceptive methods. The aim of the second study (Boglione et al., 1988) evaluated clients' knowledge about health reform and sociosanitary services in a local health district. A secondary aim of the study was to examine clients' knowledge and attitudes toward different modes of gathering information and their validity.

There are many studies which explore the social perception of the professional nurse. A longitudinal study was conducted in Veneto eliciting the views and perceptions that young people have of nursing education and nursing as a profession and on students' main motivations in choosing to enroll in nursing schools (Agostini, Poletti, Zanotti, & Vian, 1989). The results showed that at an earlier stage the major motivations to be a nurse are idealistic and humanitarian, while the social and professional perception of the nurse is poor. The study also explored young persons' reasons for dropping out of nursing school and the perceived positive or negative characteristics of nursing schools among young persons in Veneto.

Sirago (1990) analyzed the inhabitants of Basilicata's perception of the nurse with a randomly chosen sample of 3,422 people. The image obtained was only partly positive. Those interviewed said that they would not choose the profession because of the numerous difficulties. Another study, concerning student's motivation and the role of nursing schools, analyzed a sample of students in Piemonte through a 3-year educational process (Garbolino, 1995). Berto and Taricco (1994) presented their findings using Kelman's theory as framework, which describes the learning process as characterized by compliance, identification, and internalization. However, the authors did not provide references about the framework.

Pessina (1996) used a self-administered questionnaire to study consumers' (*n* = 320) level of satisfaction with accessibility to their provider, quality of health care provided, and level of relationship with their general practitioner.

A multivariate analysis showed that relationships existed between satisfaction levels and age of client and frequency of use of provider services. The author concluded from the information that the overall relationship between the general practitioner and the client is the critical issue perceived by users.

EVALUATION AND FUTURE DIRECTION

To date, nursing research in Italy has focused most of its energies in the clinical area, particularly in evaluating the quality of care and care for the chronically ill. Another major focus has been systems analyses of varying hospital, day care, and healthcare organizations. The majority of the research, by far, is still limited in its sophistication, utilizing most often data gathered through various survey methods. Most other studies are descriptive and omit the manipulation of any variables. Studies that did entail interventions were usually involving some type of patient education and the measurement of effects with a pre-post test design. Statistics that venture beyond the basic descriptive are rare.

Much of the current research is being carried out by nurses who have little or no research training. It has only been since 1994 that nurses with advanced education in research (i.e., PhDs) have begun to enter the healthcare market in Italy. Important now for the development of research in nursing is the continued education of student and practicing nurses in the process and value of research. In order for this to happen, nurses with clinical and academic expertise must continue to pursue higher degrees in order to supply the discipline with the much-needed source of this training. Areas of research that emphasize and validate both nursing's current role and potential contribution to the care of patients in the form of experimental and quasi-experimental outcome studies are essential for the continued growth of nursing as a profession in the healthcare system among its peers and colleagues.

Currently there is a growing movement to restructure and redefine the role of the nursing profession within Italian society and its healthcare system. This is partly the result of the changes taking place that have been discussed in this chapter. It is anticipated that the turn of the century will hold many new opportunities and challenges for nursing in Italy. Over the next 10–20 years, given the better opportunities provided by an increased educational level and more funding from the European Commission for research, Italian nurse researchers will make a significant contribution to the growth of nursing scientific knowledge at national and international levels.

REFERENCES

Acquafredda, V., Cuccu, G., Fassina, G., Fassi, D., Fontana, M., Liistro, I., Gazzetti, A., Liber, A. M., Fabbro, G. M., Paladino, S., Papico, C., Padico, G., Ricotta, A., Ronchi, R., & Tommasini, P. (1987). Livelli di assistenza e carichi di lavoro in un reparto di medicina [Care levels and work loads in a medical unit]. *Rivista dell'Infermiere, 2,* 91–101.

Agostini, A., Poletti, P., Zanotti, R., & Vian, F. (1989). Perchè si iscrivono alla Scuola per Infermieri? [Why do students enroll in a school of nursing?]. *Rivista dell'Infermiere, 1,* 28–29.

Alborghetti, A. (1992). Indagine sull'identità professionale dell'infermiere in rapporto alla riorganizzazione dei modelli assistenziali nelle unità di degenza [Enquiry on the nurse's professional identity in relation with the re-organization of care models in hospitals]. *Professioni Infermieristiche, 45*(2), 36–46.

Ambrogio, U., & Gori, C. (1997). Bisogni degli anziani e assistenza domiciliare [Needs of the elderly and home care]. *Prospettive Sociali e Sanitarie, 15–16,* 14–19.

Andreoli, G. B., Cirigliano, F., Gabutti, G., Flego, G., Forte, C., Mentore, B., & Pietrantoni, C. D. (1997). La tubercolosi in ospedale: Studio delle caratteristiche dei ricoverati in un ospedale genovese nel periodo 1990–1995 [Tuberculosis in the hospital: A study of the characteristics of hospitalized patients in a Genova hospital from 1990–1995]. *Quaderni ANIPIO, 10,* 13–18.

Apostoli, M., Fenotti, A., Bravo, M., Archetti, A. M., Magazza, A. R., Pedersoli, F., Cosio, R., Zappa, S., & Candiani, A. (1988). Osservazioni sull'epidemiologia e la profilassi delle lesioni da decubito in rianimazione [Observations on the epidemiology and on prophylaxis of bedsores in the intensive care unit]. *Rivista dell'Infermiere, 1,* 18–22.

Arciero, L., Denti, M., Franchi, S., Gallani, D., Ghezzi, L., Mottola, E., & Toscani, F. (1993). Malato oncologico terminale ospedalizzato e privacy: Bisogni del paziente e percezione da parte dell'infermiere professionale [The terminal oncological patient in the hospital and his privacy: Patients' needs and nurses' perception]. *Rivista dell'Infermiere, 1,* 8–15.

Arduini, L., Di Giulio, P., Franchi, M., Nebuloni, G., Pianosi, G., Sisti, P., Torre, L. D., Valioni, V., & Ottone, M. (1989). Indagine campionaria in sei ospedali lombardi sulle conoscenze possedute dagli infermieri sui rischi associati alla esposizione accidentale al sangue dei pazienti [Sample survey in six hospitals in Lombardia on nurses' knowledge about risks caused by casual exposure to patients' blood]. *Rivista dell'Infermiere, 2,* 84–92.

Bagnis, C., Gabella, P., Gigliotti, E., Mariano, C., Petrosino, G., Poggio, G., & Ramondetti, A. (1996). Dialisi peritoneale automatizzata: É ancora una schiavitù dell'uomo dalla macchina? [Automated peritoneal dialysis: Is man still enslaved to machine?]. *Infermiere Formazione, 3*(1), 16–17.

Bedendo, M., Marchetto, S., & Stievano, A. (1986). L'organizzazione di un centro antidiabetico [The organization of an anti-diabetic center]. *Rivista dell'Infermiere, 4,* 208–216.

Bedin, M., Bergamin, I., Bertolini, P., Onestini, C., Piazza, L., Rotini, M., Silvestri, C., Lacquaniti, L., Carraro, R., & Verlato, R. (1988). Ricerca sulla realtà Italiana delle terapie intensive [Research on the Italian situation of intensive therapies]. *Scenario, 3,* 31–34.

Berto, P., & Taricco, M. (1994). L'influenza della scuola per infermieri professionali sull' apprendimento degli allievi [The influence of a professional nursing school on students' learning]. *Infermiere Informazione, 9*(1), 7–27.

Bertolotto, N. R., Biagi, S., Burlando, S., & Olcese, S. (1996). Relazione infermiere parente in una rianimazione aperta [Relationship between nurse and relatives in a critical care open unit]. *Scenario, 4,* 24–29.

Bertoni, B., & Coato, L. (1994). Gli allievi infermieri e l'evento morte: Una ricerca sui vissuti e sui bisogni di formazione [Nursing students and death: A research on experiences and education needs]. *Rivista dell'Infermiere, 13,* 153–156.

Bettiolo, E., Coccato, P., Fanelli, L., Lucato, O., Rigo, D., & Santinello, M. (1993). Caposala e conflitti [Head nurse and conflicts]. *Rivista dell'Infermiere, 12,* 85–90.

Bianchet, A., Camerin, F., Cancian, P., Candusso, M., Copetti, S., Jus, C., Pasquon, L., Rangan, D., Schiratti, C., Trazzini, C., Lattuada, L., & Urli, N. (1993). Indagine sulle condizioni di vita dell'anziano nella realtà del Sandanielese [Survey on the life conditions of elderly people in the San Daniele area]. *Professioni Infermieristiche, 46*(2), 43–48.

Biancoli, S., Carletti, N., Gulini, C., Quercia, D., Raspadori, C., Zecchin, L., Gentili, A., Mungo, G., Grossi, G., Nastasi, M., & Gelli, G. F. (1989). La canulazione venosa centrale: Metodiche di nursing e prevenzione delle complicanze infettive [The central venous canulisation: Nursing methodologies and prevention of infectious complications]. In *VIII ANIARTI National Congress: Man and the critical area* (pp. 217–220). Bologna, Italy: ANIARTI.

Boccagni, F., Prencipe, M., Ravelli, A., & Trecate, F. (1991). Oltre la dipendenza: I risultati di un'analisi in un reparto di lungodegenza per anziani [Beyond dependence: The results of an analysis in a long stay ward for elderly people]. *Prospettive Sociali e Sanitarie, 2,* 12–14.

Boglione, M., Di Sanza, M., Paradiso, S., Saglione, G., Testo, S., Tuninetti, T., & Verzino, E. (1988). Conoscenza ed utilizzo dei servizi socio-sanitari: Indagine sulla popolazione del distretto di Racconigi [Knowledge and use of social and health services: Study on the population of the Racconigi district]. *Infermiere Informazione, 3*(1), 26–29.

Bonannini, S., Mannelli, G., Guizzotti, S., Montini, A., Manfredi, S. G., & Arcangeli, A. (1996). Prodotti di pasticceria per diabetici: Una possibile alternativa [Sweets for diabetics: A possible alternative]. *Il Diabete & l'Infermiere, 4,* 95–96.

Borsarelli, L. (1994). Orientamento dell'A.F.D. nella realtà lavorativa: Proposta di un modello per il settore ospedaliero [A.F.D's orientation in work situations: A proposal for a hospital area model]. In *Ricerca Professionale Infermieristica: Vol. 16. Education Series* (pp. 186–192). Veneto Region, Italy: Regional Committee, Health Council Department.

Borsarelli, L., Galizio, M., Pastorutti, V., Schirru, M. A., & Vittone, T. (1994). Indagine conoscitiva sull'organizzazione e la gestione del personale afferente all'ufficio dell'operatore professionale dirigente [An exploratory survey of the organization and management of personnel under the supervision of the professional manager]. *Infermiere Informazione, 9*(8), 4–27.

Bovino, A., & Zanotti, R. (1985). Un'indagine sull'impegno informativo degli operatori infermieristici [An inquiry on nursing workers' educational engagement]. *Rivista dell'Infermiere, 4,* 140–151.

Brandi, A. (1990). Strategie e metodi di valutazione della qualità dell'assistenza: Studio della incidenza delle infezioni urinarie nei pazienti sottoposti a cateterismo vescicale [Methods and strategies of assessing care quality: A study on the frequency of urinary infections in patients with a vesical catheter]. *Professioni Infermieristiche, 43*(2), 36–40.

Brandi, A. (1991). Organizzazione e analisi del lavoro. Le mansioni improprie nelle attività infermieristiche [Organization and work analysis. Improper functions in nursing activities]. *Professioni Infermieristiche, 44*(2), 35–43.

Brandi, A. (1992). Ruolo formale e sostanziale dell'infermiere: Quale lo scostamento. In ANIARTI *Responsabilità dell'Infermiere Professionale: Proceedings of the XI National Congress* (pp. 53–59). Firenze, Italy: *Scenario, 2,* 53–59.

Brivio, E., & Gamba, A. (1989). Efficacia e difficoltà in un programma di assistenza domiciliare per i pazienti con cancro in fase avanzata [Efficiency and difficulties of a home care program for patients with advanced cancer]. *Rivista dell'Infermiere, 8,* 190–196.

Brosolo, A., Constatini, O., Gallo, C., Pozzobon, A., Cecchetto, A., Bacchion, G., & Rosato, L. (1989). Organizzazione di un gruppo di lavoro per la prevenzione delle lesioni da decubito [Organization of a work group for prevention of bed-sores]. *Rivista dell'Infermiere, 4,* 179–189.

Buttan, R., Fanari, F., Fronteddu, G., Meroni, A., Pecora, C., & Pierazzi, D. (1985). Gli infortuni sul lavoro in ospedale: Indagine nell'ospedale Fatebenefratelli e Oftalmico di Milano [Work accidents in hospital. Inquiry on Fatebenefratelli and Oftalmico hospitals in Milan]. *Rivista dell'Infermiere, 4,* 195–201.

Buzzai, P., Gasparini, M., Glavina, S., Lenhard, S., & Sema, L. G. (1991). Le cadute evitabili dei pazienti ricoverati in ospedale [The avoidable falls of hospitalized patients]. *QA, 4/5,* 46–49.

Capodaglio, E. M., Capodaglio, P., & Bazzini, G. (1997). Una valutazione ergonomica del carico fisico dell'attività infermieristica [An ergonomic evaluation of the physical load of nurses' activities]. *Nursing Oggi, 3,* 23–30.

Caron, R., Florianello, F., & Oltolina,V. (1992). Ecco come affrontare l'assistenza quando le corsie si tingono d'argento [How to face care when wards are grey-coloured]. *L'Infermiere, 36*(4), 57–65.

Casati, M., Nicoli, M. T., Fiocchi, R., & Milesi, M. I. (1994). Indagine sugli aspetti relazionali tra il soggetto trapiantato di cuore e la famiglia del donatore [A study of the relationship between the patients who have undergone a heart transplantation and the donor's family]. *Rivista dell'Infermeire, 2,* 66–69.

Caspani, P., Lattarulo, R., & Mantegazza, T. (1989). Punture accidentali con aghi usati: Cinque anni di osservazioni in un ospedale lombardo [Accidental sticks with used needles: Five years of observations in a hospital in Lombardia]. *Rivista dell'Infermiere, 8,* 142–144.

Cavestri, R., Buontempi, L., Arreghini, M., Laviola, F., Mazza, P., Tognoni, G., Roncaglioni, C., & Longhini, E. (1996). Accesso alle risorse riabilitative in una popolazione ospedaliera non selezionata di pazienti con ictus in fase acuta [Access to rehabilitation programs for acute phase stroke patients not selected for therapy]. *Rivista dell'infermiere, 15,* 184–189.

Cecchetto, D. G. (1995). Epidemiologia della routine assistenziale: Dati e ipotesi a partire da una lungodegenza per anziani [The epidemiology of routine assistance: The resulting data and a hypothesis based on a long stay unit for elderly patients]. *Rivista dell'Infermiere, 14,* 173–179.

Ceroni, C., Di Furia, G., Giovanni, D., Notari, & Orsini, B. (1989). Rapportarsi ai pazienti: Valenza e significato delle abilità sociali nel nursing [Referring to patients: Valence and meaning of nursing social abilities]. *Rivista dell'Infermiere, 1,* 6–11.

Chiari, P. (1982). L'infermiere insegnante: Risultati e implicazioni di un ricerca su 31 scuole della regione Lombardia [The nurse who teaches: Results and implications of a study of 31 schools in Lombardia]. *Rivista dell'Infermiere, 1,* 61–70.

Cirillo, R., Okely, F., Orlandi, C., Pisoni, L., Stefanizzi, L., Zandona, S., Zanotto, G., & Zanni, R. (1987). La diffusione delle conoscenze sui metodi contraccettivi [The diffusion of knowledge about contraceptive methods]. *Rivista dell'Infermiere, 3,* 172–180.

Collareda, G., Gomitolo, O., Pellizzari, G., Corradin, H., & Erle, G. (1995). L'assistenza domiciliare al diabetico nell'ambito del progetto-obiettivo: Progetto pilota integrato per la tutela della salute del diabetico, Regione Veneto [Home care for diabetics: An integrated pilot project to keep diabetics healthy, conducted in the Veneto region]. *Rivista dell'Infermiere, 14,* 131–137.

Colli, R., & Mazzitelli, C. (1987). Tirocinio: Un intervento di educazione alimentare svolto nelle scuole elementari [Training: Educational intervention on learning in some elementary schools]. *Professioni Infermieristiche, 40*(2), 122–137.

Cornaglia, M., Mecca, G. M., & Miglioranza, E. (1990). Professioni in crisi: Indagine tra gli infermieri delle dialisi in Piemonte e Valle d'Aosta [A profession in crisis: A survey of dialysis nurses in Piemonte e Valle d'Aost]. In *EDTNA (European Nursing Dialysis and Transplant Association) and ERCA (European Renal Care Association). Proceedings from the Ninth National Meeting* (pp. 11–23). Genova: EDTNA-ERCA.

Cosi, A. (1997). L'ansia nei bambini sottoposti ad intervento di chirurgia elettiva: Indagine descrittiva [The anxiety of children undergoing elective surgery: A descriptive study]. *Rivista dell'infermiere, 16,* 144–150.

Cossu, S., Costantini, D., Didone, I., Fabiani, P., Massa, M., Triulzi, M., & Zunino, C. (1988). L'organizzazione di un Day Hospital [The organization of a day hospital]. *Rivista dell'Infermiere, 7,* 81–87.

Cultural Nursing Association of Catanzaro. (1992). Le conoscenze sulla terapia farmacologica di un gruppo di infermieri calabresi [The knowledge of pharmacological therapy of a group of nurses from Calabria]. *Rivista dell'Infermiere, 11,* 71–80.

D'Andrea, N., Tamburlini, G., Tonchella, C., Sione, M. G., Petrina, D., Perobelli, S., Mastella, G., Paldan, A., Tettamanti, A., Codamo, T., & Parente, C. (1988). Organizzazione e rapporti di lavoro nel reparto pediatrico [Organization and working relationships in a pediatric ward]. *Rivista dell'Infermiere, 3,* 135–142.

Deana, P., Baldassi, C., Fiorino, M. R., Lacuzzi, E., Pavan, A., Tat, L., & Liva, C. (1993). Uso di un dispositivo per lo spostamento dei pazienti allettati [Utilisation of a transport device for bed ridden-patients]. *Q.A., 1–2,* 43–45.

Dellai, M., & Zampieron, A. (1996). I giovani e l'obesita: Diffusione del fenomeno e comportamento alimentare negli studenti della scuola infermieri [Childhood obesity: The spreading of the phenomenon and eating behavior of nursing students]. *Il Diabete & l'Infermiere, 4,* 21–28.

Delli, R. (1994). Studio trasversale retrospettivo sul servizio di assistenza infermieristica domiciliare nel distretto di Empoli [A cross-sectional retrospective study on the home care service in the district of Empoli]. *Professioni Infermieristiche, 47*(2), 7–16.

Demichelis, O., Gruppo, A., & Marchisone, D. (1990). Abuso sessuale: Indagine sulla conoscenza del fenomeno e dei possibili interventi dell'infermiere professionale [Sexual abuse: A study on the information about the phenomenon and on the possible interventions of the nurse]. *Professioni Infermieristiche, 43*(1), 26–28.

Deriu, P. (1997). L'analsi organizzativa con il metodo delle congruenze: Sperimentazione in Piemonte [An organizational analysis using the congruence method: An experiment in Piemonte]. *Nursing Oggi, 2,* 38–45.

Di Cristofano, A. (1989b). Prevenzione delle malattie allergiche in neonati a rischio [Preventions of allergic illnesses in newborns at risk]. *Professioni Infermieristiche, 42*(1), 17–23.

Di Cristofano, A. (1989a). La vaccinazione contro il morbillo in bambini allergici all'uovo [Measles vaccination in children who are allergic to eggs]. *Professioni Infermieristiche, 42*(1), 24–30.

Di Giulio, F. (1988). Carichi di lavoro e fabbisogno di personale infermieristico in un Day Hospital [Work loads and need of nursing personnel in a Oncology Day Hospital]. *Rivista dell'Infermiere, 7,* 23–30.

Di Mauro, A. (1991). Confronto di conoscenze sulla Thalassemia tra un gruppo di studenti della scuola media inferiore degli allievi del III anno della provincia di Siracusa [Knowledge about the Conemia in nursing students versus high school students]. In: *Ricerca Professionale Infermieristica: Vol. 14. Education series* (pp. 527–531). Veneto Region, Italy: Regional Committee, Health Council Department.

Fanton, S., & Zanotti, R. (1992). La formazione al ragionamento diagnostico [Diagnostic reasoning education]. *Salute e Territorio, 81,* 57–60.

Farina, L., Morra, M. R., & Bruziches-Bruziches, D. (1997). La prevenzione dei rischi lavorativi [The prevention of work-related risks]. *Professioni Infermieristiche, 50*(3), 37–43.

Ferrari, F., Di Giulio, P., Franchi, M. A., Fiorica, E., & Tognoni, G. (1982). Conoscenza e pratica della terapia farmacologica [Knowledge and practice of the pharmacological therapy]. *Rivista dell'Infermiere, 3,* 138–148.

Fiorni, A., Manzoli, N., Forlani, M., Bertelli, S., Bonazzi, M., Orlandi, B., Passarelli, R., Gamberoni, L., Gaiani, R., Polesinanti, C., & Soffritti, A. (1994). Efficienza ed efficacia infermieristica in endoscopia digestiva il parere dell'utenza in una indagine conoscitiva mediante questionario [Nursing efficiency and efficacy in digestive endoscopy: A questionnaire based study on client's opinions]. *Professioni Infermieristiche, 47*(1), 30–32.

Garbolino, I. B. (1995). Dall'analisi organizzative alla valutazione del fabbisogno di assistenza infermieristica nel DRG 430 (psicosi): Progetto di ricerca in tre S.P.D.C. della regione Piemonte [From organizational analysis to nurse care needs, assessment of DRG 430 (psychosis): A research project in three S.P.D.C. of the Piemonte region]. *L'Infermiere Dirigente, 2*, 25–48.

Gattolin, F., Marangon, M., Martini, F., Santinello, M., & Zannoto, R. (1992). Stress e lavoro infermieristico. Confronto dei livelli di burnout tra reparti chirurgici e di terapia intensiva [Stress and nursing work: Comparison between burnout levels in surgical wards and intensive care units]. *Rivista dell'Infermiere, 1*, 10–14.

Geatti, S. (1993). L'organizzazione del servizio infermieristico nei centri dialisi in Italia [The organization of nursing service in Italian dialysis centers]. *Rivista dell'Infermiere, 12*, 235–244.

Gerbino, P., & Frascotti, A. (1995). Opinione pubblica e trapianti: I risultati di un'indagine [Public opinion and transplants: The results of a study]. *Rivista dell'infermiere, 14*, 67–70.

Ghizzoni, A. M., & Agostino, M. B. (1996). Indagine conoscitiva sul docente infermiere nei corsi di diploma universitari in scienze infermieristiche [An explorative survey of nurse-teachers at a university-based diploma school of nursing]. *Professioni Infermieristiche, 49*(3), 41–52.

Grazia, L. & Pozzi, A. (1990). La C.A.P.D. nell'anziano: problematiche assistenza e sociali [C.A.P.D. with the elderly: Caring and social problems]. In *EDTNA (European Nursing Dialysis and Transplant Association) and ERCA (European Renal Care Association). Proceedings from the Ninth National Meeting Proceedings from the Ninth National Meeting* (pp. 31–36). Genoa: EDNTA-ERCA.

Gruppo infermieri Ospedale S. Carlo-Milano. (1990). Carichi di lavoro ed organico di reparto [Work loads and ward staffing]. *Q.A., 1*, 44–53.

Gruppo di Ricerca di Matera. (1996). Epidemiologia dell'ansia in ospedale. *Rivista dell'Infermiere, 15*, 83–87.

International Institute of Nursing Research. (1991a). Caposala e relazioni interpersonali [The head nurse and interpersonal relationships]. In *Ricerca Professionale infermieristica: Vol. 14. Education series* (pp. 481–482). Veneto Region, Italy: Regional Committee, Health Council Department.

International Institute of Nursing Research. (1991b). Una indagine sulla operativitá degli infermieri nel Veneto [Nursing system in Veneto]. In *Ricerca Professionale infermieristica: Vol. 14. Education series* (pp. 465–466). Veneto Region, Italy: Regional Committee, Health Council Department.

Kaldor, K., Deconi, O., & Pitacco, G. (1994). Indagine sui livelli di burnout del personale inferieristico in un ospedale pediatrico [Inquiry on nursing personnel's burnout levels in a pediatric hospital]. *Scenario, 2*, 40–51.

Lolli, A. (1987). Ricerca sull'identità professionale dell'infermiere: Analisi di uno dei possibili agenti di cambiamento: La formazione permanente [Research on the identity of the professional nurse. Analysis of a possible change agent: Continuing education]. *Professioni Infermieristiche, 40*(4), 338–342.

Lombardo, S. (1991). Utilizzo degli infermieri nei servizi sanitari pubblici [Nurses' employment in the public health service]. *L'Infermiere, 35*(3–4), 73–81.

Longhitano, E., Cavicchioli, A., & Petrillo, C. (1991). Valutazione del processo assistenziale per la prevenzione ed il trattamento delle lesioni da decubito: Approccio metodologico [Evaluation of a care process to prevent and treat bedsores: A methodological approach]. *Q.A., 3,* 46–52.

Maccari, C., Ricci, F., & Valeri, A. (1995). Terapie intensive e rianimazioni: Le visite ai pazienti ricoverati [Intensive care and reanimation Units: The visits to the patients]. *Rivista dell'infermiere, 14,* 125–130.

Mammarella, L., Mennilli, S., & Di Renzo, M. (1992). Condizioni di lavoro e di vita del personale infermieristico nei centri di Nefrologia e Dialisi della Regione Abruzzo [Nursing personnel's work and life conditions in nephrologic and dialysis centres in Abruzzo]. *Professioni Infermieristiche, 45*(3), 23–30.

Mannocci, A. (1987). Il lavoro infermieristico per piccole équipe di assistenza: Un' esperienza organizzativa in ambito ospedaliero [Nursing work for small care teams: An organizational experience in a hospital]. *Salute e Territorio, 57,* 61–63.

Marchini, M., Zanzani, G., Bernardi, R., Antimi, C., Morri, S., Cupioli, M., Fastosi, G., Cappella, P., Cangini, G., Ronconi, C., Bartoletti, A., & Casadei, M. (1989). L'assistenza familiare per la prevenzione dei disturbi comportamentali dell'anziano ricoverato in una unità di terapia intensiva cardiologica [Family's assistance to prevent behavioural disturbances of age patients in a cardiology intensive care unit]. *VIII National Congress: Man and the critical area* (pp. 91–96). Firenze, Italy: ANIARTI.

Mariotto, A., Bonavina, M. G., Favarett, C., Haymar d'Ettory, R., Castoro, M., & Padovan, M. (1992). Monitoraggio delle cadute dei pazienti per la valutazione della qualità dell'assistenza: Studio prospettico nell'ospedale di Padova [Monitoring of patients' falls in order to evaluate the quality of care: A prospective survey in the hospital of Padova]. *Q A, 4/5,* 43–47.

Martini, G., & Pigato, G. (1987). Le infusioni venose nell'assistenza infermieristica [Venous infusions in nursing]. *Rivista dell'Infermiere, 6,* 10–19.

Masera, G., Tognoni, G., Jankovic, M., Adamoli, L., Corbetta, A., Fraschini, D., Labrozzi, D., Giulio, P. D., Lia, R., Pertici, S., & Riboldi, D. (1996). La valutazione della soddisfazione delle famiglie in oncologia pediatrica [The evaluation of families' satisfaction in the pediatric oncology unit]. *Rivista dell'Infermiere, 15,* 5–13.

Mele, M. G. (1987). L'informazione ai genitori di bambini pretermine: L'esperienza in una clinica universitaria [Information to parents of prematurely-born babies: The experience of a university clinic]. *Professioni Infermieristiche, 40*(2), 138–156.

Metthews, D. B. (1986). *Metthews Burnout Scale for employees.* Orangeburg, SC: State College.

Milan, R., & Targa, M. T. (1992). Vivere la morte in ospedale [Experience death in a hospital]. *Rivista dell'Infermiere, 4,* 206–211.

Milan, S., Bernardinello, M. E., Bedendo, M., Chiarion, L., Capitozzo, M., Lippi, C., Marchetto, S., Perari, D., & Stievano, A. (1989). Proposta di verifica del ruolo educativo dell'infermiere professionale con il paziente diabetico [Evaluation proposal on the educative role of professional nurses with diabetic patients]. *Rivista dell'Infermiere, 2,* 93–103.

Mislej, M. (1984). Le lezioni di educazione sanitaria come interazione delle conoscenze-esperienze del singolo e del gruppo e le conoscenze teoriche sull'argomento [Lessons on health education seen as a knowledge-experience interaction of an individual or a group, and the theoretical knowledge on this subject]. *Professioni Infermieristiche, 37*(2), 97–100.

Molinaro, C., Martini, S., Sacchetti, S., Lucchetti, G. L., Mastini, M., Bracci, L., & Torelli, R. (1991). Problemi di interazioni personali in un centro di dialisi [Personal interaction problems in a dialysis center]. In *EDTNA (European Nursing Dialysis and Transplant Association) and ERCA (European Renal Care Association): Proceedings from the Tenth National Meeting* (pp. 19–29). Genova: EDTNA-ERCA.

Monesi, G., Marchetto, S., Chiarion, L., Manunta, R., Stievano, A., Perari, D., Lipi, C., Mollo, F., & Lisato, G. (1992). Intervento educativo di gruppo sul piede diabedico: Obiettivi, strategie pedagogiche, contenuti di conoscenza, risultati [A group educational intervention on the diabetic foot: Objectives, pedagogic strategies, knowledge and results]. *Rivista dell'Infermiere, 2,* 81–88.

Moro, F., & Spangaro, S. (1994). Monitoraggio della terapia eparinica endovenosa dopo trombosi: É possibile una gestione infermieristica? [Monitoring on the endovenous heparin therapy after thrombolysis: Is a nursing management possible?]. *Rivista dell'Infermiere, 8,* 190–196.

Nebuloni, G. (1986). L'anziano ospedalizzato: Problemi e proposte [The hospitalized elderly: Problems and proposals]. *Rivista dell'Infermiere, 5,* 232–236.

Nicastri, N., Poletti, P., Torsello, C. T., & Vian, F. (1991). Infermiere e lingua inglese: Bisogni e risposta [Nurse and English language: Need and answers]. In: *Ricerca Professionale Infermieristica: Vol. 14. Education series* (pp. 264–271). Veneto Region, Italy: Regional Committee, Health Council Department.

Paschini, P. (1985). Studio del metodo direzionale dei capisala [Study of the head nurse's directive method]. *Professioni Infermieristiche, 38*(1), 37–40.

Pasquot, L. (1986). Cartella infermieristica computerizzata [Informatics and nursing: Computerized nursing file]. *Professioni Infermieristiche, 39*(4), 386–374.

Pegoraro, C., & Bertarelli, P. (1995). La qualità assistenziale ai fini di un ottimale reinserimento sociale della persona sottoposta a trapianto [The quality of care received by post-transplant patients reintegrating into social life]. *Scenario, 3,* 43–46.

Pegoraro, C., & Bertarelli, P. (1996). La valutazione della qualità di vita da parte della persona sottoposta a trapianto di fegato [An evaluation of the quality of life of liver transplant patients]. *Nursing Oggi, 2,* 18–22.

Pessina, G. (1996). La qualita percepita dall'utente nella medicina di base: Valutazione dell'accessibilità e del gradimento della popolazione afferente ai Servizi Sanitari di base del mandamento di S. Vito al Tagliamento [Perceived quality by consumers of community services: An evaluation of accessibility and satisfaction in the S. Vito al Tagliamento area]. *QA, 7,* 171–178.

Piccini, G., & Hoffer, C. (1997). Rifiuti in ospedale: Sicurezza dei lavoratori [Waste disposal in the hospital: Workers safety]. *Rivista dell'Infermiere, 16,* 12–14.

Piras, A., & Sansoni, J. (1997). Quali sono i disagi riferiti alla sfera sessuale vissuti dagli anziani istituzionalizzati e quali sono le conoscenze del problema da parte degli operatori di assistenza? [Institutionalized elderly person's discomfort about sexuality and caregivers' knowledge of the problem]. *Professioni Infermieristiche, 50*(1), 15–20.

Poletti, P., Vian, F., & Zanotti, R. (1991). Gli atteggiamenti di infermieri e medici nei confronti del piano di nursing [Nurses and physicians' attitudes toward the nursing process]. In *Ricerca professionale infermieristica: Vol. 14. Education series* (pp. 130–138). Veneto Region, Italy: Regional Committee, Health Council Department.

Poletti, P., & Vian, F. (1986). Informazione informatica per la formazione e la ricerca nel nursing [Information and informatics for nursing education and research]. In *Informazione Informatica e Nursing. Vol. 5. Education series.* Veneto Region, Italy: Regional Committee, Health Council Department.

Poletti, P., & Vian, F. (1992). *Il sistema infermieristico Veneto [The nursing system in Veneto]: Vol. 16. Education series.* Veneto Region, Italy: Regional Committee, Health Council Department.

Poletti, P., Vian, F., Vittadello, F., & Zanotti, R. (1994a). Insegnare metodologia della ricerca e statistica nelle scuole infermieri: Prima parte [Teaching research methods and statistics in nursing schools: Part one]. *Rivista dell'Infermiere, 13*(3), 144–152.

Poletti, P., Vian, F., Vittadello, F., & Zanotti, R. (1994b). Insegnare metodologia della ricerca e statistica nelle scuole infermieri: Seconda parte [Teaching research methods nd statistics in nursing schools: Part two]. *Rivista dell'Infermiere, 13*(4), 228–242.

Poletti, P., & Zanotti, R. (1992). La formazione permanente degli infermieri educatori [Continuing education for nurse teachers]. *Salute e Territorio, 81,* 42–46.

Preiata, L. (1986). I problemi psico-emotivi e sociali dei malati in situazione critica [The psycho-emotional and social problems of people in critical situations]. *Scenario, 4,* 7–15.

Proli, A. (1997). Verifica della concordanza tra gli operatori sanitari di un pronto soccorso nell'assegnazione dei codici di priorità (triage) [A comparison of triage evaluations between professionals of an emergency room]. *Rivista dell'Infermiere, 1,* 8–10.

Randi, M. (1997). Indagine rivolta ad analizzare l'abitudine al fumo in operatori sanitari ospedalieri [A survey analyzing the smoking habits of hospital personnel]. *Professioni Infermieristiche, 50*(1), 25–30.

Rasero, L., Errico, A., & Bertelli, A. (1997). Misure per la prevenzione delle complicanze infettive in pazienti sottoposti a trapianto di midollo osseo [Measures for preventing infection in bone marrow transplants]. *Rivista dell'Infermiere, 16*, 139–143.

Rasero, L., Errico, A., Puccetti, M., & Tellarini, G. (1996). Ruolo delle pratiche igieniche personali nella prevenzione degli episodi infettivi nel trapianto di midollo osseo autologo [The role of personal hygiene procedures in preventing infection in autologous bone marrow transplant patients]. *Rivista dell'Infermiere, 15*, 127–130.

Ricci, A., Suzzi, R., Bassi, N., Corazza, G., & Rainaldi, F. (1996). Smaltimento dei rifiuti organici: Introduzione di un nuovo sistema monouso [The disposal of organic waste: The introduction of a new method of waste disposal]. *Quaderni ANIPIO, 4*, 9–19.

Roggi, D. (1987). L'emergenza extraospedaliera [Extra-hospital emergency]. *Scenario, 2*, 11–19.

Rolando, S., Pizzo, L., Caratti, G. P., Materossi, L., Lazzarin, A., Salvatico, M. T., Porro, G., Borghino, L., Tedde, A. R., Mari, S., Castagna, G., Favata, L., Negrini, N., Obinu, G., & Tavellin, G. (1992). Le infezioni ospedaliere in terapia intensiva: Un problema, un indicatore per valutare la qualità dell'assistenza [Infections in intensive care units: Problem and an indicator of quality of care]. *Infermiere Informazione, 7*(5), 187–192.

Sabbadin, S., Caon, C., Giacometti, R., Lavezzo, P., & Volpato, A. (1991). Sperimentazione del modello "Bisugni" per la diagnose infermie ristica: a) Div. Neurologica castelfranco; b) Div. Neurologica roviga [Sperimentation of the model "Human Needs" for nursing diagnosis in : a) Neurological ward of Castelfranco; b) Neurological word of Rovipa]. In *Ricerche Professionale Infermieristica, 16*, 323–331.

Sacco, M. P., & Renis, F. (1997). Indagine sulla soddisfazione degli utenti del pronto soccorso psichiatrico del Policlinico di Bari [The satisfaction of patients receiving emergency psychiatric care at Policlinic d'Bari]. *Prospettive Sociali e Sanitarie, 21*, 11–16.

Salmaso, L., Scaggiante, R., Cadrobbi, P., Orsini, A., & Favaretti, C. (1992). AIDS: Razionalizzare e umanizzare i servizi [AIDS: An enumeration and rationing of the facilities]. *Prospettive Sociali e Sanitarie, 2*, 8–14.

Sansoni, J. (1991). Il dirigente dell'assistenza: Insegnante o dirigente? [Care managers: Teachers or managers?]. In *Ricerca Professionale Infermieristica: Vol. 14. Education series* (pp. 252–257). Veneto Region, Italy: Regional Committee, Health Council Department.

Sirago, B. (1990). Percezione che i cittadini hanno della figura infermieristica [Citizens' perceptions of nurses]. *Professioni Infermieristiche, 43*(4), 28–29.

Spada, P. A., Bonfoco, E., Bonzi, E., Boscolo, M., & Giroletti, A. (1991). Indagine descrittiva dei dati essenziali delle strutture di area critica della Regione Lombardia [Descriptive survey on the structure of the critical area's essential data, in Lombardia]. *Scenario, 4*, 10–16.

Sposito, D., Ringo, D., & Villani, S. (1989). Studio di incidenza dei traumi cranici dopo l'applicazione della legge sull'obbligatorietà dell'uso del casco [A study of the incidence of head trauma after the institution of a law making helmet use mandatory]. *Scenario, 1,* 12–14.

Torre, R. (1994). Test multicentrico sul primo disostruttore per tubi endotracheali [Multicentre test on the first disobstruent for endo-tracheal tubes]. *Scenario, 2,* 9–13.

Tosco, S. (1997). Carichi di lavoro: Opportunità di confronto [Workload: Opportunity for comparison]. *Nursing Oggi, 2,* 22–30.

Viganó, G., Villa, L., & Corvi, C. (1994). Infortuni in ospedale e sorveglianza del rischio da gas anestetici: Un modello di prevenzione [Accidents in hospital and control of anaesthetic gas risks: A prevention model]. *Infermiere Informazione, 9*(94), 4–13.

Vignali, A., Grifone, M., Di Renzo, P. M., Mammarella, L., Zuppini, C., & Di Giuseppe, D. (1990). Scuola e salute: La salute nelle scuole per infermiere professionale della Provincia di Chieti [School and health: Health in nursing schools of Chieti]. *Professioni Infermieristiche, 43*(1), 23–28.

Villa, A., DeGobbis, M., Capuzzi, M., Esposito, A., Zanotto, G., & Confalonieri, F. (1994). Conoscenze sull'infezione da HIV in un gruppo di allievi infermieri professionali [Knowledge of the HIV infection of a group of nursing students]. *Rivista dell'Infermiere, 13,* 16–22.

Work Group. (1990). Epidemiologia e culturea dell'assistenza sanitaria in gravidanza in una realtà urbana italiana degli anni '80 [Epidemiology and culture of health care during pregnancy in an Italian urban situation of the 1980s]. *Rivista dell'Infermiere, 1,* 5–13.

Zanotti, R. (1992). Nuovi approcci nell'organizzazione e nell'intervento assistenziale [New organizational and caring approaches]. In *Il Servizio Infermieristico Domiciliare e L'Ospedalizzazione a Domicilio, the First Triveneto Convention* (pp. 36–45) Castlefranco Veneto: ULSS 13 press.

Zanotti, R., & Bini, B. (1994). Apprendimento del processo diagnostico infermieristico da parte degli studenti infermieri [Learning of the diagnostic nursing process by nursing students]. *Rivista dell'Infermiere, 13,* 80–89.

Zucchetti, E. (1996). L'infermiere dentro il cambiamento: Sintesi di un'indagine sui mutamenti professionali e le implicazioni formative [The nurse inside of change: A synthesis of the study of professional change and the educational implications]. *Nursing Oggi, 4,* 23–34.

Index

Page numbers in *italics* indicate figures.
Page numbers followed by "t" indicate tables.

323

Contents of Previous Volumes

ORDER FORM

Save 10% on Volume 18 with this coupon.

___Check here to order the ANNUAL REVIEW OF NURSING RESEARCH, Volume 18, 2000 at a 10% discount. You will receive an invoice requesting prepayment.

Save 10% on all future volumes with a continuation order.

___Check here to place your continuation order for the ANNUAL REVIEW OF NURSING RESEARCH. You will receive a prepayment invoice with a 10% discount upon publication of each new volume, beginning with Volume 18, 2000. You may pay for prompt shipment or cancel with no obligation.

Name _____

Institution _____

Address _____

City/State/Zip _____

Examination copies for possible adoption are available to instructors "on approval" only. Write on institutional letterhead, noting course, level, present text, and expected enrollment (include $3.50 for postage and handling). Prices slightly higher overseas. Prices subject to change.

Mail this coupon to:
SPRINGER PUBLISHING COMPANY
536 Broadway, New York, N.Y. 10012